Praise for
BODY, SOUL, AND

"Body, Soul, and Baby is both a practical sourcebook and an inspiring companion to help all women access the inner wisdom available during pregnancy and birth."
—Christiane Northrup, author of *Women's Bodies, Women's Wisdom; The Wisdom of Menopause;* and *Mother-Daughter Wisdom*

"Dr. Gaudet's book *Body, Soul, and Baby* provides an up-to-date review of the issues, changes, and medical needs for a successful pregnancy. However, much more is covered: how to have a 'conscious pregnancy'—the ability to pick up important clues about potential problems; the opportunities to optimize the health of mother and baby and make better self-care choices. It teaches the reader to connect the dots between body, soul, and baby—a truly revolutionary way to view birth and all that leads up to it." —Charles B. Hammond, M.D., E. C. Hamblen Professor of Obstetrics and Gynecology, Duke University Medical Center

"Having a baby? At last, a book that addresses all your concerns and supports all your hopes. *Body, Soul, and Baby* is a must-have for every woman who not only plans to give birth but wants to become a mother in the fullest, most complete sense of the word."
—Rachel Naomi Remen, M.D., author of *Kitchen Table Wisdom*

"This is exactly what a pregnancy guide should be—up-to-date and comprehensive information about the medical aspects of pregnancy combined with what every mom-to-be needs to know about the rest of her body, mind, and soul. Pregnancy is indeed about more than what is going on in the uterus." —Alice Domar, author of *Self-Nurture*

"Dr. Gaudet shows how to turn pregnancy into a mindful experience resulting in health and well-being for mother and child." —Ellen Langer, author of *Mindfulness* and *On Becoming an Artist: Reinventing Yourself Through Mindful Creativity*

"From the first thought of getting pregnant to the magic of motherhood, this book celebrates every stage of the extraordinary process of giving birth. It's the perfect gift for any expecting mom or dad!"
—Cheryl Richardson, author of *Stand Up for Your Life, Life Makeovers,* and *Take Time for Your Life*

Also by Tracy W. Gaudet, M.D.,
with Paula Spencer

CONSCIOUSLY FEMALE
How to Listen to Your Body and Your Soul
for a Lifetime of Healthier Living

Body, Soul, and Baby

A Doctor's Guide to

the Complete Pregnancy Experience,

from Preconception

to Postpartum

TRACY W. GAUDET, M.D.

Executive Director of Duke Integrative Medicine

with Paula Spencer

Original Drawings by Michael E. Leonard

Bantam Books

This book is designed to help you make informed choices; it is not meant to replace consultation with a physician or other licensed health care provider.

BODY, SOUL, AND BABY
A Bantam Book

PUBLISHING HISTORY
Bantam hardcover edition published February 2007
Bantam trade paperback edition / February 2008

Published by
Bantam Dell
A Division of Random House, Inc.
New York, New York

Book design by Patrice Sheridan

Library of Congress Catalog Card Number: 2006043077

Bantam Books and the rooster colophon are registered trademarks of Random House, Inc.

ISBN 978-0-385-33575-1

Printed in the United States of America
Published simultaneously in Canada

www.bantamdell.com

BVG 10 9 8 7 6 5 4 3 2

For my son, Ryan, with love

Acknowledgments

I would like first to acknowledge my best teachers, my patients, who have shared their most intimate experiences with me. I honor you and I thank you. I am also deeply indebted to the many people who trained me in the art of obstetrics and gynecology—particularly the nurses, the faculty, and my fellow residents at the University of Texas in San Antonio; and Dr. Charles Hammond for his mentorship, which began in medical school.

My heartfelt thanks to Elly Xenakis, Barbara Schroeder, and Mark Funk for their support and love, and also for their contributions to the manuscript. I thank Ruth Quillian-Wolever, Greg Hottinger, and Diana Dell for sharing their invaluable input and for their friendship, Paul Vick for his great help in the end stages, and Joanne Kurtzberg for her expertise.

I am deeply indebted to Paula Spencer, whose writing talents enliven and inform this book and whose hard work and perseverance were crucial throughout its gestation. My thanks, too, to my agent, Doe Coover, and her associates, Frances Kennedy and Amanda Lewis, for doing whatever it took to keep things on track; and most especially to my editor at Bantam Books, Beth Rashbaum, for enduring this process and staying committed to making this the best book it could be. To the rest of the Bantam team—Barb Burg, Theresa Zoro, Nita Taublib, and Irwyn Applebaum—thanks for having confidence in me.

I want to thank Michael Leonard for his beautiful and elegant (and accurate!) artwork. It was a pleasure working with you.

Finally, my love and gratitude to my friends and family for supporting me through the process of writing this book, and simultaneously supporting me through: being caught in the coup in Haiti with my infant son for three months, my first surgery, my separation, my second surgery, my divorce, and the launch of our new Center for Integrative Medicine at Duke. Special thanks to my sister Wendy Williams, my niece Jessica Novotny, my mother-in-law Edie Liebowitz, the Grochowski family, Lillian Kathungu, Christy Mack, Paul Vick; the awesome men friends in my life—Mark Gaudet, John Tarrant, Steve Forrest, David Thorne, Roger Kirkpatrick, and Todd Welch; and the Cool Women—Dottie Williams, Colleen Grochowski, Ruby Moon, Dagmar Ehling, and Nancy Bernstein. Deep gratitude to my colleagues at DCIM, and especially to Marshall Adesman for his support and help.

And lastly to my son, Ryan—thank you for sharing your most amazing life with me. You are a beautiful, wise, and loving soul, and I am honored to be your mother.

—Tracy Gaudet, M.D.
Durham, North Carolina

Contents

Introduction

∞

You Have an Opportunity Like No Other

Returning from a trip, Jessica realized that she was late for her period—nearly a week late, she guessed. As soon as her home pregnancy test read positive, she made an appointment with her ob-gyn. From that first visit, when she was six weeks along, she dutifully had her prescriptions filled for prenatal vitamins and had all the recommended screenings and tests. She found a pregnancy diet in a book and followed it faithfully. At work, she cruised along on autopilot, downplaying her condition under loose shifts and blazers and negotiating an eight-week leave. She smiled through baby showers and at strangers who asked when she was due.

The idea of a baby was so overwhelming that Jessica preferred not to dwell on it. The idea of herself as a mother was practically unimaginable. And the idea of labor was so scary, she tried not to think about it at all.

At 38 weeks, her baby was in a breech position (feet down, rather than the head-down position desired for a safe vaginal delivery), so Jessica's doctor suggested a C-section for the following week. That sounded good to Jessica, who was getting tired and a little impatient. Her baby, a boy, was perfectly healthy. She was relieved that pregnancy was over, and a little astonished to find herself a mother. Almost before she knew it, she was home alone with Adam, everything having unfolded just as it should.

Or did it?

Jessica went through the *event* of bearing a child. But did she have the *experience*? Compare her pregnancy to Sarah's.

Like Jessica, Sarah received the conventional medical care. But that was only part of her preparation for birth and motherhood. Sarah took a few minutes each day to check in with herself, to get a handle on what was happening with her body as well as with her inner self—her soul. When her body told her it felt more tired than usual, she napped or put her feet up. When Sarah felt worried about what kind of mother she'd be or felt scared about the prospect of labor, she did some simple exercises to help her address those fears and make them less scary. And because bonding begins long before birth, she checked in with her baby, too, talking to it and rubbing her belly. She reflected on the significance of this amazing transition in life.

In this way Sarah attended to her daily self-care routines, too. Instead of simply taking prenatal vitamins and "eating healthy," she considered all five of the dimensions that make up good health—nutrition, physical fitness, the state of her mind, spiritual and social supports in her life, and sexuality and sensuality (senses). Each day she tried to tune in to her physical and emotional needs within these areas: Was she craving something salty? Did she need a little time alone? Did she feel like prenatal yoga today, or dancing? By tuning in, she was able to self-manage her stress levels and her weight gain, as well as her everyday aches and pains.

Like Jessica's, Sarah's baby was breech. She carefully considered her options and decided she wanted to try some alternative therapies to turn the baby around before delivery, which proved successful. During labor, however, an unexpected emergency led to her daughter's delivery by Cesarean after all. Although Sarah was disappointed, her nine months of working in partnership with her doctor led her to trust the doctor's instincts. She had felt very connected to her body during the hours of labor and appreciated that this was the right choice under the circumstances. Holding baby Eva, she marveled at what her body had been capable of doing. She felt ready for motherhood, a continuation of the amazing journey she had begun nine months earlier.

Two women, two seemingly similar outcomes—but two very different approaches. And this made for two very different passages to motherhood. One woman experienced pregnancy as an incredible life experience; the other as a medical event. Having a baby is something that half of humanity can never do. It happens only once or twice in a lifetime for most American women. And it's unlike any other opportunity life has to offer. To have a baby is to see your body change—your shape, your hormones, your nutritional health, and the inner workings of your muscles, organs, and joints. To have a baby is to feel your psyche change, too. Your soul is to your nonphysical self what your body is to your physical self; it includes your feelings, your intuition, your emotions, your beliefs, your instincts, and your spirit. To have a baby is to be transformed in a thousand ways between your initial thoughts of a possible child and the tumultuous first weeks at home with a newborn snuggled in your arms.

That's tremendous—and there's more. Creating a new life is also an amazing opportunity to "connect the dots": to align your body and your soul in a way that puts you in a balanced and optimally healthy state, enriching both you and your future child. Pregnancy is an opportunity to forge a deeper relationship with yourself even as you're creating a relationship with the growing life within.

I'd call conceiving and carrying a baby one of the richest, most potent, most dynamic experiences a woman can have.

Not that most doctors talk about it this way. Our culture—and our medical establishment—rarely see pregnancy as a journey of self awareness, self-discovery, and self-enrichment. We're fixated almost exclusively on the outcome—a healthy baby—and seldom bother to look within.

My perspective is very different. I consider it central to your health, as well as your baby's, to look inside yourself and become fully aware of the multidimensional changes taking place.

After all, mother and baby are completely intermingled. When you're pregnant, your breathing provides the oxygen for your baby and your blood transports everything essential for life to your baby's blood. Your hormones, what you eat, your stress level, and your health habits all directly affect the baby. And the baby is changing you, too, from your physical profile to the contours of your mind, heart, priorities, and plans. It's only logical—only natural—to pay attention to this symbiotic miracle and to use that insight to nurture you both.

I want to show you a way back to connecting with yourself—connecting those dots between body and soul—throughout this important transition. Being truly *aware* of what's taking place within allows you to make much better choices to support your ever-changing needs.

I also want to guide you through the labyrinth of confusing and often conflicting medical advice out there—advice that isn't always the best match for the unique demands of pregnancy. Once you're tuned in to your body and your soul, and once you understand the "whys" behind medical advice, you can make much better choices to support your ever-changing needs. You can filter this information through your personal experience and become fully proactive in your own care.

Awareness of both these dimensions—personal insight and medical insight—will help you best navigate all the important fertility–pregnancy decisions before you: Am I ready for a baby? Who should provide my care? What should I eat during pregnancy? How do I handle nausea? Amnio or no amnio? To induce or not to induce? Breast or bottle? The choices are endless. Consciousness is critical.

That's why I want to change the very framework through which we approach this tremendous life transition. To use the best of modern medicine, without losing the sacredness of the experience. *Body, Soul, and Baby* is the first physician-written guide to a *conscious* conception, pregnancy, delivery, and postpartum recovery.

WILL YOU TUNE IN . . . OR MISS OUT?

I see each of my patients not as the passive recipient of my care, her uterus merely a Portacrib for a baby-to-be. I see them—I see *you*—as embarking on a wonderful adventure.

There are many ways in which approaching this adventure with your eyes and ears open—with consciousness and intention shaping your care and your decisions—can reshape your pregnancy experience.

In a conscious pregnancy,

- you pick up important cues from your soul about how you're feeling, what you're believing, and what is right for *you* (not your sister, your mom, your best friend, or your care provider)
- you pick up important cues from your body about what it needs— cues that can alert you to early signs of problems or simply keep you in touch with the constant, dramatic demands of pregnancy
- you can optimize your health by knowing what you require to be in the best possible condition for conception, pregnancy, and childbirth
- you make better self-care choices, nurturing your mind, your

nutrition, your movement, your spirit, and your sensuality and sexuality

- you make more fully informed choices, reflecting both your gut feelings and a broad range of facts, rather than just relying on one person's opinion, and feel more at peace with your choices
- you enter a world of increased self-awareness, self-discovery, and self-enrichment
- you begin to bond with your child not on the day he or she is born, but right from the start of life, which leads to a smoother transition to motherhood, a deep mother–child relationship, and a more balanced life
- you fully experience the miracle of creation, the good and not-so-good, and find it all rewarding
- becoming a mother happens not as a sudden, one-day event, but gradually, and deeply, as a life-altering experience.

WHY INTEGRATIVE MEDICINE IS IDEAL FOR PREGNANCY

My ideas rise from my dual background as both an obstetrician-gynecologist and a pioneer in the fast-growing field of integrative medicine. Integrative medicine isn't another way of saying "alternative medicine." Integrative medicine *integrates* the best of conventional Western medical practices with a careful selection from a range of other, less mainstream therapies. These complementary and alternative practices (known collectively as CAM), large in number and diverse in their therapeutic approaches, have been categorized by the National Center for Complementary and Alternative Medicine (NCCAM) at the National Institutes of Health as follows:

- biologically based therapies, including botanicals, supplements, and vitamins
- manipulative and body-based therapies, including chiropractic and massage
- mind-body–based interventions, including relaxation techniques, hypnosis, and imagery
- energy therapies, including therapeutic touch and Reiki
- alternative medical systems, including Oriental medicine, acupuncture, and homeopathy

I have been able to incorporate many of these therapies into the care I offer pregnant women, as well as take advantage of the tremendous advances of modern medicine. In 1935, there were 582 maternal deaths per 100,000 live births in the US; by 1985 that number had fallen to 8, a drop in large part due to medical advances. In practicing integrative medicine, I offer my patients the best of both worlds. As a board-certified obstetrician-gynecologist, my ideas are grounded in standard ob practice. But when circumstances are right, I often steer my patients toward alternative therapies that I feel will benefit them. I believe in integrative medicine because it is:

- healing-oriented rather than disease-oriented
- focused on the whole person—body, mind, and soul
- proactive rather than reactive
- self-directed rather than physician-directed
- committed to the use of low-tech, low-cost methods wherever appropriate

At the Duke Center for Integrative Medicine, which I direct, I see women seeking help for all kinds of health issues. As a practicing ob-gyn who has treated thousands of women of all ages, I have a specific interest in and understanding of reproductive issues including fertility and pregnancy. Of all the specialties of medicine, the integrative perspective is a particularly perfect match for pregnancy. Here's why:

Pregnancy is not a disease state. Conventional medicine does an incredible job of saving lives and fixing problems—if I'm having a heart attack, get me to the ER, stat! But pregnancy is not a medical problem, it's a natural part of life. To optimally manage life cycles and their times of transition, especially pregnancy and birth, requires a different perspective and awareness than disease management.

Pregnancy is a holistic experience. Carrying a child involves more than your uterus. Nearly every organ is affected, not to mention your muscles, your appearance, and your psychological and emotional states. Every aspect of your life undergoes a shift. When conventional medicine practitioners deal strictly with the medical aspects of pregnancy, they're considering only a fraction of the woman's full experience.

Pregnancy is a natural process. A miraculous one! Integrative medicine respects—and indeed presumes—the natural power of the human body and its wondrous capacity to heal. Honoring these capabilities allows both patient and care provider to work with, rather than against, nature.

Pregnancy is usually best cared for by the least invasive approaches. Out of concern for the fetus, the general rule is to use noninvasive treatments first. Noninvasive alternative approaches can often offer better relief than conventional approaches. They can also delay or negate the need for more invasive approaches. Many of the common concerns of pregnancy—headaches and back pain, for example—can be effectively treated without medications. CAM therapies can also be used with conventional medicine to manage chronic conditions during pregnancy, such as asthma, depression, lupus, and arthritis.

Pregnancy is a condition that requires optimal health. The growing fetus highlights in a dramatic, recognizable way the significance of its mother's lifestyle choices. Tobacco, alcohol, and drugs can cause fetal damage. Both the lack of certain nutrients (such as folic acid) and the excess of others (such as extremely high concentrations of bio-flavonoids, which are synthesized from soy and found in some dietary supplements) are linked to birth defects and serious problems. A lack of folic acid increases the risk of spina bifida, for example, while a high concentration of bioflavonoids has been linked to early-childhood leukemia. Stress in the mother's life significantly increases the risk of preterm delivery, the leading cause of death in newborns. Proper nutrition, exercise, relaxation, and support all make for a healthier pregnancy as well as a healthier baby. Pregnancy is therefore a golden opportunity for behavioral changes. A woman often finds the motivation to make choices on behalf of her baby that she might not make for herself. And she may continue this improved lifestyle throughout her life.

HOW THIS BOOK IS ORGANIZED

Body, Soul, and Baby begins by helping you learn how to "pay attention." This, for me, is the most crucial skill a woman can bring to childbearing. Regardless of whether you're already pregnant or not, or how far along you are in your pregnancy, start with Part One: Equip Yourself for a New Life Phase. This part includes practical stratagems you'll use over and over: ways to grow more aware of your body, your soul, and your baby, as well as a daily health planner to use as a blueprint you will embellish and alter throughout your pregnancy.

Part Two: Preconception is for readers who aren't yet pregnant. Parts Three through Five: The First Trimester, The Second Trimester, and The Third Trimester explain, trimester by trimester, what you'll be experiencing and what you need to be concerned about in early, mid, and late pregnancy. Parts Six and Seven, Labor and Delivery and Postpartum, take you through the life-altering and life-giving experience of labor, and on to the first weeks of motherhood.

Except for Part One, which is intended to be a starting point for every reader regardless of your condition or stage of pregnancy, each part of the book from Preconception through Postpartum contains these basic sections:

1. *Reflection and Observation.* Start by checking in. How do you feel this week, this day, this moment? The exercises in this section invite you to explore what your changing body, your changing soul, and your changing baby have to say to you.

2. *The Inside Scoop.* Insight isn't enough, especially at such a dynamic phase of life. To understand what you're experiencing and why, as well as to make fully informed choices, you need to understand the realities of reproduction. Here I present what's happening to you on a physiological, anatomical, and hormonal level and what's happening to the child growing within you.

3. *Medical Care.* Then, from an integrative medicine perspective, I walk you through the medical issues that you'll encounter regarding standard prenatal care, as well as other issues you may encounter. This approach means I'll always present the "whys" so you can make well-informed choices that are right for you, rather than just saying, "At X weeks, do this," without encouraging you to take your individual circumstances into consideration.

4. *Self-Care.* It's not all up to the doctor. So for each phase of pregnancy, I'll tweak the core advice offered in the Chapter 4 Basic Self-Care Plan to show how you can best nurture yourself while taking into account the changing needs of this dynamic time of life.

Although my perspective and advice are different from what you'll find in other pregnancy books, rest assured that I cover all the basic issues every woman faces on the road from preconception to postpartum. I share every care provider's—and every parent's—universal goal of a healthy baby. However, I also want you to have a rich, multidimensional experience that puts you in touch with a deeper, more authentic part of yourself than you may ever experience again.

Part One

Equip Yourself for
a New Life Phase

————————— ∞ —————————

Start Here! A Fresh Framework

for Thinking About Pregnancy

Chapter 1

A Better Way

∞

*Will pregnancy just happen to you or
will it become a part of you?*

You have a choice in the way you approach having a baby. You can do so consciously, with a nonjudgmental awareness of where you're starting from, what you need, and who you are, body and soul, inside and out. Or you can remain tuned out, going about on autopilot and ignoring the insistent whispers (and sometimes shouts) of your body, your soul, and your baby. Living unconsciously means living as though events are not really happening to you. You go through the motions, but you are disconnected physically and/or emotionally.

And so you miss out. This is so common that many women aren't even aware it's the case for them. In living unconsciously, you risk missing the real experiences of your own life. We are so good at dwelling on the past or the future that we often miss the present altogether.

That's the funny thing about being disconnected—we're oblivious to what we're missing. A lack of awareness can be particularly problematic in pregnancy. Conversely, being fully conscious at this time of your life will yield tremendous rewards—in terms of improving your baby's health, as well as your emotional and spiritual state.

THE RISKS OF BEING TUNED OUT

Let's consider some of the ways that approaching your pregnancy unconsciously can play out:

- *You miss important cues from your soul.* At her first ob visit, Cassie tells me she's "great," everything is "fine," she feels "fabulous." When I ask what's the hardest thing for her about this pregnancy (pointing out that mixed feelings are common even in a desired pregnancy), she starts to cry. Only then does she reach beyond the social expectation of maternal bliss to confide what's really on her mind—that she's hugely stressed by her new job and doesn't feel ready for parenthood. As a matter of fact, not only do many women miss the opportunities that pregnancy and delivery create, many are actually traumatized by the experience. In fact, studies have found that 3 percent of women who had a "normal" birth and 33 percent of those who had a difficult or complicated birth met the criteria for post-traumatic stress disorder. Something is seriously wrong here.

- *You miss important cues from your body.* Sami doesn't notice her swelling feet and hands and ignores her frequent headaches until her preeclampsia has reached life-threatening proportions. Tess can't tell me the last time she felt her baby move—"maybe a week ago?" Bridgette delivers a healthy daughter but afterward ignores her own loss of appetite, sleeplessness, and other symptoms of serious postpartum depression.

- *You miss opportunities to optimize your health.* Mandy is so out of touch with her body that she doesn't realize she's pregnant until her fourth month—missing, among other things, the opportunity to have supplemented her diet with folic acid, a known preventive of spinal defects when taken in the first weeks of pregnancy. Keira conceives unintentionally, before her recently diagnosed diabetes is under good control—placing her unborn baby at a heightened risk for birth defects. Shauna continues running on caffeine and little sleep without taking any basic steps to optimize her health habits. It's not that she doesn't care about her baby; she's not really aware of her habits and their potential effects in the first place.

- *You make poor self-care choices.* By her eighth month, Amber is on track to gain more than 60 pounds in her pregnancy, largely as a result of her unconscious eating habits. Marnie continues working a 60-hour week, leaving little time for her to explore her changing feelings, let alone her changing body. Nan worries obsessively about her baby but fails to nurture herself adequately, and spends winter and spring with chronic colds and flu.

- *You make uninformed choices.* Carmen suffers through nausea and vomiting so severe she must be hospitalized; she's unaware of effective noninvasive treatments such as acupuncture and hypnosis. Chelsea's bias is for a "natural" pregnancy, so she takes only herbal medications, many of which have not been tested for use in pregnancy, and does not tell her doctor.

- *You regret choices you make.* Shanti quickly tells me no, she doesn't want amniocentesis. Then she spends the rest of her pregnancy fretting about birth defects. Bethany agrees to a repeat C-section for her second delivery without considering that this ensures that all her future deliveries will be C-sections, too—a decision she later regrets.

- *You miss opportunities for personal growth and bonding with your child.* Grad student Lorna studies so hard throughout her pregnancy that she remarks, "Sometimes I'm shocked to look down at my stomach and remember I'm pregnant." Elle watches a movie during her labor. Her epidural is so effective that when I tell her it's time to push, she says, "Oh, not yet—can I just watch this part?" After Shannon delivers, she says she feels no connection to her baby. "It's like a stranger," she complains.

- *You have the event—but not the **experience**.* Li thought that, at 41, she was "too old" to have a baby, so she wrote off her pregnancy symptoms as perimenopause and never had them checked out until the 18th week of her term. Sheila, too, missed half her pregnancy; she was so focused on work, she didn't realize the "flu" was a baby. And every ER doc can tell you a story about a woman who did the ultimate disconnect and came to the emergency room with abdominal pain ("I think I have food poisoning"), only to deliver a full-term baby!

I see such examples all the time. Unfortunately, in giving short shrift to conception, pregnancy, and postpartum, women shortchange themselves, and often their babies and partners, too.

HOPPING OFF THE "CONVEYOR BELT"

Unfortunately, unconsciousness is the rule on the modern Fertility Pathway. It's not part of standard prenatal care to encourage patients to be more conscious, much less teach them how. Doctors almost never present these months as a journey of self-awareness and self-discovery. (Indeed, even female ob-gyns who have been through pregnancy firsthand rarely hold such a view themselves.) The perception very often is that we now know so very much about pregnancy and delivery, and the entire process has been so neatly figured out by modern medicine, that the expectant mom need not worry about a thing or even be much involved! She should just do as she is told by the experts and all will probably be well. This approach ignores the fact that while doctors may be medical experts, you are the expert about *you*—if you tune in and become conscious.

Modern pregnancy can feel like a streamlined, automated conveyor belt of "do this, don't do that" advice and high-tech management of your "condition." You hop on it when your pregnancy test turns positive (and seldom any earlier). The ride peaks in a labor that's often anything but natural, and then you are sent back home some 24 to 48 hours after your delivery, alone with the object of those nine months of scrutiny, until one last postpartum checkup six weeks later.

Surprisingly, the concept of consciousness doesn't even show up in most childbirth education classes, despite the fact that being truly "in the moment" can often make the difference between a positive birth experience and one tinged with self-reproach and regret, or even trauma.

Our whole culture discounts this important idea. Most of the focus during pregnancy is on the baby. The mother is congratulated and patted on the belly. She's feted with showers and given a comfortable seat in her doctor's waiting room. After the delivery, the spotlight turns to the baby: names, the layette, diapering, feeding, and "sleeping when the baby sleeps." There's very little emphasis on what the woman herself is feeling and how she is being transformed—before, during, and after motherhood. There's an old saying, "The world doesn't want to hear about the labor pains. It just wants to see the baby." Sadly, it's too often true. In fact, there's little support, medically or socially, for excavating beneath the superficially perfect and happy facade. Especially in pregnancy, though it's perhaps the most dynamic life transition of all, there's little public tolerance for the dark side of things. But, of course, even pregnancy has a shadowy side; all of life does.

Interestingly, this disconnect is as true of women who prefer a "natural" pregnancy full of organic food, botanicals, acupuncture, and yoga classes, as it is for those following a more conventional approach. Whether you veer toward the conventional or the alternative end of the spectrum, you can unconsciously wind up following some culturally (or counterculturally) sanctioned version of what to do, without ever exploring your deepest feelings. In any scenario of pregnancy care, few care providers are asking, "What are you really feeling? How are you processing the remarkable number of changes coming at you every single day, every hour?" We just don't go there.

A time of internal wonder has been reframed almost entirely as a time for external worry. You may be bombarded with warnings and advice about your every action, from eating fish to crossing your legs properly, but no one will ask you what your greatest worry is. You can find information on whether to use Botox or eat sushi, but not on how to steer around self-reproach, guilt, or panic.

The natural capabilities of a woman's body have been ignored in favor of a medical model of childbirth. In some circles, in fact, a "natural delivery" simply means a vaginal one featuring the often useful but unnatural procedures of epidurals and episiotomies. The rate of induced labors has more than doubled since 1990, from 9.5 percent to 20.6 percent of all deliveries in 2003. More than one in four women (27.5 percent) delivers surgically, by C-section, which is an all-time high, and the rate in some hospitals approaches one in three. Meanwhile, vaginal births after a previous C-section (VBACs) are at an all-time low. Elective C-sections—chosen when there is no medical indication—increased 25 percent from 2000 to 2002, and first time C-sections in women with very low risk has increased 67 percent from 1991 to 2001. The percentage of preterm babies (12.3 percent in 2003) and low birth weight babies (7.9 percent) continue to rise. Preterm labor has been clearly linked to stress, yet questions about an expectant mom's stress level are not even part of the traditional ob exam, nor do doctors generally have the time to ask. Postpartum depression and breastfeeding success have both been linked to the quality of maternal support, yet new moms routinely go home without any further contact with the medical system for four to six weeks. The conveyor belt is front and center, rather than the woman herself.

This is backward! The pregnancy is not something that is happening to you; it is happening *within* you. It *is* you. And if you become conscious of these inner movements—not just of your body but of your heart, soul, and baby—you can tap in to all the wonder of this life-altering event.

Chapter 2

Where Pregnancy Begins

∞

The starting place for a healthy pregnancy isn't a date,
it's a mind-set

A conscious pregnancy doesn't begin with your first trimester, last menstrual period, first prenatal exam, or a positive home pregnancy test. I believe that for a truly healthy, happy pregnancy, a different starting place is in order. I want to start with where *you* are.

Do you know?

By "where you are," I mean in all the many different dimensions that comprise you: physical, emotional, and psychological—in your work, in your relationships, and in your heart and soul. They're all interconnected and relevant to your well-being. Where are you, as an individual, as you approach this new path in your life? A conscious pregnancy begins with developing awareness about yourself.

WELCOME TO THE FERTILITY PATHWAY

Whether or not you are now pregnant, the fact that you've picked up this book indicates some interest in becoming a mother. And that's the real starting place of a pregnancy. You are at a time and place in a woman's life I call the Fertility Pathway. It's a season of your life marked by a distinct set of experiences and choices surrounding the active desire to have a child. A woman who is menstruating and does not hope for a child or is not pregnant is in the life phase I call Cycling. She has different experiences and concerns. You may go back and forth between Cycling and the Fertility Pathway more than once. Eventually you reach the Transition Pathway, which marks the shift out of your reproductive years and into perimenopause and then menopause.

My goal is to help you reframe the way you think about your time on the Fertility Pathway, planning and/or experiencing pregnancy and childbirth. In order to do that, you need to reframe the way you think about yourself.

Wait a minute, you may be thinking. *I just want to know about having a healthy baby!*

Of course you do. And I will tell you all about it. But first you need to appreciate this reality: Having a baby isn't all about the baby. It's also about you, and the relationship between the two of you.

THE REFLECTIVE INVENTORY

When I first work with a new patient, I use an exercise I call the Reflective Inventory. It's basically a series of questions designed to help her take inventory of her whole self. You can do the same thing on your own. As a physician, I am not looking for "correct" answers; I am simply encouraging you to shift your attention to various important dimensions of your health and see what they bring up for you.

I've designed a home version of the Reflective Inventory to help you create a self-portrait of where you are right now. Ideally, you should do this exercise before continuing on with the tools and care plans in the following chapters, because the information you discover can inform all of your decisions throughout your pregnancy, from how to best care for yourself every day to how to work most effectively with your doctor.

You don't need to write anything down. This is an emotional exercise, not an intellectual one, and thus different from the forms you're asked to fill out at your doctor's office, or the health and medical history your care provider takes. All you need to do is skim the questions and, without dwelling on them, give them brief consideration. This simple act will increase your awareness. I sometimes call the Reflective Inventory a "soul magnet," because it attracts bits and particles of insight floating around inside you and pulls them to the surface. Notice which topics seem to stick in your mind afterward; that's an indicator that you may want to spend time reflecting on them later.

Before beginning:

Find quiet time and space. It's easier to turn your attention inward when you feel relaxed and safe. There are several ways to do this. First, find a time when you're not likely to be interrupted. Let your physical surroundings help shift your attention, too, by going somewhere you feel comfortable, such as your peaceful back deck or in a favorite chair, where you can snuggle up under an old quilt. Most important, find such a space anywhere by making a mental transition from your busy day to a quieter place in your head. Get comfortable and relaxed. Use any relaxation technique that works for you; try experimenting with several if you don't already have one you use to center yourself. (See Chapter 4, pages 36–42, for some suggestions.) Yoga, meditation, or simple deep-breathing works well for many people.

Be honest. There are no "right" or "wrong" answers here. There are only *your* answers.

Dare to peer into the shadows. This exercise is meant to provide a snapshot. And to continue this metaphor, a photograph, technically, is light captured on paper. Without degrees of both lightness and darkness, there would be no image. The same applies to capturing a picture of where you are right now in your journey to motherhood. Both light and dark are part of the journey. When a woman tells me that she's "not afraid of anything" or "not worried about anything," or that she feels "nothing but joy and happiness" about her pregnancy, I have to wonder if she's repressing something. We all have fears and worries, especially about a great life change that is as full of unknowns as this one is.

Be aware of the "judging mind." That's the little voice in your head that editorializes your own thoughts and feelings. "You shouldn't think that way," it chastises. Or, "You must be a bad person if you do this or believe that." Simply notice that you are having such thoughts, recognize them for what they are—judgmental commentary—and set them aside. Just say, "Oh, there's that voice again." Then move on.

Understand that your answers change every single day. As a living, breathing human, you're not designed to live in static, robotic sameness. And, especially as a pregnant woman, you couldn't possibly.

Every day will bring changes. That's why it's so critical to have an ongoing awareness when you're pregnant.

The Reflective Inventory Questions

Scan through the following questions and see what areas you are drawn to, and what answers come to mind. You don't need to respond to every single question. Remember, the purpose here is to bring these topics to the forefront of your awareness.

Your Mind

- How much stress do you experience? What are the main sources? How much is stress from things you enjoy (a challenging job you love, for example), and how much is stress from negative life circumstances (overwork, financial worries, or a death in the family, for example)?
- How do you usually cope with stress? Do you sleep more or less? Eat more or less? Exercise more or less? Do you feel that you have enough coping strategies? Enough support?
- Has your stress level changed now that you are on the Fertility Pathway? For example, are you worried about how your pregnancy or a baby will affect your work situation or your finances?
- Do you have time in your day when you can "unplug"? How do you relax in the course of a normal day?
- Do you remember your dreams? Have they changed since you began this pathway?

Your Nutrition

- What kind of eater are you? Do you eat three meals a day? Do you graze? Binge? When do you eat? Has it changed since you've been on the Fertility Pathway?
- What's your relationship with food, and how has it changed over time? Are you conscious of *why* you eat as well as *what* you choose to eat? Is mealtime a special time or do you eat on the run?
- Have you ever had an eating disorder? If so, how does it affect you now?

- Are you happy with your weight? In the past has your weight been fairly consistent, or do you have a pattern of gaining and losing?
- What are your beliefs about eating or nutrition in pregnancy? Are you excited about "eating for two"? Concerned?
- What are your feelings regarding gaining weight in pregnancy? Are you concerned that the weight will be hard to lose afterward? Or do you see it as a great opportunity?

Your Movement

- What movement brings you joy? When was the last time you experienced that kind of movement in your life?
- What about exercise? Does the very word make you cringe, or is it something you look forward to? Do you have an exercise routine built into your day or week? How often do you usually exercise?
- What kind of exercise do you usually do? Aerobic? Strength training? Stretching and flexibility work?
- What are your beliefs about movement and exercise in pregnancy? Do you believe you will be more active or less active?

Your Relationships

- What in your life allows you to feel connected to things outside of yourself? When was the last time you did something that made you feel connected in that way?
- What brings you joy and a sense of fulfillment? When was the last time you experienced that feeling? What do you do well? What are you proud of? How do you express your gifts?
- What gives you a sense of meaning and purpose in your life? How palpable is that for you, and how has it shifted over your life? Does it feel as if it is shifting in any way as you think of bringing a new life into the world?
- Who are your friends? Do you have friends to whom you can say anything? Do their experiences with their fertility help you feel more connected to them, or less?
- Who in your family makes you feel most supported and in what ways? What are your relationships to your parents and your siblings like (whether they are living or not)? What does

your experience of family life bring up for you when you think of starting a family of your own?

- How is your relationship with the father of your baby-to-be? What are the qualities of this relationship? How do you imagine that pregnancy and a child will impact it? Or if there is no father-to-be in the picture, how do you feel about that? Do you feel isolated? Or do you have a partner or a strong network of friends who will give you support?

Your Sensuality and Sexuality

- Are you sexually active now? Is the frequency of sexual activity what you want it to be? Do you want more? Less? Or just something different?
- How has your sexuality changed since you've been on the Fertility Pathway? For you? For your partner? How has your sensuality changed?
- Are you comfortable in your sexuality? Do you feel free about expressing yourself sexually? Are your needs met? How has that shifted over time? What role does body image play in your sexual life? Do you feel you know what you want sexually? How has this changed on the Fertility Pathway?
- What are your hopes around sexuality during pregnancy? What are your fears? Your concerns? What about postpartum?
- What about sensuality in your life? How do you define your sensuality? What kinds of experiences do you consider sensual? Are there enough of these experiences in your life? How does your sensuality relate to your sexuality? How has your sensuality shifted since you've been on the Fertility Pathway?

Your Feelings About Childbearing and Childrearing

- How do you feel about being on this pathway—honestly? What are the best things about it? What are the worst? What are most exciting? What are most scary?
- Have you ever been pregnant, miscarried, or had an abortion before? What was that experience like? Do you feel at peace with the experience or are there unresolved feelings?
- Do you feel "ready" to become a mother? Does it feel real to you? Abstract?

- What are you most excited about with this pregnancy? What are your concerns or fears?
- Where do your images of childbirth come from? What do you most look forward to about delivery? What do you fear or worry about?
- What are your expectations about becoming a mother? What will your partner be like as a parent? How do you think becoming parents will alter your relationship?

BEGINNING YOUR JOURNEY TO A CONSCIOUS PREGNANCY

Your answers will influence the choices you make as the coming months unfold. Reflecting on these questions often stirs the subconscious or the unconscious. Notice which questions seem to stay in your mind or heart, and spend more time reflecting on them. Some will resonate because they surprise you, or because you've never thought about them before. Others may trigger a strong response, whether joyful, sad, fearful, or merely mystifying. You can write about these topics in a journal, or share your thoughts with your partner or a close friend. This is a good time to pay particular attention to your dreams, which are a voice of your unconscious mind.

Remember that bringing consciousness to your life and your choices is all part of the process of getting to know yourself. The Reflective Inventory is just the beginning.

Chapter 3

Ten Tools for Tuning In

∞

Ways to gather insight and info about your body, soul, and baby

The growth and changes that result from pregnancy take place within three different dimensions: 1) your body; 2) your soul; and 3) your baby. In this chapter you'll learn about tools that will enable you to pay closer attention to all three. Throughout the book, I'll refer to these basic tools, suggesting ways to use them at every stage of your journey to birth and beyond. They're so easy to learn, they can quickly become second nature. The insights they provide will help you make choices that are not just medically sound, but personally right for *you.*

This is not a book filled with reductionistic lists of symptoms matched up mechanically with ready-made "cures." I want to teach you a whole new approach to your pregnancy, an approach based in a holistic understanding of the interrelatedness of your body, your soul, and your baby. By increasing your awareness of what is happening within you and learning to listen to your own wisdom, you will be able to take advantage of the body's innate ability to heal. The stronger and healthier your whole system, the better able you will be to navigate the changes and challenges of pregnancy. This care plan teaches you strategies to fuel your whole self. In so doing, you will be the healthiest you can be.

My emphasis on awareness is one major way this book differs from any other pregnancy guide. I believe that many of the "aches and pains" common to pregnancy can best be alleviated (and sometimes avoided) by being tuned in to your body and soul in the first place. Doing so can help you detect the earliest signs of potential trouble and often take steps that allay the problem or prevent it from developing further—whether that means noticing the earliest signs of a headache, and using stress reduction techniques and Tylenol to remedy it before it becomes a full-blown migraine; or, more seriously, noticing changes in fetal movement that could indicate problems with the well-being of your baby so that you can seek help quickly. More important, increasing your awareness allows you to be proactive in optimizing your health. Knowing what aspects of your well-being are running on empty allows you to take steps to refuel. Good health is multidimensional. Set aside the granola-and-yoga connotations often associated with the word "holistic" and consider what it really means: wholeness, or looking at your health across all the dimensions that make up the whole of you.

DEVELOPING BODY AWARENESS: FOUR TOOLS

Your body speaks to you every day. A twinge in your back might say "I didn't like that bike ride yesterday," or it may be a signal of preterm labor. A general lack of energy might signal a need for more sleep, or something deeper, such as a general response to an overstressed pace at work. A heightened sex drive in the second trimester, feeling fetal movement, a burst of "nesting" energy—these all tell you something about what's happening within. Yet women are often disconnected from the biological blockbuster of effects taking place inside their own bodies. They may notice the most dramatic "shouts," such as morning sickness or the first kick, but miss all of the whispered clues, complaints, and quiet requests their body also continually makes.

To bring a new level of awareness to the skin you're in at this time is tremendously fun. It's a wonderful opportunity to marvel at and understand your body. I'm always awestruck when I reflect on the amazing changes the human body undergoes to support new life. And you will be, too, as you learn to tune in to these perfectly orchestrated capabilities. Besides, there are practical benefits to tuning in. You will be better able to nurture yourself because you'll have a keener sense of your needs. You'll also be better able to recognize signs of problems because you are more attuned to what's normal for you and what's changing.

TOOL #1: BODY QUICK PIC

This exercise is a quick method of assessing how you are at any given moment. Think of it as taking a mental snapshot of your body. Because it's portable, you can do it anywhere. Because it's so easy and fast, you can do it as often as you like.

To do a Body Quick Pic:

- Pause and close your eyes. Take a few deep breaths to relax. You can be standing or sitting.
- Take a moment to tune in to your body. How is it feeling right now? What do you notice? Are there places that warrant attention or have needs?

That's it! The mere act of connecting with your body, of paying attention even for a few moments, brings it to the fore of your consciousness. It's like asking, "Hey, how're you doing?" If we don't stop to ask, many things go unnoticed. When something comes up that is troubling—for example, "I'm so exhausted! I don't think I can do this!" or "I'm uneasy"—then you can explore that feedback further with other tools. Using a complementary tool, such as Dialoguing or Dreamagery (see below), is a great way to get a handle on the source of such feelings.

Try It: Do a Body Quick Pic now. It's less a way to notice every little sensation than to connect with the overall feeling of your body. But its beauty is its speed; simply taking the time to do it at all allows you to connect in a way you might not otherwise.

TOOL #2: BODY SCAN

A Body Scan is a more methodical means of assessing how you are at any given moment. Find ways to incorporate it into your daily routine—such as doing a Body Scan right after you shower or before you leave the house—so it becomes a habit.

To do a Body Scan:

- Sit or lie down and close your eyes. (Lying down is easier, but don't lie flat on your back after the fourth month of pregnancy because your uterus presses against the aorta, which can reduce blood flow to the baby.) Take a few deep breaths or use another centering technique that works for you.

- Turn your attention to your body. Is there any part that draws your immediate notice? If so, just be aware of this for now.
- Turn your attention to the very top of your head—your scalp. What do you notice? Do you feel any tension? Any pain? Or do you feel that these muscles are relaxed and doing fine? Move down to your forehead, your eyes, your nose/sinuses, your mouth and jaw. What do you notice? Any discomfort? Pain?
- Now continue to mentally scan your whole body, part by part, all the way down to your toes. Be aware of your breasts, your uterus, your skin—just notice what you notice.
- Once you've completed the scan, return to the parts that give you concern and spend a little extra time considering how they might warrant further attention.

Some people, especially those who are visual thinkers, like to do this exercise while actually picturing their body, as if giving themselves a mental CT scan.

Try It: Conduct a Body Scan now. What do you notice? Do you feel tension? Pain? Calm? Build an awareness of any "unhappy spots" that merit closer attention.

TOOL #3: DIALOGUING
(WITH YOUR PHYSICAL SELF)

To dialogue is to have a conversation. And that's exactly what this exercise does—it gives you a forum for having a conversation with yourself. This tool is a useful way to explore in greater depth a topic that might come up during your Quick Pic or Body Scan. For example, you might be plagued with a chronic symptom such as backaches or headaches. Dialoguing is a way to "talk" to your back or your head to explore what's going on. What does your body have to say about this symptom? What would you like to say to your body? Dialoguing also works with bigger-picture issues that concern your physical self, such as your fertility or your feelings about labor.

Dialoguing is essentially a structured form of introspection. It's a playful tool, a way of giving yourself an opportunity to hear the voice within you. Your conscious mind poses a question, and you wait for answers to come.

Here's how it works:

1. Set the stage. Give yourself time in a quiet place where you are not likely to be disturbed. Start with some slow, deep breaths or another relaxation exercise to focus yourself.
2. Think about what body part or issue you will converse with. Dialoguing employs imagination and is a kind of bridge between your conscious mind and your subconscious. In order to have a two-way conversation, it's helpful to have some mental idea of who (or what) is on the other end of the line. You don't need to "picture" anything, although some people find it useful to personify the body part or problem (or whatever you are Dialoguing about).
3. Begin the conversation in your mind. Ask the topic you're Dialoguing about what it wants to say to you. Is there anything it needs from you? Is there anything you need from it? What do you want to say or ask it? Let these questions be a starting point, and feel free to continue wherever the conversation leads.

This exercise works best if you approach it in a light, open manner. Don't get hung up on the feeling that you are talking to yourself—because that's exactly what is happening. Your conscious mind is probing your unconscious mind. See if you can suspend critical thinking and just go with it. Do the exercise a second time if the first time was difficult, and see what kinds of answers spring to mind. Remember, your body is in partnership with you, and has its own perspectives to share.

Remember, too, that you are only one half of the conversation. Allow space for your body to "talk back" to you. Most women find that answers simply "pop" into their heads. Even if it feels like you are "making it all up," run with it. Pay attention to the tone of the response, too. Is it angry? Sad? Overjoyed? Frustrated?

Try It: Start Dialoguing by imagining a conversation with your reproductive system. At the most basic level, that's the physical dimension that you're in the closest relationship with on this journey to having a baby. Dialoguing with your reproductive system is a good way to gain a fuller picture of your health concerns now and bring complex feelings to the fore.

1. Find a quiet place when you won't be interrupted.
2. Now think about your reproductive system—that is, think of it not as a static "thing" but as an entity to interact with.
3. In your mind, ask your reproductive system what it wants to say to you. Is there anything you want to say to it? Is there anything it needs from you? Is there anything you need from it?
4. Accept the first answers that come to mind. Ask follow-up questions as they occur to you, such as "Can you tell me more?" and "How long have you felt this way?" Remember that you can return to this particular conversation, or Dialogue on other topics, as often as you like.

TOOL #4: BODY MONITORING

Never in your life is it more thrilling to be conscious of the state of your body across time than in the nine months of pregnancy. It's ideal to start Body Monitoring before conception, or shortly thereafter, because it will be easier to assess changes and needs if you have a solid sense of what your baselines—your personal norms—are. A baseline is not an ideal or a goal; it's simply what is normal for you. By tuning in to yourself, you'll become intimately familiar with your baselines. And then you can more effectively monitor changes (positive ones and negative ones, as well as changes that are neither positive nor negative, but simply the normal developments of pregnancy) and plan action steps in response to them.

The easiest way to learn how to monitor yourself is within a structure. Follow these steps until the Body Monitor idea becomes second nature. You may choose to use this tool every day after you step out of the shower, or once a week on a leisurely weekend morning.

1. Weigh yourself. Knowing your weight is important during pregnancy so that you can track your rate of gaining. It can be an indicator that all's well, or that there are possible problems. Being conscious of

your weight—in a nonjudgmental way—also helps you be aware of whether you are gaining too quickly or too slowly. Lots of women have baggage around the whole issue of weight, so it's helpful if you can shift to simply thinking of the scale as a routine part of neutral Body Monitoring.

2. Stand naked in front of a full-length mirror. That request alarms many of my patients who are unaccustomed to their own nudity or have body-image issues. If so, start with what makes you comfortable. Wear as little clothing as you're okay with, but with the intention of becoming increasingly aware of your body and working up to standing there in just your skin.

3. Assess your general appearance. What do you notice? How is your coloring, your energy level, your posture? Pediatricians know that mothers are often the first to notice when a child isn't feeling well, even without taking a temperature. Mothers are used to observing their children—whether they are pale or listless, for example. I think we generally observe others, especially our loved ones, very closely. Learn to focus that loving attention on yourself.

4. Notice your face. Having a baseline familiarity with its shape and coloration will be important as time goes on to assess swelling. Look into your eyes, what do you see? Excitement? Sadness? Fatigue? Joy?

5. Inspect your skin. Become familiar with the markings, freckles, moles, and scars. It can be hard to do your back—use a mirror. Over time, look for changes in the shape and size of these markings. Report anything out of the ordinary to your doctor.

6. Get to know your breasts. I purposely did not say "examine" your breasts. Rather than focusing on looking for a problem, as in a breast self-exam, this exercise asks you to become very familiar with a part of your body that is particularly dynamic during pregnancy. What do you see in the mirror? How is the color and tone of each breast and its areola? Touch them all over, from the nipple up to your armpit, as well as any part of the breast that may rest against your rib cage. How do they feel, both on the surface of the skin and beneath? Is there any discharge? Feel free to use lotion if that makes it more comfortable, easy, or enjoyable.

7. Review your belly/abdomen. It's especially fun to notice how this changes across pregnancy. Look at it from the front, and in profile. Notice its dimensions and shape, and how it feels to your touch.

8. Do a vulvar self-exam. Many women have never even heard of this, but it's based on the same idea as getting to know your own breasts. It's hard to see anything without a hand-held mirror and bright light. First wash your hands, then try straddling a mirror placed on a closed toilet seat, so you'll have both hands free, or sitting on a towel on the floor facing a mirror. What do you notice about your pubic hair? The color and surface of your labia? What does the skin feel like? Do you notice any lumps or bumps?

9. Look over your extremities—arms and legs, hands and feet. Do they seem to be normal temperature, or cold? Do you notice any swelling or knots under the skin? What do the nails and nail beds look like?

Try It: Do an initial Body Monitoring to get a baseline familiarity with your body. If helpful, you might want to write down what you find to keep track of how things change across time.

DEVELOPING SOUL AWARENESS: THREE TOOLS

Pregnancy is one of the times in a woman's life when her inner voice is particularly close to the surface and brimming with things to say.

You may have experienced this on a lesser scale during the premenstrual phase of your cycle. When women pay close attention to their physical, emotional, mental, and spiritual changes from day to day during their menstrual cycle, they usually notice the following pattern: In the first half of their cycle (from the first day of menstruation to ovulation), they feel sharper, more energetic—most "like themselves." During the second half of the cycle, leading up to their periods, most women begin to feel less sharp, more tired, increasingly emotional, even moody—the classic symptoms of PMS. Our soul-level feelings and thoughts seem closer to the surface then. This phase of our cycle doesn't *cause* the moodiness and emotionality; rather it lifts the curtain of unconsciousness that is ordinarily drawn between the body and the soul. We gain access to the inner workings of our soul more easily.

We've been conditioned to view premenstrual weepiness or blues as "bad," but I see them as potentially very good. Instead of dismissing these emotions as "just hormones," think of them as messages. With your usual insulating defenses dulled a bit, issues that are very real for you may surface during this time—issues that you are better able to repress and ignore at other times in your cycle. Maybe the very feelings you are pushing away are those that most need your attention. If you can tap in to these innermost fears and desires, you're much better able to align your conscious choices with your unconscious needs.

If your period offers a peephole into your soul, pregnancy is a veritable picture window. A lot is stirring in you at this time—making it a wonderful opportunity to uncover and explore matters that may have been buried. You're predisposed to be—indeed, designed to be—receptive to new life, new creation, and new discoveries. You are "wired," if you will, for this very kind of self-exploration.

TOOL #5: SOUL QUICK PIC

What is your soul saying to you? This exercise is a quick method of assessing what's "on your soul" at any given moment. Like the Body Quick Pic, it provides a fast snapshot.

- Pause and center yourself, closing your eyes or taking a few deep breaths.
- Turn your attention to your soul. What's its state right now? Is there anything it needs? Anything it wants? Is there anything you need or want from it?

That's it! By turning your attention to your soul, you glimpse what's brewing deep within you. The more you practice this speedy check-in, the more quickly and clearly the observations will come in.

Try It: Do a Soul Quick Pic now. Remember to do a warm-up—such as taking a few deep breaths and closing your eyes—before using any reflective tools to help yourself relax. This helps you transition from action to reflection, so you can better hear the messages within.

TOOL #6: JOURNALING YOUR JOURNEY

Keeping a journal is a wonderful way to access the tremendous changes taking place within you. Some women groan at the idea. Others are thrilled. Maybe you already keep a diary, or have considered keeping a diary specifically about pregnancy.

The journal I am asking you to keep is a mechanism for exploring, so keep in mind:

- *This journal is for your eyes only.* It's not intended to be an experience you share with your partner, or a diary of impressions that you are preserving for your future child. You need to feel free to record what is truly in your heart, without the self-editing that happens when we suspect that someone else might be digesting the information as well.

- *It's okay (and sometimes preferable) to destroy the pages once you have written them.* Some women prefer to burn or shred their ruminations after getting them down on paper. That's fine. If any part of you is concerned—even a little bit—that someone might read what you have written, get rid of it. This journal is a tool in a discovery process; it's not a product or keepsake.

- *Journaling can lead to self-awareness whether or not you're "good" at writing.* If you hate to write, think of Journaling as "off-loading" rather than writing. The act of putting pen to paper helps bring inner thoughts to the surface. Even if you don't think of yourself as particularly verbal, you can be sure you'll find plenty to say. You need not write long paragraphs or even full sentences. Journaling for you may consist of thoughts, phrases, lists, and even sketches.

- *Pick a journal that appeals to you.* Find a notebook that makes you want to touch it and write in it. It can be loose sheets that you store in a folder or handsomely bound, acid-free pages. The size doesn't matter, although portability is a plus so that you can always have it close at hand. The key prerequisite is plenty of empty pages.

Try It: Write a little bit about what you're feeling about pregnancy at this particular moment. Try to regularly set aside at least a few minutes of quiet time each day in a comfortable place to Journal.

TOOL #7: DIALOGUING
(WITH YOUR NONPHYSICAL SELF)

This tool works exactly the same way as tool #3, Dialoguing (with Your Physical Self). It's listed here separately mostly as a reminder that you can use the Dialoguing exercise to explore any issue, whether it's related to your body or to your soul. Below I've suggested the issue of becoming a mother, since it's such an obvious one to start with.

Try It: Practice Dialoguing now.

1. Find a quiet place where you won't be interrupted. Remember to make some mental space for reflection, using techniques such as deep breathing.
2. Now think about yourself being a mother.
3. In your mind, ask this mother "self" what she wants to say to you. Is there anything you want to say to her? Is there anything she needs from you? Is there anything you need from her? How does your soul feel about the possibility of motherhood? Does it have any reservations or concerns? Any advice? Any requests?
4. Accept the first answers that come to mind. Ask follow-up questions as they occur to you.

DEVELOPING BABY AWARENESS: TWO TOOLS

Pregnancy—imagined or real, planned or unintended—is different from every other part of your life in that there's a third dimension, beyond your own body and soul, to consider when making decisions: your baby. By being on the Fertility Pathway, you've invited another entity into that intimate sanctum that is your self. And you have a relationship with it, even before the baby is a ball of cells or a kicking fetus, even when it is still just a hope or a wish. Develop that relationship right from the beginning, rather than waiting until the umbilical cord is cut and you can hold him or her in your arms.

TOOL #8: BABY QUICK PIC

What is your baby saying to you? This exercise is a quick method of acknowledging and assessing your baby (real or prospective) at any given moment. It's convenient to do it together with the Body and Soul Quick Pics; many expectant mothers enjoy doing it on its own more often.

To do the Baby Quick Pic:

- Pause and center yourself, closing your eyes or taking a few deep breaths.
- Turn your attention to your baby. How is it doing today? What is its state right now? Is there anything it needs? Anything it wants? Is there anything you need or want from it?

This tool has psychological benefits in preconception and in the first half of pregnancy. By the second half, it also has enormously practical benefits, as you'll see.

Try It: Do a Baby Quick Pic now. Give it a little time, especially if you're not yet pregnant, to get used to the concept. What comes up for you?

TOOL #9: DREAMAGERY

This tool is an expansion of Dialoguing, though turned up a notch: It's a tool of insight that taps the active imagination. Its name ("DREAM-a-jry") is a combination of "dream" and "imagery." Dreamagery relies more heavily on imagery than Dialoguing does. It's a deeper, more visual conversation with your subconscious.

I love this tool. I've used it hundreds of times in a variety of settings and circumstances. Everyone comes away with deeper insights. Pregnancy is an especially wonderful time because not only is there so much roiling within, but moms-to-be tend to be in an especially receptive, creative, and visual state, even when they might not normally describe themselves this way.

When most of my patients first hear the word "imagery," they tend to think of visualization. That's imagery that's used to alter an outcome, such as imagining crossing the finish line of a race or powering through a contraction in labor. Cancer patients use imagery to imagine healthy cells gobbling up cancerous ones in their bodies, for example. That type of imagery is a terrific low-tech, high-reward therapeutic tool that enables the mind and body to participate in healing in a very empowering way.

The kind of imagery in Dreamagery is slightly different, however. We'll be inviting images to reveal personal insights, to gain understanding, and to build your relationship with your baby. You can use this tool to access information that might otherwise go unnoticed by your crowded conscious mind.

You can use Dreamagery, like Dialoguing, to explore any issue; here I have somewhat arbitrarily focused on using it to relate to your unborn child, but you'll find it useful in many other contexts.

Here's how Dreamagery works:

1. Allow yourself 15 to 20 minutes of uninterrupted time for this exercise. Get centered and relax using any tool you enjoy.

2. Invite an image of a relaxing, safe place to come to mind. It can be a place you are familiar with, or one that you make up. Notice as many details as you can about the place. Involve all your senses. How does it look? How does it smell? Are there sounds? Spend a few moments enjoying being there. This step deepens your relaxation and level of engagement.

3. After you're comfortable in this imagined place, invite an image to come to your mind that represents your unborn (or not yet conceived) child. "Represents" is the key word. Accept the first image that comes to mind; it may not be an actual baby or child, and that is absolutely fine. (In fact, for most women with whom I've done this exercise, the image is nothing baby-related.) Notice all the details you can about the image. Can you hold it? What color is it? What does it smell like? The more details you can observe, the deeper your state of relaxation will be. Be aware that the image may change shape or form during this conversation. It may also assume a different form each time you do this exercise.

4. Welcome this image that represents your baby. Ask the image what it has to say to you. Does it have any thoughts, concerns, requests, or questions to share?

5. Now you do the same. Share your own thoughts, feelings, or questions with this image. Feel free to have a back-and-forth conversation. "Talk" for as long as you would like, about whatever you would like. Don't feel you have to get everything "said" right now, though; this is just the beginning of your conscious relationship with your unborn child. You can always come back to it.

6. When the conversation feels complete for now, thank the image for coming and slowly return your awareness to the place you envisioned. Then, gradually let your attention turn back to the room you are in. Finally, make time to pay attention to what came up for you. Your journal can be a good partner in this exercise, whether you just jot down some key notes or explore the experience in detail.

Some women have an easier time than others getting the hang of Dreamagery. Those who are visual or intuitive may often find that images leap quickly to mind. Others may feel frustrated that they don't "see" anything right away; be patient and an image will come, even if you feel as though you are consciously concocting it.

I'm often asked, "But how do I know if I'm interpreting it right? Maybe it meant to say something different." It's not your job to interpret—that's your intellect crowding in. Your job in this exercise is merely to experience. The insights may reveal themselves immediately or gradually, sometimes much later while you're in the middle of doing something else. Dreamagery is not like dream analysis or tarot card reading, a riddle that you are supposed to unlock. It is simply a way to look inside yourself and see what is already there.

Try It: Invite an image of your unborn (or not yet conceived) child to come to mind. What your image looks like is not what's important. Patients have described to me images of flowers, dolls, blankets, aliens, seeds, children, inanimate objects, and more—you should run with whatever pops into your mind. It's common for the critical mind to barge in and criticize what the unconscious mind is "seeing." Acknowledge these thoughts and let them go; don't engage in dialogue with them. Get back to your image, however quirky or literal or unrelated to a baby it might seem.

The conversation that you have with that image, not the image itself, is where the unconscious mind begins to unfold.

DECISION-MAKING WITH AWARENESS

Are you ready to have a baby? How should you handle morning sickness? What will you eat today? Will you have an amniocentesis? Who will be with you during labor? How will you manage the pain of labor? There are a tremendous number of choices or decisions in pregnancy for which no right or wrong answer exists. To a large extent, what happens is up to you. I can't and wouldn't want to dictate your choices. What I can do is give you a process by which you can make conscious choices.

The Feedback Loop is a great decision-making tool that helps you arrive at the answer that's best for you. It consists of three cyclical steps: reflection, information, and action, and then picks up again with re-reflection. By running your choices—large or small—through this cycle, you can't help but live with greater awareness and intention. Net result: healthier choices.

This tool is easier to use than it may sound at first. In fact, I've done it so much and for so long that it's second nature; I can no longer *not* think in this way!

TOOL #10: THE FEEDBACK LOOP

Here's how the Feedback Loop looks:

• *First, reflection.* Start by reflecting on your personal or internal data. You can do this in many different ways, including reviewing insights from the Reflective Inventory, Journaling, Body and Soul Checks, Dialoguing, and other tools. Such data include your starting opinions, your emotions, your perceptions, your fears, and your physical sensations related to the issue you're considering.

• *Second, information.* Next, gather as much as you need to know from external data. Some people prefer to find an expert they trust (such as their ob-gyn) and use whatever information that individual provides. Others may want to supplement a consultation with second opinions or independent research. How much external data to incorporate into your decision-making is a very individual matter; some women have greater appetites for a lot of facts than others. Decide how much information you need for your own comfort level and find out how to access it.

• *Third, action.* Take a step based on both the internal and external data you have gathered. The step you take will depend on the topic being considered. It can be something relatively small and reversible (such as deciding to make an appointment for a preconception exam, if you are considering having a baby) or it can be a big step, such as discontinuing birth control (if you are considering having a baby and have already had preconception counseling).

• *Then, re-reflection.* Making a choice is not an end in itself. Reflect on the step you have taken—give yourself feedback—beginning the cycle again. How do you feel about your choice? What are your body and your soul telling you about this course of action? Does it feel right and good? Or uncomfortable and disconcerting? Your feedback is new and important information.

You can use the Feedback Loop in countless ways during your time on the Fertility Pathway. For example:

- To decide whether or not to get pregnant
- To choose your doctor or midwife
- To decide whether to have genetic counseling
- To decide whether to have a prenatal test
- To figure out when and how to get fertility help
- To cope with the diagnosis of a complication
- To decide whether you want to find out your baby's sex
- To plan the kind of delivery you prefer
- To select a method of childbirth education
- To decide whether you want to be induced
- To assess your pain-relief choices in labor
- To choose who will be present at your delivery
- To help you decide whether or how long to breastfeed
- To decide whether to circumcise your son
- To plan your maternity leave
- To plan your next pregnancy

You can even use the Feedback Loop when you're facing an irreversible choice (such as whether or not to have a surgery, procedure, or test). There's just one small difference: In these cases, you take the Action step in your head. *Imagine* that you have had that test or surgery. Live with that hypothetical choice for a few days or a week. (At least one day is a good rule of thumb if possible.) See how it feels. What do you notice? Then re-reflect on that imagined choice. Next "choose" the opposite route, and imagine it for a few more days. What do you notice? Did you feel more at peace when living with one choice? Did you have more anxiety while living with the other? Using the Feedback Loop is a great way to help work through difficult decisions that feel—and perhaps are—unchangeable.

Try It: Think of a decision you are facing, large or small, and run it through the Feedback Loop to get a feel for how this process works.

TINKER WITH YOUR TOOLS

Which tools you find most useful for gaining awareness about your body, soul, and baby is likely to change during the course of your pregnancy. So will the amount of time you probably spend on each. For example, the first trimester is such a dynamic time physically, most women are inclined to give extra focus to body awareness then. As pregnancy progresses, you're likely to continue to pay attention to your body, but find that the volume gets turned up on your soul-level concerns. As one's due date approaches, baby awareness naturally begins to dominate.

Noticing the evolution of what tools you are drawn to is part of the fun, and a further reflection of how changeable this time in your life is.

Chapter 4

Your Pregnancy Self-Care Plan

∞

How to nurture your health across your five Centers of Wellness

I wish I could offer you a magical formula for a perfect pregnancy and baby. But no such formula exists because "perfection" is a word that has no place in describing the human endeavor of childbearing. What's more, differing backgrounds, histories, tastes, habits, starting points, and so on mean that no one-size-fits-all health plan can possibly have the same effect on every person. Every birth is different, too. Sure, all female bodies are designed to gestate and give birth, but while some lucky people can just step out of the way and let the body do its thing, more often challenges arise—nausea, anemia, preterm labor—where our attention and involvement can make a difference. In addition, certain aspects of birth simply fall beyond anyone's control or understanding. We don't know why some women develop preeclampsia or why some fetuses refuse to come out of a breech position, for example. Your goal should be to move toward a lifestyle that will support *your* pregnancy in an optimal way. And that's something I *can* give you.

Whatever your starting point, this season of change is an ideal time to make some improvements in the way you take care of yourself. Whether you work to bring better balance into your life, shed unhealthy habits, or improve the good habits you already have, a child is the ultimate motivation. What's more, these benefits reverberate well beyond pregnancy and childbirth. You can create new habits that persist long after your baby is born, setting yourself up for a healthier midlife and beyond. By modeling those behaviors in motherhood, you'll send out powerful messages that shape your child's health as she or he grows, too.

THE FIVE CENTERS OF WELLNESS

Good health consists of five different (but overlapping) domains that must be individually strong as well as balanced overall.

These five Centers of Wellness are:

1. **Nutrition:** food, drink, and supplements.
2. **Movement:** exercise for fitness as well as movement that brings you joy.
3. **Mind:** the state of your mind, including your stressors and your perceptions.
4. **Spirit:** a feeling of connectedness to self, to other beings, and to an entity larger than yourself (such as God or nature), whether via spirituality, community, religion, or other vehicles.
5. **Sensation:** sensuality (the senses: touch, taste, vision, hearing, and smell) and sexuality.

It's through these five centers that you nourish your body and soul.

They're listed in no particular order of importance, because *all five are important*! Conventional medicine tends to value the first two and give a nod to the third. The last two are rarely even considered in a medical setting. But I believe all five interconnect to impact your well-being. For example, when you are eating well, you often feel less depressed, more energetic and apt to exercise more, and your relationships are also better. When you are not managing stress well, you may overeat and stop exercising, and your relationships and sex life may suffer.

What's so interesting is that your needs within a given center are constantly shifting—especially in pregnancy. The way you move, your appetites and food preferences, your stress level, your libido, your sense of connection to God or to your own mother or your friends—all will be impacted across the arc of this experience and all will vary from trimester to trimester, and even from day to day. That's why paying attention to all five of your Centers of Wellness is so important, and why you need a flexible plan that changes as you do.

The Basic Self-Care Plan for Pregnancy is simple and life-changing. In each of your five Centers of Wellness, I've mapped out a handful of daily goals. These are the minimum steps necessary to bring consciousness to that aspect of your health each day. Then I've listed a number of suggestions as to how you can attain each goal. Although the following summary of base-plan goals may sound like small steps, the ways you meet them, which I'll outline in the following pages, add up to big health changes.

BASIC SELF-CARE PLAN FOR PREGNANCY

Mind Center goals

- Try to bring awareness to your level of stress every day.
- Trigger the relaxation response at least once a day.
- Explore ways to use mind-body techniques to support the specific needs of your body and your soul.

Nutrition Center goals

- Explore and understand your relationship with food.
- Bring meal-by-meal consciousness to your food choices.
- Eliminate substances that are known dangers.
- Shift to a more pregnancy-friendly, balanced diet, with:
  - More essential nutrients
  - More fruits and vegetables
  - Healthier fats, especially omega-3s
  - More whole grains
  - Healthier proteins
  - Fewer empty calories

Movement Center goals

- Make conscious choices about the kinds of activity that your body needs and enjoys every day.

- Do a low-impact aerobic activity that you enjoy at least three times a week on nonconsecutive days.
- Strength-train at least three times a week on nonconsecutive days.
- Stretch every day.

Spirit Center goals

- Think about your sense of your life's meaning and purpose.
- Build a "sacred time" into each day.
- Do one thing every day to fuel or feed a relationship that you care about.

Sensation Center goals

- Pay attention to which of your senses you are most nurtured by.
- Actively nurture the full range of your senses and sensuality each day.
- Explore and support your sexuality as it evolves throughout your pregnancy and beyond.

THE MIND CENTER

Your mind is the interface between reality (the world, your outer life) and your body's response. I look forward to the day when this powerful connection is more routinely woven into the fabric of pregnancy care, because it so clearly impacts the health of the mother and her baby. We now know the state of your mind can influence your reproductive hormones, your blood pressure, your glucose levels, and the time and progress of your labor, among other things.

Your body responds not to the reality of the circumstances you are in but to your *perception* of those realities. If you're resting on the sofa with your feet up and a glass of lemonade in your hands after a long workday, but you're ruminating about the dish-throwing argument you just had with your husband and what shape your unsettled marriage will be in by the time the baby arrives, your body responds as if still in the middle of the fight. Your brain goes on alert and the fight-or-flight response built into your system kicks in, poising your body for action. The stress hormones cortisol and adrenaline jump, your blood pressure and heart rate increase, muscles tense, and glucose and cholesterol are released to provide quick energy. These changes are collectively known as the *stress response*.

On the other hand, you could be in the stressful throes of labor and yet, if your thoughts and breathing are aligned to a calm, relaxed mode, your body will respond accordingly and relax. This physiologic reaction is called the *relaxation response*. It can happen naturally—say, because you are actually lying there drinking lemonade and enjoying it—or you can use mind-body tools to trigger this response to counter stress.

Relaxation is to the mind what sleep is to the body. Sleep is a time when the body can truly unplug and be at rest. Your mind needs rest, too. And yet, when push comes to shove in a busy day, this center is one of the first my patients seem to ignore. Failure to relax can impact the likelihood of conceiving or of carrying a healthy baby to term.

The following are some ways to nurture this center and achieve the basic mental goals of pregnancy. (Trimester-specific advice appears in the chapters that follow.)

GOAL: Try to bring awareness to your level of stress every day.

• *Reflect on your stress level.* Whether pregnant or not, we grow accustomed to chronic stress. Our bodies adapt to it and our minds begin to consider this state normal. Over time, we keep setting our baseline a little higher and higher, so that eventually we don't even notice how stressed out we really are. Stop and bring a level of awareness to what you're feeling each day.

• *Reflect on your stress points.* Your stress points are how stress manifests itself. Notice how and where your body holds stress. Reflect on which body systems or parts of you are most affected by stress. Do you get headaches or backaches? Are you more likely to get sick? Are you simply tired or fatigued under stress? Does your gastrointestinal system take the hit (for example, changed bowel habits such as constipation or diarrhea, or indigestion)? Do you get depressed? Do your relationships suffer? Often an individual's stress points change or intensify while on the Fertility Pathway. Places in your musculoskeletal system that previously manifested stress—the lower back, for example—may be even more vulnerable, while areas that might never have given you much of a problem—your GI system, for example—may start responding noticeably to stress. Reflect on whether and how your stress responses have changed.

• *Be conscious about how much sleep you're needing and getting.* The average nonpregnant woman needs eight hours of sleep a night—and one-quarter of us don't sleep enough to be fully alert the next day. Now add in the demands of gestation. At various points in pregnancy, your body may require more sleep than what you're used to. Be aware that sleep is an arena that can change a lot on the Fertility Pathway, and throughout pregnancy. Pay attention to your individual needs, and honor what you learn. If your body is telling you it needs more sleep, then listen and get more sleep. Pay attention to sleep surroundings as well. During pregnancy, you may find that you require more space, more pillows (to support your body), different room temperature, or more/fewer blankets.

GOAL: Trigger the relaxation response at least once a day.

• *Find a form of meditation that works for you.* Essentially, meditation is a way to quiet the mind and is often done with an inner focus, in contrast to the outer-focused, preoccupied unconsciousness that we use to get through much of everyday life. Meditation is sometimes also called "centering." It's been used for centuries in the Far East as a practice for attaining spiritual enlightenment. You can learn this kind of formal meditation, which sometimes involves special postures and mantras, or you can attain a similar state of deep calm through such practices as deep breathing, meditative prayer, yoga, or other deeply relaxing pursuits. Meditation activates the relaxation response, quieting the mind and clearing it of anxiety and worry while also causing such physical changes as reducing blood pressure and stress hormones, and relaxing the muscles. Experiment with different forms of meditation until you find one that is comfortable and effective for you, then try to incorporate it into every day.

• *Practice mindfulness.* Are you connected and living in the present, or preoccupied with the future (for example, what's next on your to-do list), the past (the argument you had last night), or a different place (such as text messaging while you're lunching with a friend)? A certain amount of shifting out of the present is necessary to function, but when you find yourself doing too much of it, you tend to feel out of balance and more stressed. (Not to mention you're probably missing a whole lot of your life!) Begin to notice how much of the time you are fully present and practice this skill consciously. Put down the BlackBerry or cell, and turn all of your attention to your friend, for example, or to the food on your plate.

   • *Try breathing exercises when anxiety creeps in.* Conscious breathing is a great way to catch a few quick moments of relaxation, even in the midst of stress. Any kind of slow breathing—such as taking deep rhythmic breaths or doing the following breathing exercise—can put a brake on rising stress.

4/7/8 Breathing (Paced Breathing)

1. Rest the tip of your tongue on the ridge behind your front teeth throughout the exercise.
2. Breathe in through your nose for a count of four.
3. Hold for a count of seven.
4. Exhale through the mouth for a count of eight. With your tongue in the same position as in step 1, you should hear a *shoosh* sound as the air goes out.

Repeat four times. Do this as often as needed throughout the day.

   Try It: Take a few minutes to practice 4/7/8 breathing right now. See how easy and relaxing it is?

This simple breathing pattern, which Andrew Weil taught me years ago, has become my favorite secret sanity-saver since I became a mom. When we get really stressed, we tend to take shallow, panting breaths. Paced breathing, which is based on an ancient yoga practice, helps reverse that tendency, whether it's subtle or pronounced, and sends a relaxation message to the body.

   • *Calm your mind and relax your body with mental muscle relaxation.* We hold tension in our bodies without even being aware of it. Examples include tooth-grinding at night, or a tight back that's not in pain yet flinches when touched. This exercise—ideal to do at bedtime—relaxes major muscle groups to release stress.

Mental Muscle Relaxation

1. Sit or lie in a comfortable and quiet place with your body fully supported by a chair or the floor. (Do not lie on your back after the fourth month of pregnancy.) Close your eyes. Take a few deep breaths: deep inhale, deep exhale.
2. Begin at the top of your head, with your scalp and your forehead, noticing whether there is any tension there. Give it permission to let go.
3. Progress down your body, from head to toe, mentally assessing the muscles along the way and then mentally releasing any tension you find. Move from your head to your neck, your shoulders, your upper arms and lower arms, your fingers, all the way down your spinal column, around to your chest, your belly, your hips, your buttocks, your thighs, your knees, your calves, the arches of your feet, your toes. Let the tension go with your mind.
4. Take all the time you need. If there are places that still seem to be holding tension after you finish, return there. Only when you feel completely relaxed should you slowly bring your attention back to the present.

•   *Try progressive muscle relaxation (PMR).* Instead of patrolling for tension and then mentally letting it go, as you do in mental muscle relaxation, in this exercise you actually tense the muscle and then physically release it. PMR helps make you more aware of when your muscles are tensed and can help invite the relaxation response in your body.

Progressive Muscle Relaxation

1. Lie on your back with your arms at your sides, on a firm but soft surface such as a soft carpet or a workout mat. (A bed is too soft.) After the fourth month of pregnancy, you should sit in a chair that supports your head and neck. Loosen any tight clothing and remove your shoes.
2. Ideally, when you are first learning this exercise, you should have someone slowly read the instructions below to you, or make a tape of them for yourself.

3. First, tense the muscles throughout your body, from head to toe. Tighten your feet and your legs, tense your arms, and clench your jaw. Pull in your stomach. Hold the tension while you sense the feelings of strain and tightness. Notice the difference between how this feels and how the muscle feels when it is relaxed. Notice that as you tense the muscles, you most likely naturally hold your breath. Hold it for a few seconds more, and exhale long and slowly as you relax all your muscles, letting the tension go. Notice the sense of relief as you relax.

4. Now you will tense and relax individual major muscle groups. Keep the rest of your body as relaxed as you can. You will hold the tension for a few seconds until you get a clear sense of what the tension feels like. Then inhale deeply, hold the breath, and release the tension as you exhale.

5. Start by making your hands into tight fists. Feel the tension through your hands and arms. Relax and release the tension. Now press your arms against the surface they're resting on. Feel the tension. Hold it . . . and let it go. Let your arms and hands go limp.

6. Shrug your shoulders up tight, toward your head, feeling the tension through your neck and shoulders. Hold . . . and release. Drop your shoulders down, free of tension.

7. Now wrinkle your forehead, sensing the tightness. Hold . . . and let it go so your forehead is smooth and released. Shut your eyes as tightly as you can. Hold . . . and let it go. Now open your mouth as wide as you can. Hold . . . and let it go, letting your lips gently touch. Then clench your jaw, teeth tight together. Hold . . . and relax. Let the muscles of your face be at ease.

8. Take a few moments to tense your arms and shoulders, up through your face. Now take a deep breath, filling your lungs down through your abdomen. Hold your breath while you feel the tension through your chest. Then exhale and let your chest relax, your breath natural and easy. Suck in your stomach, holding the muscles tight . . . and relax. Arch your back . . . hold . . . and ease your back down gently, letting it relax. Feel the relaxation spreading through your whole upper body.

9. Now tense your hips and buttocks, pressing your legs and heels against the surface beneath you. Hold...and relax. Curl your toes down so that they point away from your knees. Hold...and relax, letting the tension go from your legs and feet. Then bend your toes back up toward your knees. Hold...and relax.

10. Now feel your whole body at rest, letting go of more tension with each breath. Your face relaxed and soft...your arms and shoulders loose...stomach, chest, and back relaxed...your legs and feet resting at ease...your whole body calm and relaxed.

11. Take time to enjoy this state of relaxation for several minutes, feeling the deep calm and peace. When you're ready to get up, move slowly, first sitting, and then standing up gradually.

• *Take a mental vacation.* This is one of my favorites! Get relaxed using any technique you like and then let an image come to mind of a place where you feel completely at ease and safe. It may be a place you've been before, or a place you have never been but would like to go, or an imaginary world that does not exist. Notice every detail about the scene with each of your senses: What do you see, smell, hear, feel, and taste? Who else, if anyone, is there? Spend as much time as you would like in the scene. Relax and enjoy it. And best of all, know that you can go back anytime you wish. When you feel ready, slowly return your attention to the reality around you—and don't be surprised when your body actually feels like you have been on vacation!

THE NUTRITION CENTER

I don't believe that there is one nutritional formula that is right for every pregnant woman. What if I told you broccoli were part of such a diet, and you hated broccoli? What if I prescribed eating three meals a day, or six, but nausea prevented you from keeping anything down? The risks of a formula include false hope and then guilt when you can't stick to it. The perfect diet in *your* pregnancy is one that allows you to make mindful choices that support your own physical and emotional needs, as well as your health goals—including a healthy baby.

That's why nutrition begins with reflecting on your personal relationship to food. It's a complicated issue. Food is fuel, food is sociability, food is sensual, food is nurturing, food is comforting—and in pregnancy, food can also be a source of worry or the object of cravings. Ideally, nutrition should provide you with the nutrients you need in a pleasant experience free from guilt, anxiety, mindlessness, or fear.

Another consideration: your predispositions regarding your relationship to food tend to be magnified. So if you're an obsessive label-reader, your focus on nutrients, carb counts, or calories is apt to continue with renewed zeal. If you've struggled with weight control in the past, the prospect of intentionally gaining pounds may bring old battles back, or you may feel like "giving up" since you'll be gaining weight anyway. That's why paying attention to your tendencies is so important.

You'll notice that the suggestions in this center are more detailed than in the others. This is because there is far more research on how nutrition affects body, soul, and baby. Nutrition also comprises so many different elements (food, liquid, supplements) and nutrients.

Here are some ways to nurture this center and achieve the basic nutrition goals for pregnancy.

GOAL: Explore and understand your relationship with food.

• *Reflect on your relationship with food—and how anything has changed since you've been on the Fertility Pathway.* What's your nutritional history? What has your relationship with food been like? Have you ever had an eating disorder? How about now? What do you eat on a typical day? Why do you eat? Do you ever eat when you are not hungry? Why?

• *Consider reviewing your diet with a nutritionist or other health expert.* Any eating plan other than a balanced diet incorporating all of the food groups should be reviewed in light of the special demands of pregnancy. Especially if you are a vegetarian or vegan, or follow a special diet because of allergies, diabetes, or other medical conditions, it's a good idea to ensure that you're not falling short in any of the nutrients needed for childbearing, especially folic acid, iron, calcium, B vitamins, and zinc.

• *Reflect on your weight.* Being particularly overweight or underweight can significantly impact your ability to conceive and carry a child. Discuss this issue with your health care provider. While no one should try to lose weight during pregnancy, every woman should pay attention to what she eats and how much weight she's gaining, and weight targets will vary depending on your pre-pregnancy weight.

GOAL: Bring meal-by-meal consciousness to your food choices.

• *Before eating anything, take a breath and check in with your body.* Notice if you are hungry and/or whether you are tired, worried, bored, nervous, or stressed. Other factors are often behind what we perceive as hunger. Try using a hunger scale to help you decide whether your body is truly signaling a need to eat. Ask yourself how hungry you are on a scale of 1 (very hungry) to 6 (very full). Your goal should be to eat when you feel 2 to 2.5 (moderately hungry); don't wait until you are ravenous. Stop eating at 5 to 5.5, before you become uncomfortable. By simply increasing your awareness and making your choice to eat consciously, you will find that both what you eat and how much you eat are likely to shift.

• *When you eat, take it slowly, savoring each bite and taking time between bites to let the food do its job.* Put the fork down in between bites, if that helps, or use your nondominant hand to make yourself slow down. Be sure you're in a quiet environment so you can focus on the food—take at least 20 minutes to eat a meal, and stop every few minutes to assess whether you are still hungry. Notice the smell of the food, the texture, the flavor, and how it changes as you chew and swallow. Eat mindfully.

GOAL: Eliminate substances that are known dangers.

• *Discontinue all vitamins and supplements and switch to prenatal vitamins.* Prenatal vitamins contain adequate amounts of the nutrients needed in pregnancy, especially iron and folic acid. Your doctor can prescribe them, ideally three months prior to conception. If you have morning sickness, and you cannot keep the prenatal vitamins down, try supplementing with just folic acid, which is a much smaller pill. Don't double your usual vitamin dosages, or take megadoses of any vitamin. Outside of prenatal vitamins, vitamin supplements have not been well studied in pregnancy.

✓REALITY CHECK: Botanicals and Pregnancy

Taking an integrative approach to pregnancy means considering the best of all systems of medicine. In conventional Western medicine, hard data are scarce on the use of botanicals (herbal medicine) in pregnancy, mainly because we don't like to experiment in pregnancy out of concern for endangering the mother or fetus. Yet in other systems of medicine, such as Chinese medicine, there is a long tradition of using certain herbs for the prevention of miscarriage, morning sickness, and many other pregnancy-related disorders and conditions. Unfortunately, no proof of effectiveness exists in the medical literature.

Lack of hard data doesn't mean a given botanical is unsafe, any more than it indicates it's safe. So while I recommend that you avoid botanicals unless specifically okayed by your doctor, I can also appreciate that many practitioners of alternative systems of medicine are very knowledgeable in this area. For my own patients, I ask them to discontinue all over-the-counter botanicals immediately. If they are working with an herbalist or an Oriental-medicine doctor who uses herbal teas, I ask them to avoid use in the first trimester, unless I know the substance is harmless (like ginger tea, for example). Do your homework and find someone you trust who knows what they're doing, and someone who is willing to work in collaboration with your physicians. If they are hesitant to do this, I would be hesitant about working with them.

• *Review with your doctor any botanicals you currently take.* Just because they're "natural" doesn't mean they're safe. Because there have been few studies of botanicals in pregnancy, I recommend that my patients discontinue taking them completely unless given the green light by their care provider. (See box.) If you are receiving care from anyone prescribing botanical medicine, be sure to let your conventional provider know, and continue to share information freely.

- *Stop drinking alcohol.* It's not yet known if there is a safe limit for pregnancy, so it's best to eliminate it completely. Although there is no evidence regarding alcohol and conception, the multitude of data linking alcohol to low birth weight and birth defects (many of which occur in the earliest weeks after conception) makes it advisable to stop while you're trying to conceive. What's more, alcohol increases estrogen, which can interfere with your normal hormonal cycles. That said, there's no reason to skip an occasional glass of wine or beer before you conceive, provided you drink consciously—which means drinking no alcohol at all around the time of ovulation, and limiting alcohol to one glass on days you're certain you're not pregnant, such as during your period or immediately after. I'd avoid heavy drinking at any time on the Fertility Pathway just to be safe.

- *Decaffeinate your diet.* Caffeine stimulates the central nervous system and can cause insomnia, nervousness, gastric irritation, nausea, and vomiting. It can shorten the stress response, increase heart rate, increase blood pressure, quicken the respiratory rate, and, in great excess, cause tremors and convulsions. There are suggestions that it could take less than one cup of coffee a day to interfere with conception and implantation. More than one cup of coffee a day has been associated with an increased risk of miscarriage. Women who have more than three to four cups of coffee or its equivalent (about 375 mg of caffeine) are more than twice as likely to miscarry. Therefore it's best to have very little caffeine in your system from the earliest points of pregnancy. If you're a pot-a-day drinker, for example, don't wait until your home test turns positive to wean yourself. Because withdrawal can cause headaches, some women find it easier to eliminate it from their diet before they become pregnant. Try starting with half-decaf in your cup and gradually decreasing the amount that's caffeinated. Better still, experiment with drinking caffeine-free teas (such as herbal teas) or water (plain or flavored) in place of your usual java breaks. Instead of caffeinated sodas, drink decaf brands or, ideally, switch to water, flavored with lemon or lime if desired. (I advise patients to steer clear of the new fortified and vitamin waters, however, as some contain herbals, which I don't recommend in pregnancy.)

Although caffeine is also found in chocolate, the amount is so low you generally needn't worry; if, however, you consume huge amounts of chocolate—which is not ideal for other nutritional reasons—check the labels and add up caffeine-content totals.

HOW MUCH CAFFEINE?

You can see how quickly the milligrams add up,
depending on your drink of choice:

Beverage	Caffeine (milligrams)
Brewed coffee (8 oz.)	60–120 mg
Instant coffee (8 oz.)	90–110 mg
Espresso (1 oz.)	45–100 mg
Mountain Dew (12 oz.)	55 mg
Black tea (8 oz.)	50 mg
Coca-Cola (12 oz.)	35 mg
Green tea (8 oz.)	30 mg

• *Quit smoking.* Smokers have been found to have reduced fertility (nearly one-third the conception rate of nonsmokers). Smoking also increases your chances of miscarriage, stillbirth, prematurity, low birth weight, and birth defects such as cleft palate—just to name a few of the proven unfortunate side effects. Quitting is seldom simple, but it is easier before you're pregnant, when you can safely use nicotine-replacement therapies such as patches or gums. (They are not recommended for use in pregnancy.) Other methods to check out include hypnosis and acupuncture.

• *Limit consumption of mercury-rich fish.* Mercury is a toxin that can cause long-term neurological and developmental problems in developing fetuses and growing children. Because mercury can accumulate in your bloodstream over time and take up to a year to leave your system, it's wise to follow this guideline even before you conceive. Avoid fish with high levels of mercury, including shark, swordfish, tilefish, and king mackerel. You don't need to cut out all fish, however, and you shouldn't. Many fish are a good source of nutrients such as omega-3 fatty acids, which are important for the developing fetus. The most common fish and shellfish that are relatively low in mercury, according to the FDA, are shrimp, canned light tuna, salmon, pollock, and catfish; pregnant women are advised to eat up to 12 ounces (about two regular meals) per week of these. Because albacore ("white" canned) tuna and tuna steak (not canned) tend to have higher levels of mercury than the regular light kind, the FDA recommends that women of childbearing age consume no more than 6 ounces of these types per week. The presence of mercury in freshwater catches (such as lake trout) or in coastal catches depends on the individual lake, river, or coast; you should follow local health department recommendations or avoid such fish if in doubt about their source. The FDA says one meal per week of such fish is probably safe if there are no such advisories out, and if you eat no other fish that week.

• *Forgo raw or unpasteurized products.* In the interest of safety, put a hold on raw milk, raw-milk cheese, and unpasteurized cider or juice, which can contain bacteria such as *Listeria* or *E. coli.* Pregnant women are 20 times more likely than other adults to get listeriosis, a foodborne illness that can cause miscarriage and stillbirth. About one-third of listeriosis cases occur in pregnant women. Bid sayonara to sashimi and sushi containing raw fish, raw shellfish, soft cheeses (feta, Brie, blue, Camembert, queso blanco fresco), runny eggs, and meats cooked rare or medium rare. Cream cheese is safe, though not especially nutritious.

• *Discontinue any use of diet pills.* Aside from being a generally unhealthy way to shed pounds, they are specifically not recommended for pregnant women or those trying to conceive.

FEAR: I've eaten food past the sell-by date!
FACT: While you want to bring awareness to the freshness, quality, and safety of the food you eat, try not to become too obsessive. That only invites stress, which more or less cancels out the good gained by eating healthfully.

GOAL: Shift to a more pregnancy-friendly, balanced diet, with:

More essential nutrients
• *Get sufficient folic acid.* This B vitamin reduces the chance of neural tube defects affecting the spinal cord and brain, such as spina bifida and anencephaly. The neural tube (which later becomes the spinal cord and brain) is formed in the first 28 days of development. Without sufficient folic acid in the blood, the neural tube can fail to close properly. About 70 percent of neural-tube defects can be

✓ REALITY CHECK: Medications in Pregnancy

Consult with your doctor about all medications, before taking them and before going off them. Certain prescription medicines can cause severe birth defects, such as the acne product Accutane (isotretinoin), which is linked to newborn heart abnormalities; tetracycline; lithium (used to treat manic depression); and tamoxifen (used to treat breast cancer). Others indicate no fetal risk, according to the Food and Drug Administration, including insulin and the sleep aid Ambien. Many over-the-counter (OTC) products have been pronounced safe in pregnancy, including Tylenol, Benadryl, and Imodium. Cold remedies, however, should be avoided until after the first trimester. And new research is coming out all the time. A study published in February 2006 showed that newborns whose mother used a type of antidepressant called SSRIs, such as Prozac and Zoloft, had a significantly higher risk of developing a heart and lung disorder called persistent pulmonary hypertension. Be certain to talk to your obstetrician about the most recent research regarding any medications you are taking.

prevented by adequate folate consumption. Ideally, you should begin consuming at least 400 to 800 mcg (micrograms) of folic acid every day for two to three months before conception. You may be especially low in folate, magnesium, zinc, and vitamin C if you recently used the birth control pill or other hormonal contraception. A prenatal vitamin can provide this. Folic acid is also found naturally in spinach, brussels sprouts, avocado, egg yolks, lentils, peanuts, wheat germ, liver, strawberries, oranges, and orange juice. Since 1998, many grain products (breads, cereals, pastas) have been fortified with folic acid.

• *Review your iron status with your doctor and supplement as necessary.* Iron helps form red blood cells, which carry oxygen to your baby. Some evidence indicates that supplementing 30 mg of iron daily may increase fertility. A simple blood test (part of the standard preconception or prenatal workup) can determine your iron levels. Fortify your iron levels with diet as well as supplements, if prescribed.

The best dietary sources of iron include beans, lentils, fish, shellfish, dried fruits, and egg yolks.

• *Be certain to get adequate calcium in your diet.* In a large study published in March 2006, when women who consumed less than 600 mg of calcium a day were supplemented with 1,500 mg, they had far fewer complications of preeclampsia, including preterm delivery. Pay attention to your diet and choose calcium-rich foods.

• *Add choline-rich foods.* This vitamin-B-like compound exists in eggs, beef liver, chicken liver, soybeans, and wheat germ. Choline is beginning to get a lot of attention because it's thought to play a critical role in fetal brain development and may lower the risk of spinal cord defects. Few women are normally deficient in choline, since it's found in so many common foods, but during pregnancy the body's stores are taxed as it's pumped into the placenta for fetal use. While there is no evidence to support supplementing choline, it's important to have enough in your diet. Good sources include beef liver (418 mg/g), eggs (251 mg/g), wheat germ (152 mg/g), bacon (125 mg/g), and dried soybeans (116 mg/g). Vegetarians or anyone who eats a minimal amount of milk, eggs, and meat should try to get 450 mg of choline a day through wheat germ and soy.

More fruits and vegetables

• *Aim for at least seven and ideally 10 servings of fruits and vegetables every day.* This is not as much as it may seem if you understand portion size: A serving is one cup of raw vegetables or one half cup cooked; one medium-sized piece of fruit or half a banana; or four ounces of juice. *Every day* some of these 10 servings should include dark green vegetables (broccoli, greens, spinach, salad mix) and orange vegetables (carrots, sweet potato, cantaloupe). Fruits and vegetables such as these, especially, are packed with the nutrients your growing baby needs.

Healthier fats

• *Increase omega-3 fatty acids in your diet.* Your baby uses omega-3 fatty acids in the development of the central nervous system and this is especially true in the third trimester. They also help prevent chronic diseases such as heart disease and arthritis. But American diets are notoriously lacking in omega-3s, so begin to incorporate them as soon as you can. There is evidence that children born to mothers who have a diet rich in omega-3s have better visual acuity when they are toddlers. Increased omega-3s may have a protective effect on post-partum depression. While flaxseeds contain only one of the three types of omega-3s, they are also a great source of fiber. Try buying it whole and grinding it as needed with a coffee grinder or blender. Store in the refrigerator and sprinkle it on cereal, salads, or vegetables. Also high in omega-3s: such fish as salmon, sardines, bluefish, herring, mackerel, and tuna. (See fish warnings above.) The following table shows some of the best sources of omega-3s, which are of three major types: alpha-linolenic (ALA), eicosapentaenoic (EPA), and docosa-hexaenoic (DHA). Most research showing general health benefits is on EDA and DHA.

OMEGA-3 FOODS

Aim for 7 to10 grams of omega-3s weekly

Source (3.5 ounces fish)*	ALA	EPA	DHA	Total (grams)
Flax oil (1 teaspoon)	2.7			2.7
Mackerel, Atlantic		0.9	1.6	2.5
Mackerel, king (mercury concern)		1.0	1.2	2.2
Herring, Pacific		1.0	0.7	1.7
Flaxseed (1 tablespoon ground)	1.6			1.6
Herring, Atlantic		0.7	0.9	1.6
Tuna, bluefin (mercury concern)		0.4	1.2	1.6
Tuna, skipjack (mercury concern)		0.4	1.2	1.6
Trout, lake		0.5	1.1	1.6
Salmon, chinook		0.8	0.6	1.4
Anchovies		0.5	0.9	1.4

Source (3.5 ounces fish)*	ALA	EPA	DHA	Total (grams)
Tuna, albacore (mercury concern)		0.3	1.0	1.3
Bluefish		0.4	0.8	1.2
Salmon, Atlantic		0.3	0.9	1.2
Salmon, sockeye		0.5	0.7	1.2
Salmon, chum		0.4	0.6	1.0
Salmon, pink		0.4	0.6	1.0
Sardines, canned		0.4	0.6	1.0
Bass, striped		0.2	0.6	0.8
Salmon, coho		0.3	0.5	0.8
Trout, rainbow		0.1	0.4	0.5
Sea bass, Japanese		0.1	0.3	0.4
Halibut, Pacific		0.1	0.3	0.4
Bass, freshwater		0.1	0.2	0.3
Carp		0.2	0.1	0.3
Catfish, channel		0.1	0.2	0.3
Cod, Atlantic		0.1	0.2	0.3
Perch, ocean		0.2	0.1	0.3
Pike, walleye		0.1	0.2	0.3
Flounder		0.1	0.1	0.2
Haddock		0.1	0.1	0.2
Snapper, red		Tr	0.2	0.2
Sole		Tr	0.1	0.1

*USDA Nutrient Database

• *Avoid trans fats.* Also known as hydrogenated fats, these man-made fats are created when hydrogen gas reacts with oil, usually to give a product a longer shelf life. There is a proven and direct relationship between diets high in trans fats and high levels of LDL (low-density lipoprotein) cholesterol, aka "bad" cholesterol, which increases the risk of coronary artery disease. Trans fats are found in many fried fast foods and in processed foods such as crackers, doughnuts, muffins, cookies, and microwave popcorn. Check food labels; information about a food's trans-fat content has been required since 2006.

• *Move your diet away from saturated fats.* Saturated fats are another known link to high levels of LDL cholesterol and therefore another heart-health risk. Aim for fewer than 15 grams daily. Saturated fats are the kind in most cheeses, butter, ice cream, whole milk, beef, and processed foods. For example, one cup of vanilla ice cream with 16 percent fat contains 14.8 grams of saturated fat.

• *Choose healthy oils.* Replace polyunsaturated kinds (vegetable oils, corn oil, sunflower oil, soybean oil) with monounsaturated kinds (olive oil, canola oil, organic peanut oil). Be aware that peanut oil is just as potent an allergen as peanuts themselves if you have such an intolerance. Be sure to check any labels before using blended oils.

• *Eat more healthy fats.* Fats derived from plants and fish tend to be good choices. Plant fats include nuts, seeds, seed butters (peanut, almond, tahini), avocado, and olives.

More whole grains
• *Focus on fiber, more than on carbs or calories.* Most women don't get enough. Fiber-rich foods include fruits and vegetables, beans and legumes (including chickpeas, kidney beans, lentils), flaxseeds, whole-grain breads, and higher-fiber cereals such as oatmeal or those with a bran base.

• *Swap white grains for whole grains.* Look for the words "100 percent whole wheat" on the label of wheat bread; you can't always tell by the color of the bread. Bagels, pastries, white pasta, and baked goods contain little fiber, and even when they purport to be whole grain this isn't always the case; look for "whole grain" as one of the first ingredients on the label. Whole-grain foods promote intestinal regularity, reduce cholesterol, and offer vitamins and protective antioxidants. Other good whole-grain choices include whole oats and oatmeal (including instant), whole rye, brown rice, and pearl barley. Try making pancakes, muffins, and baked goods with half whole-wheat and half white flour if all-whole-wheat products are not to your liking.

• *Fry not.* Stay away from french fries, fried chicken, and snack chips that are fried rather than baked.

Healthier proteins
• *Choose low-fat animal proteins.* Examples include chicken breast, turkey breast, egg whites, fish, lowfat yogurt, lowfat cottage cheese, and lowfat milk.

• *Reduce high-fat animal proteins.* Eat less red meat, which is high in saturated fat. Avoid cured or smoked meats (bacon, hot dogs, sausage, luncheon meats such as salami or bologna) altogether because they contain not only saturated fats but nitrates, which are linked to cancer-causing compounds. These guidelines are relevant whether you are pregnant or not.

• *Eat fewer animal proteins and more fish as well as soy and other protein-rich foods.* Examples: soy-based veggie burgers, tofu, ethnic meals (Indian, Thai, Chinese), hummus, vegetable stir-fry, and whole-bean burritos.

Fewer empty calories
• *Plan your indulgences.* Nobody enjoys (or can stick to) a rigid diet that leaves them feeling deprived and cranky. Consciously build occasional decadences into your eating. What that means is up to you. It could mean whole-wheat bread warm from the bakery and dipped in olive oil. Or it could mean a dish of your favorite ice cream on occasion.

While the list above tells you to avoid or minimize consumption of many different substances, avoid demonizing foods. It's true that you want to move away from eating processed foods, highly sugared foods, and the "bad" fats, but you'll find that when you develop the habit of making conscious choices about nutrition you will just naturally start eating—and enjoying—the more healthful foods. You'll also discover that you will take great pleasure in their colors, their smells, their tastes.

FEAR: Nonorganic food is inferior to organic.

FACT: It makes sense to avoid any unnecessary additions to your food such as hormones and pesticides. Given the choice, eating whole, natural, organic foods is ideal. On the other hand, without getting into the politics of agriculture, you shouldn't worry too much if you lack the access or budget for an all-organic diet. Most nonorganic foods eaten in the course of a normal diet don't put a fetus at any added risk. And while organics are grown pesticide-free, pollutants and toxins are everywhere, including in the air and water used to grow them. Organic and nonorganic foods have similar nutritional profiles. Bottom line: Eat organic and hormone-free when feasible, but don't stress if it's not.

THE MOVEMENT CENTER

There's a reason I don't call it the "Exercise Center." That label is too narrow. Too often we associate Movement with calorie-burning drudgery and overlook the pleasure it can bring. Movement is any kind of activity, both the gym-workout kind and milder purposeful efforts such as walking the dog, gardening, or taking the stairs instead of the elevator. Movement also encompasses things we do just because they feel good or make us happy, like dancing or stretching. The body likes to move. It's designed to move. If you root your Movement choices in the joy that comes with moving your body, you'll be more likely to do them. And if your body is moving, it's reaping benefit.

In fact, there is no drug, vitamin, mineral, or botanical that offers as many health benefits as exercise. Being fit and active eases stress, lifts mood, improves the quality of your sleep, and helps you feel empowered in your body at a time when so much else that is happening to your body is beyond your control. There is no hard evidence that exercise in pregnancy leads to a shorter, easier labor or creates a healthier baby. But fit women are more likely to cope well with labor's demands, have fewer complications, and have a faster and smoother postpartum recovery. Recent research at McGill University confirmed that active pregnant women were less depressed, less irked by daily hassles, and less likely to suffer from anxiety and stress than sedentary women. Women who develop gestational diabetes have been shown to reduce or eliminate their need for insulin when strength training is part of their pregnancy routine.

Developing the exercise habit during pregnancy, even if you haven't had it previously, will make you more likely to continue it afterward, when Movement can help you lose weight, gain energy, and feel better primed to handle the challenges of parenthood. What's more, benefits to your baby may include improved fetal stress tolerance, advanced brain maturation, and lower amounts of body fat later in life. A study in *Clinical Sports Medicine* found that the children of women who exercised in pregnancy were leaner than others at five years of age.

"Confinement" is a term that went out with the bustle. Yet our sedentary modern lifestyle, combined with the physical demands of pregnancy and our concerns about harming the baby, make it a real challenge to incorporate a healthy amount of Movement into our daily lives. Even active women often wonder how much they should cut back, if at all, or how to alter their usual routines in a baby-safe way.

Here are some ways to nurture this center and achieve the basic Movement goals for pregnancy.

GOAL: Make conscious choices about the kinds of activity that your body needs and enjoys every day.

• *Reflect on movement in your life.* When has moving your body been fun or given you a sense of joy? When is the last time you did this? When in your life have you felt most fit? What was your routine then? What do you do now for exercise? Do you enjoy it (whether you do it regularly or not)? What do you not like to do?

• *Make sure your movement choices are balanced.* Aerobic exercise, flexibility (stretching), and strengthening (weight training) should all have a place in your Movement Center.

• *Start a new or different routine, if that feels right to you.* The advice is often given not to embark on a new fitness regimen in pregnancy, but there's no medical reason not to if you choose your activities wisely, proceed mindfully, and have no medical or obstetrical impediments. Even a sedentary woman can begin exercising, such as walking and/or working with free weights, in pregnancy. And if you are not yet pregnant, all the better! It's a perfect time to start a new routine.

• *If you do have a fitness routine, evaluate what kinds of changes you will need to make to adapt it to pregnancy.* Some sports, including scuba diving, waterskiing, and platform diving, should be abandoned. Others, including contact sports, skiing, horseback riding, and running, may or may not be suited to pregnancy, depending on how long you've been doing them, your fitness level, and the nature of your pregnancy, which you don't know at this point. Still others, like yoga, can be continued, but with modifications. You may not need to make any changes yet, but it's wise to be alert now so you can plan ahead.

• *Review your exercise wardrobe.* You'll be able to do more if you're comfortable. You may find that you're hotter than before, so layers can be useful. You may need a more supportive athletic bra than previously and more stretchy, elastic waistbands as pregnancy progresses. Check the fit of your shoes periodically, too, since the ligaments of your feet loosen, making them wider.

• *Consider activities that you can sustain across the pregnancy-postpartum year.* Water aerobics and swimming are good matches for pregnancy, for example, because they are non-weight-bearing exercises and there is little risk of falls. A water workout is also cooling and refreshing. Yoga and Tai Chi help increase body awareness and balance, excellent when your body is changing rapidly and your center of gravity is shifting.

• *Move just for the sake of joy.* Ideally, this is a time of free-flowing energy and creativity. (What could be more creative and exciting than making a new life?) Look for ways to move that both express and enhance this idea. For example, dance around the house to music that you love. If you enjoy the feeling of your body moving through water, get yourself to a pool or body of water and just enjoy feeling your body move through and with the water (as opposed to dutifully swimming laps). And sex, of course, is a joyful kind of movement, too!

GOAL: Do a low-impact aerobic activity that you enjoy at least three times a week on nonconsecutive days.

• *As a general guideline, aim for 30 minutes or more of moderate exercise most, if not all, days of the week.* That's what the American College of Obstetricians and Gynecologists recommends for women who have no medical or obstetrical complications. Low impact means such activities as walking, cycling (until late pregnancy), swimming, or stair-climbing. If you are accustomed to doing a highly aerobic activity, such as running or spinning, and wish to continue it, limit it to every other day, with milder workouts in between.

• *Don't be afraid to work up a sweat.* There's no evidence that the increase in body temperature from hard exercise places the fetus in danger.

• *Monitor yourself as you go.* Check in during the middle of any workout, but especially an aerobic one, to see how your body is doing. You have less oxygen available for aerobic exertion during pregnancy, so you may need to modify the intensity of your workouts. Stop when you're tired, and never exercise to exhaustion. Take frequent breaks.

• *Be sure you can talk while exercising.* That's a good rule of thumb to avoid overexertion.

• *Drink water.* Pregnancy limits the capacity of your bladder, so you may need to hydrate more often and urinate more often than usual while exercising.

GOAL: Strength-train at least three times a week on nonconsecutive days.

Strength-training (working with weights) is good for your general health, improving muscle tone and bone strength. It also may help prevent the normal aches and pains of pregnancy. Backaches, for example, which are a common by-product of being pregnant, can be minimized by strong, healthy muscles.

• *Use relatively light weights.* Light weights with moderate repetitions help you maintain flexibility and muscle tone while minimizing the risk of injury.

• *Don't forget Kegels.* Pelvic-floor exercises (their name comes from the doctor who promoted them) strengthen the muscles that support your urethra, bladder, uterus, and rectum. They may not raise a sweat, but they do count as a strengthening exercise. Having a strong pelvic floor is always important, but particularly when so much more weight will be placed on those muscles throughout pregnancy and in labor and delivery. You can do Kegels while you're driving or watching TV, or anytime throughout the day. To do a Kegel, tighten the muscles of your vagina as if you were interrupting the flow while urinating. Hold five to eight seconds and release. One regimen I like: Start doing sets of 10 and over time increase the number, aiming for three or four sets throughout the day. (Don't do this exercise while actually urinating, however, because it can lead to urinary tract infections.)

GOAL: Stretch every day.

• *Always avoid positioning yourself flat on your back.* This compresses a vital vein from about the fourth month on, and it's best to avoid the habit from the start.

• *Warm up before workouts and stretch afterward.* An exercise basic whether you're pregnant or not.

LISTEN TO YOUR BODY

Stop exercising and seek medical attention if you experience:

∽

• vaginal bleeding
• suspicious leakage (possibly amniotic fluid)
• shortness of breath before you begin
• dizziness
• headache
• chest pain
• muscle weakness
• calf pain or swelling (signs of possible blood clot)
• contractions
• decreased fetal movement

THE SPIRIT CENTER

Spirit is about connecting with something larger than yourself. It's a feeling that life is about more than you: You are also part of a family, part of a lineage, part of a community, part of a culture and a country, part of the fabric of humanity, part of the vast universe. It's little wonder that most women find this center—which too often goes woefully underserved in the busy buzz of everyday life—to have intensified meaning and to be complexly rewarding in pregnancy.

To nurture this center is to explore your relationship to yourself, to others, and to what most people call God, or a higher power, your sense of something much greater or larger than yourself.

Many studies support the protective benefits of connectedness. For example, socially connected individuals live longer than those who are isolated. Other studies have revealed that those who attend religious services live longer and that those who pray regularly have lower blood pressure, reduced incidence of coronary artery disease, and a lower incidence of depression. I'm especially intrigued by the evidence supporting the importance of the Spirit Center to fertility. In one study of 100 women undergoing fertility treatments, 54 percent of those belonging to a support group conceived, compared with 20 percent in a control group who did not. While this is a small study, the results are significant, especially in a patient population (infertility) where an over 50 percent pregnancy rate is unheard of. If a drug had shown these results, the study would have been repeated in large populations and, if corroborated, quickly implemented in centers around the country. Feeling connected and supported is essential.

GOAL: Think of your sense of your life's meaning and purpose.

• *Reflect on what spirituality means to you.* All human beings are spiritual beings in some way. What are your beliefs in this area? For you, Spirit may refer to conventional religious faith (whether you are currently active in a religious community or not). Spirit may also, or alternately, be found in your communion with the natural world, the experience of transcendence through artistic endeavors, or in a direct feeling of relationship with a higher power.

GOAL: Build a "sacred time" into each day.

• *Define a window of time for religious or spiritual reflection.* Deciding you will spend a small bit of time—I recommend at least 15 minutes a day—with this intention is a step in itself. Try to build the time into your daily routine—perhaps by reflecting on a spiritual passage such as a Bible verse or a Rumi poem every morning over breakfast, or stopping to smell the roses in a garden near your office during lunch, or listening to music that moves you before you go to bed. Incorporating this step into your routine will help you remember to make this center a priority.

• *Make your "sacred time" a period that renews you and speaks directly to your soul.* One of my patients alternated between reading poetry that she loved and reading a book on mindfulness in parenting that she found meaningful. Another closed her eyes and listened to music with total attention. On days when she had more time, she visited her favorite chapel and just spent time alone there, taking time to walk in the surrounding gardens and woods afterward. The point is to use the time in a way that has real meaning for you.

GOAL: Do one thing every day to fuel or feed a relationship that you care about.

Reflect on who truly nurtures you, and deepen your connection with that person or people. Conversely, you may realize you need to distance yourself from relationships that are not nurturing.

• *Strengthen your relationship with the baby's father.* Commit to a weekly date, where the focus is simply each other—use this transition in your relationship from partners to parents intentionally.

• *Reflect on the family you were brought up in.* This has a powerful influence on the ways you will choose to parent. Sometimes you will find unresolved issues that you wish to confront, or ones that you choose not to confront but simply to acknowledge as a part of your life. Think about what you liked and did not like about the way you were parented. What do you hope to emulate? What do you want to avoid?

• *Connect with your parents.* Talk to your mother about the experience of being a mother. Ask how she feels about becoming a grandmother. Have similar conversations with your dad, too. Do this even if your parents are no longer living. Simply have the conversation with them in your mind. (You may want to do this using Dialoguing or Dreamagery, too.)

• *Look around for new sources of support—and not just at the "obvious" places.* Sometimes the best support arises where you least expect it. For example, reach out to that woman at work who you always thought was nice but never had a real chance to get to know, especially if she's also pregnant or a mother. Ask if she wants to have lunch sometime; initiate a conversation.

• *Look online for support.* There are many great websites that let you connect with other women who are trying to conceive or who are pregnant and have due dates at the same time as you. Many women form fast ties with their online "pregnancy pals," even though these women are virtual strangers. You might choose to spend part of your day or week engaging in online relationships.

• *Forge your relationship with your baby.* In addition to your daily check-ins with your baby, spend time making this new relationship more real in other ways. Many women converse with their fetus or stroke their bellies, for example, long before the baby's hearing has developed or the baby can be felt moving. Two wonderful books with amazing images of the developing fetus that can help make this new life seem more real for you are the classic *A Child Is Born* by Lennart Nilsson and Lars Hamberger (Delacorte Press, fourth edition) and *From Conception to Birth: A Life Unfolds* by Alexander Tsiaras and Barry Werth (Doubleday).

THE SENSATION CENTER

Why do I include sensuality and sexuality in a wellness plan? Aren't they just the dressing, the ribbons on top of a healthy package? Absolutely not. Women are sensual and sexual creatures. It's part of our biological makeup, not to mention part of the procreative system that puts us on this Fertility Pathway of life in the first place. When you're unaware of the richness of your senses, including your sexual nature, something's out of sync in your life. When Sensation needs are unmet, a vital part of both body and soul goes unnourished.

Sensuality refers to the senses: seeing, hearing, tasting, touching, and smelling. Sexuality is heavily (though not exclusively) dependent on sensuality. Think of sensuality as the appreciation and indulgence of the senses. Sensuality can exist outside of sex—and vice versa—or they can fuel each other. The relationship between these two dynamics can shift a lot now. You might find sensual pleasure (or aversion) where you had never registered it before, such as in the smells, tastes, and textures of certain foods; in the feeling of certain fabrics on your skin; or in the sounds coming in through your window at night. There may be times when you feel far more sensual, and yet far less sexual than previously, or vice versa. At times the volume of both will be turned way up (often in the second trimester) or way down (such as during severe morning sickness or if you're two weeks past your due date in the middle of August in the Deep South!).

Your needs in this center can change dramatically in pregnancy. The sense of smell is heightened during this time. Food likes and dislikes intensify. Sexuality is especially dynamic. While trying to conceive, you may feel freer and sexier than ever now that the need for birth control has vanished. If conception takes longer than you'd hoped, however, sex can become more mechanical and fraught with anxiety. Morning sickness in the first trimester can squelch amorous thoughts, while soaring hormones in the second trimester make some women more desirous and orgasmic than ever before in their lives.

For all its benefits, ironically, this is a center that women most often overlook—at a time when they would most benefit from taking care of it.

Fortunately, most of us don't need to add any extra to-do's on our daily list to address this domain. What we need to do is bring more awareness and intention to the sensual and sexual activities that we already partake in. This center is not only essential to a really balanced sense of self—it's really fun.

GOAL: Pay attention to which of your senses you are most nurtured by.

One by one, reflect on each of your senses. What are the textures that you love? Which smells? What are the sounds that you are drawn to—music, sounds in nature, or sounds like a clock ticking or a train whistling? What are the tastes that make you moan? And visually, what do you find yourself drawn to—what colors, what scenes? Each

of our senses is powerful, and for many women, some are more intimate than others. Notice what brings you the greatest sense of relaxation and joy, and simply do more of it!

**GOAL: Actively nurture the full range of your senses and sen-
suality each day.**

• *Bring consciousness to the sensuality of at least one ordinary activity in your day.* It could be brushing your hair, taking a bath, or cook-
ing dinner. Really focus on the way the brush glides through your hair.
How does your scalp feel? What is your breathing like? Turn all of
your senses to the shower you are taking, the smell of the shampoo,
the feel of your wet skin, the sensation of the water hitting your body.
Are there simple things you can do to make this everyday activity
even more pleasurable and sensual? Maybe in a bath you can light
candles or add bubbles. Take your usual nap, but do it on fresh sheets
next to an open window and drift off to sleep while doing relaxing
breathing. The point is to fully focus on the activity with all your
senses and do it consciously. Doing this doesn't have to take any more
time than you would normally give to the activity; the difference is in
how you spend that time. When you can, design a special sensual
event for yourself. Treat yourself to a trip to a favorite store or farm-
ers' market, get a massage, prepare a meal of your favorite foods, or
plan some other activity that pampers you and invites your senses to
be "on."

**GOAL: Explore and support your sexuality as it evolves
throughout your pregnancy and beyond.**

• *Protect intimate time with your partner.* Sex is not just a physical
act. Many things influence sex: your mood, your mind, your sense of
connectedness, your stress level, and the moods and realities your
partner brings. Sensuality and sexuality are interwoven. If intercourse
is not what your body and soul want, find other ways to be together.
Holding and caressing each other, for example, can bring wonderful
new levels of connection and intimacy.

• *Invite your partner to be part of your body's dynamic changes as
well.* A focus on conception or a growing belly can sometimes intimidate one partner or another. There's a feeling that sex-for-fun is not

appropriate once sex is about procreation or once a baby is growing. Rather than shying away from sexuality at this time, it's a perfect time to fully embrace it. Bring nonjudgmental awareness to how things are now. Have fun with it. Get adventurous with different positions—an expanding abdomen and carrying a baby inside you may make innovation necessary. One of the greatest gifts you can give to your partner is to share your own body awareness with him. Invite him to explore the ways your body is changing in a way that feels good to you. This will create a deeper bond between you at a time when your partner may feel a bit left out, and will also make physical intimacy more natural and inviting for you both.

• *Don't be afraid to talk to your health care provider about sex.* If you have any questions regarding what's safe for your specific situation, speak up. It's what we're here for. You may be advised to curtail intercourse or orgasm during pregnancy for different medical conditions, depending on your specific situation. This could include being diagnosed with placenta previa, a history of miscarriage or preterm labor, carrying multiples, or an untreated sexually transmitted disease. Don't take this list as a blanket no-sex rule; always understand what's appropriate for your individual case.

• *Don't douche.* For some women this habit is associated with feelings of cleanliness. Not only is there no medical benefit to the practice, but douching interferes with the natural environment of the vagina and can even contribute to infection such as pelvic inflammatory disease, which increases the risk of ectopic pregnancy and infertility.

FEAR: Sex is dangerous to the fetus.
FACT: Although you and your partner may be hyperaware of the new life inside you, intercourse poses no risk to the fetus. He or she is safely protected, floating within a sac of water in a very thick-walled muscular organ deep inside your pelvis. The fetus is well out of reach of the deepest penile thrusting. (Although this may mentally make you feel better, remember that you should do only what feels comfortable to you physically.)
   The main sexual precaution: Your partner should avoid blowing air into the vagina during oral sex, because if air

gets into the circulatory system it can cause an embolism, a rare but very serious condition resulting in the possibility of a stroke. This is a potential problem because the blood vessel walls get much more "leaky" in pregnancy and air can get pushed (or blown) into them. Be aware that it's a pretty unlikely scenario. Ordinary cunnilingus (oral sex) is perfectly safe.

FEAR: I've heard I should stay away from long, hot baths.

FACT: A hot bath is probably harmless, though you should get out of any hot place if you feel dizzy or experience any discomfort. It's almost impossible to raise your core temperature in an ordinary bath to the level that would cause fetal risk. Do avoid saunas, hot tubs, and whirlpools. Though a short stay is not likely to cause damage, extended exposure to high temperatures has been found to increase the risk of miscarriage or fetal spinal cord damage, so you may feel less guilt or worry if you avoid them entirely.

FEAR: The electricity in my electric blanket could be a hazard to my unborn child.

FACT: I don't think we fully understand the way that energy works in the body. We do know that the body has an electromagnetic field. While electric blankets are probably safe with regard to female fertility, we don't fully know the impact of electrical energy on fetal development. This form of heat has been linked to male infertility, and a study of women who used an electric blanket during early pregnancy showed that they were 1.7 times more likely to miscarry than those who did not. I recommend indulging in the warmth of natural fibers such as cashmere or wool, or the heft of down or feather quilts instead. (Or rely on body heat!)

Chapter 5

A Team Approach to Pregnancy

∞

*How complementary and alternative medicine
can supplement your care*

A truly integrative approach to optimal pregnancy care may involve people besides your doctor or midwife. As your pregnancy progresses, you may choose to work with other care providers in addition to your primary one, and if you are like most of my patients, you will benefit greatly. Specialists drawn from the worlds of complementary and alternative medicine (CAM) can make a tremendous difference, especially when there is a specific area you wish to focus on for relief (such as backache or migraines or the common yet annoying side effects of pregnancy) or when a problem arises (such as debilitating nausea or a fetus in breech position). You may end up using supplemental care just once or twice in your quest for a healthy baby, or create a team that you work with consistently throughout.

CAM treatments are especially useful in pregnancy because they fill in gaps left by conventional medicine. Many of the daily aches and pains women experience and discuss with their obstetricians tend to get dismissed. For example, if you have skin changes or nausea, you're liable to hear, "Don't worry; it's normal." After all, conventionally, the "job" of the physician is to assess the symptom and determine whether there is any cause for concern—in other words, any underlying problem or disease. If no problem is present, we are trained to think our task is done, even if we do nothing to ease the symptom. In pregnancy, especially, we are often left offering little more than reassurance, given that we are appropriately conservative when it comes to doling out drugs.

Complementary and alternative approaches, on the other hand, stem from a more health-based philosophy. This means that they can often help with the garden-variety aches and pains of pregnancy in ways that go beyond the limitations of the average obstetrician's tool bag. Examples include massage, acupuncture, hypnosis, and professionally guided imagery. What's more, if you develop a complication such as hypertension or hyperemesis, drawing from a wider pool of proven resources in addition to conventional treatment can provide reinforcement that sees you through the experience in a way not otherwise possible, in a way most fully supportive to your body, soul, and baby.

THE WIDER WORLD OF CAM

Medical research on the approaches included in complementary and alternative medicine (CAM), which are described on page xvii of the Introduction, is all over the map. At this critical time in your life, you should use only those that have been sufficiently tested to validate their safety and effectiveness. Some areas have relatively strong evidence in their favor (or disfavor), while other areas have almost no research. For acupuncture and mind-body medicine, we have a significant number of randomized, controlled trials to draw upon as evidence of effectiveness, for example. Many culturally based practices such as shamanism and curanderismo (Mexican folk healing), on the other hand, have virtually no research basis. This doesn't mean they are not valuable, only that they have not been studied and we cannot draw any scientific conclusions about their safety or effectiveness. Spiritual healing and homeopathy have a growing number of trials but remain controversial in the medical community, because there is not a clear, biomedically based understanding of how they work.

Your team should be personalized to your pregnancy (i.e., what, if any, issues you are dealing with or what you may be at increased risk for), your preferences (approaches you feel comfortable with, have had good experience with, or feel drawn to), and the professionals who are available in your community. How often you use your team can vary tremendously, based on your pregnancy, your pocketbook, your preferences, and your needs. Putting together a three-person team does not necessarily mean that you will use them extensively throughout your pregnancy. Also, while most insurance companies do not routinely cover many of these services, this is changing. You should check with your insurer, and ask your physician to get involved. This can be particularly useful if you are having a problem for which your physician could prescribe a given therapy (acupuncture for hyperemesis, for example).

Not all conventional physicians will refer you to other care providers, so you may have to do some investigating on your own. Do, however, always tell your primary doctor when you are using other forms of care. Since the goal is integration of your care, finding a physician who is open to a whole-person approach and incorporating other qualified professionals is important. If your physician is resistant, explore why this is. If the answer does not satisfy you, you may want to find another physician. Likewise, if a CAM provider is unwilling to work hand-in-hand with your conventional provider, this is a red flag. In my opinion, any practitioner who is committed to your health and best outcomes will *want* to be integrated into your health team and will be willing to share and receive information about your care.

Possible Members of Your Pregnancy Care Team

Obviously you can make it through pregnancy and delivery beautifully with only your obstetrician (and, many would argue, without!). But if you are interested in exploring an integrative team, there are many different kinds of practitioners you may turn to. (To locate and learn more about these services, ask your doctor for references and also check the Internet Resources at the end of this book.)

Based on my knowledge and training, as well as my personal experience and those of my patients, I encourage any of the following:

• A massage/bodywork expert. Massage is a powerful tool for relaxation and pain relief. It can provide tremendous help with many of the physical changes and discomforts of pregnancy. Find someone who has experience doing bodywork in pregnancy. Avoid deep muscle work.

• An exercise physiologist. Someone who specializes in or has experience with pregnancy can help you start on a course of exercise in the healthiest possible way or can help you modify your current activities, whatever they are—yoga, strength-training, swimming, aerobics—to take into account the specific needs of pregnancy.

• A nutritionist. Pregnant women who have special dietary challenges, such as diabetes or a history of an eating disorder, or are starting the pregnancy journey overweight, often find it beneficial to work with someone who can offer very personalized nutritional advice.

• A mind-body practitioner. This is someone who is trained in a variety of mind-body techniques, such as guided imagery, mindfulness-based stress reduction, biofeedback, and hypnosis. Mind-body practitioners can be physicians, nurses, therapists, counselors, hypnotherapists, or other professionals.

• A hypnotherapist. Hypnosis can help you harness the power of your mind to relieve stress; decrease nausea and vomiting; quit smoking or give up alcohol; minimize pain, including labor pain; and address any fears you may have. A hypnotherapist leads you to a state of deep relaxation, between being awake and being asleep, in which your mind is more receptive to the power of suggestion. Ask that the therapist tape the session, so that you can use it daily at home. Hypnotherapy then becomes a central part of your self-care plan, and doesn't necessitate frequent visits. You can simply return as new phases or issues arise that you would like to address with hypnosis. You can also be trained in self-hypnosis techniques, sometimes with the assistance of a tape, to aid relaxation throughout pregnancy and also during labor. Hypnosis isn't a parlor trick that can cause you to make a fool of yourself or engage in inappropriate activities. You are aware of everything that goes on during hypnosis and can come out of it at any point you wish. (This will be obvious if your session is taped for you to play back later.)

• An Oriental-medicine practitioner. Oriental medicine typically combines any or all of the following: herbal treatments, acupuncture (the use of needles to free energy that is believed to flow through the body along meridians), acupressure (the use of pressure to stimulate the acupuncture points in the body where energy flows), Tai Chi (a mind-body relaxation exercise consisting of intricate exercise sequences), and moxibustion (applying heated herbs to acupuncture points). Very mild electrical stimulation can also be applied to the needles (electroacupuncture). Some conventionally trained physicians have taken courses in acupuncture and are called medical acupuncturists, and this is not the same as practicing Oriental medicine. For the most part the services described above are provided by specialists who have studied Oriental medicine broadly. Be sure that anyone you are considering using has specific experience in working with pregnancy.

TO FIND AN ORIENTAL-MEDICINE PRACTITIONER

The most important thing to look for is a Licensed Acupuncturist. These practitioners will use LAc after their name. Individual states vary in their requirements for licensure, but it does provide for some standards. You may also want to look for diplomate status in Chinese herbal medicine (Dipl CH) or in Oriental medicine (Dipl OM), which is granted by the National Certification Commission for Acupuncture and Oriental Medicine (NCCAOM). (Some states also require passing the NCCAOM Chinese herbal exam.) Note, though, that even that degree does not necessarily mean that the person has specific training or experience with pregnancy. Aside from credentials, you can look into experience levels; it's a good sign if a practitioner has at least three to five years of clinical experience. Another factor I always take into account is the practitioner's relationship with conventional medicine; you should choose someone willing to communicate with your obstetrician.

• A labor doula. Greek for "woman caregiver," or one who "mothers the mother," a doula is a professional labor assistant, an increasingly popular option for support during labor. She works with the mother during labor to provide support and also provides follow-up care and breastfeeding help once you are back home after delivery. A doula is not a midwife; she does not monitor the fetus and is not responsible for delivering it. Nor is she meant to replace the father in the delivery room, although she may share or take over labor-coaching functions.

Rather, a doula is an expert on helping the mother labor. She watches your progress and makes suggestions for easing discomforts, and provides hands-on care such as rubbing your back or wiping your forehead with a cool compress. Using a doula can be a particularly good choice if this is your first pregnancy, if your partner is hesitant or unable to perform these labor-support functions, if your partner has been unable to take childbirth classes with you, or if you do not have a partner.

It's been well documented that particularly in first-time mothers, doula-assisted childbirths are less likely to require Pitocin or pain anesthesia; they are also shorter, have fewer complications, and a lower rate of C-section and forceps or vacuum delivery, and higher rates of breastfeeding. If you are contemplating a natural childbirth, a doula can improve your odds of making this happen. But for any mother, this kind of support can make childbirth a less stressful and more positive experience. In the past 10 years, labor doulas have become more widely available and can be found in nearly every community.

• A lactation consultant. This is a breastfeeding instructor and support person who can provide instruction and preparation advice while you are pregnant, or be on call for advice and assistance after you deliver should you run into a problem.

• A postpartum doula. This is a doula who specializes in providing care for the mother after she's delivered and gone home. She typically goes into the home to provide help with breastfeeding, mother care, newborn care, and general household support in the first weeks. These can be especially welcome services if you do not have family living close by. Among the advantages are an increased chance of successful breastfeeding, a reduced risk of postpartum depression, and increased confidence in your parenting skills—not to mention a welcome extra pair of hands and an increased chance of getting decent sleep! Some postpartum doulas also do light housekeeping and provide nutritious hot meals. Services are usually billed by the hour. Some labor doulas also provide postpartum care.

• A spiritual counselor. In this category may be anyone from a life coach or mental-health counselor (such as a psychotherapist) to a person of some religious background (clergy, rabbi, Zen roshi, etc.)

who is committed to exploring your spiritual life with you. In many communities, you can find people who call themselves "spiritual counselors"; be sure to find out what their background is and what kind of work they do. As always, make this a conscious choice based on your awareness of your needs and desires.

• A therapist. Pregnancy and new motherhood can be a time when you gain tremendous insights into your life, and you may want to explore some of them more deeply. Or you may want to make significant changes in your life to respond to issues that have arisen, whether they are relationship issues with your own parents, changing roles in your marriage, or your parenting style. Sessions with a social worker, counselor, psychologist, or psychiatrist (aka "talk therapy") can help achieve those goals. Some women find that an expressive arts therapist, who uses art as well as mind-body techniques, is a beneficial, if less conventional, alternative.

Deciding Whether CAM Is Right for You

Here are three questions to ask when exploring CAM options:

• **Is the approach of value for the goal you are working toward?**
Not all alternative practices are alike. Look for those that have been studied in pregnancy or have a long history of use in pregnancy, and avoid those that don't. Use the information in this book, and check with your physician and with the CAM provider regarding their success in treating the concern you have.

• **Can you access a provider who has these skills, and who also aligns with your philosophy and is willing to have a team approach?**
Not all types of CAM are readily available everywhere, although this is changing rapidly as a healing-based model of care catches on. Both the person providing the therapy—whether we're talking massage or acupuncture—and your primary care provider must have a team mentality. It sometimes surprises me that there can be as much resistance from certain alternative practitioners to work with conventional M.D.s as vice versa; practitioners at both ends of the spectrum can be stuck in their ways and nonintegrative in spirit. If someone isn't willing to work synergistically, keep looking.

- **What are you drawn to personally?**

This is the conscious part. If you are intrigued by the concept of hypnosis, for example, be aware of that and let that be a useful factor in choosing your care. Conversely, if the very idea of hypnosis creates strongly negative feelings for you, pay attention to that as well. Bring both your personal reflections and factual information about the technique to the decision-making process. That's the only way you can create a pregnancy-care plan that works best for *you*.

In the following chapters I'll highlight the areas in which CAM practices have proven, safe benefits for pregnancy.

Kim's Story: How a Team Approach Works

Kim, 37, had been the picture of health until her first pregnancy. She was extremely sick throughout it, vomiting 8–10 times per day in her first trimester, 5–6 times per day in her second trimester, and continuing to do so 1–3 times per day until she delivered. Prior to delivering, she developed a severe form of preeclampsia (pregnancy-induced hypertension), and underwent an emergency C-section at 32 weeks. Indeed, her complications had been so severe that her daughter had to be delivered early to save her life.

"Before this pregnancy my feeling had been that my body never does wrong. Now I was being told that my body was 'having a reaction to my baby,' " Kim told me when she came to see me at the Duke Center for Integrative Medicine when she learned she was newly pregnant again and was filled with anxiety and fear. The good news was that although her daughter, Bethany, weighed only four and a half pounds at birth, she was now a thriving three-year-old. The less-good news was that after Bethany's birth, Kim had been diagnosed with an immune disorder called antiphospholipid antibody syndrome (APS), and she had had a series of miscarriages.

Kim felt incredibly apprehensive about what her rocky reproductive history would mean for this child. Her goal was "to carry this baby to at least 32 weeks—more would be great, too." It became clear in talking with her that a large part of accomplishing this depended on her processing how fearful she was about being pregnant again. She had such conflicting feelings about it, from hope and excitement to abject terror over what had happened before and a real loss of faith in her body.

I felt that a broad team approach would best support Kim's myriad physical and emotional needs. Anyone can benefit from a team approach, but Kim's example nicely illustrates how the various providers can complement one another.

Her core team consisted of me as her obstetrician and an Oriental-medicine provider with expertise in pregnancy, who I recommended because of Kim's history of nausea and vomiting, which I knew conventional medicine could only partially manage. We both saw Kim throughout her pregnancy with varying frequency, depending on how she was doing and how far along she was. I also consulted with our maternal-fetal-medicine department for their perspective, which had the added benefit of making Kim familiar with these care providers should she need to be transferred to their care in the event of complications. (If so, I would continue to consult.) Additionally, I recommended that she draw upon the expertise of other CAM practitioners:

* A hypnotherapist worked with her weekly at first and then monthly. She made hypnosis tapes reinforcing desired outcomes—for Kim these included general good health, no nausea/vomiting, and carrying the baby for as long as possible.
* An expressive arts therapist, over a few visits, used both art and mind-body techniques such as imagery and Dialoguing to work on healing from the trauma of her first pregnancy and delivery as Kim had never really expressed or explored her deep fears. (Expressive arts therapists would not be part of the typical pregnancy team, but they can be an excellent resource in the event of prior trauma. Kim's arts therapist was also a licensed counselor experienced in using talk therapy.)
* Trainers at her gym were enlisted to help her continue her prepregnancy routine of strength-training and elliptical. This was important to help Kim stay connected to her body, which she was at risk of distancing herself from, and to encourage feelings of strength and vitality.

Kim did extremely well. At 26 weeks she noted that she felt entirely different from her first pregnancy, connected and tuned in. She had only mild and occasional nausea in the first trimester and no vomiting. Neither did she develop preeclampsia this time, though she had cultivated enough consciousness of her body that she would have been alert to its very first signs. She went on to deliver a full-term, healthy infant—after a pregnancy during which she felt deeply connected to her body, her soul, and her baby. I felt honored to be part of the process, which was a loving and moving one for all concerned.

Part Two

Preconception

---∽∽---

Preparations You Can Make

Before You Conceive

Chapter 6

Preconception:
Reflection and Observation

∞

Checking in with body, soul, and baby before you conceive

Bringing awareness and intention to pregnancy even before you conceive is ideal for you and your baby. Unfortunately, that's not quite
the norm in America: Almost half of pregnancies are unplanned. And
those that *are* planned are usually driven by external circumstances.
For example, a woman turns 30 and feels time is running out. Or her
husband is eager to start a family. There's nothing wrong with either
scenario, but bringing greater consciousness to the process offers a
multitude of benefits to you and your baby.

"But those home pregnancy tests are so good, I'll know almost immediately if I'm pregnant. I'll be able to take good care of myself right
from the start," patients sometimes tell me. That's not the point. In reality, few things that a woman does (even drinking a glass of wine or
taking a couple of birth-control pills) in the first days of her pregnancy are likely to cause her unborn child lasting harm. But imagine
how much more is available for you to experience if you enter this
new time in your life fully present, fully aware. With planning, you're
more likely to conceive once you're optimally ready—physically, psychologically, emotionally, mentally, financially, and professionally.

A conscious conception means taking time to explore your motivations and desires, your hopes and fears, all of which have a direct effect on how the coming months, and beyond, unfold for you. It also means allotting time to fine-tune problematic health habits, lose weight, address chronic conditions, get your immunizations in order, and do other things that can improve fertility and directly lead to a healthier pregnancy. By aligning your body with your soul, you truly create fertile ground for this new experience in life.

This chapter walks you through a series of reflective exercises to help you understand where you are. Armed with these data, you'll be able to explore if this is really the "right" time for you to conceive.

CHECK IN WITH YOUR BODY

Many women make the decision to get pregnant based on maternal emotions ("Suddenly babies seem so cute to me!") or considerations around timing ("The clock is running out!"). That's fine, but they never consider the full spectrum of feelings surrounding this decision. How, for example, does your body feel about the decision? Few women think to stop and ask, even though they'd certainly appreciate its cooperation, largely because our culture doesn't look at the body in this way. It only seems right to check in with the entity that literally bears the burden of a pregnancy.

Please review the detailed instructions in Chapter 3 on how to use the following tools.

SUGGESTED TOOLS:

DAILY:

Body Quick Pic (tool #1)
Use this throughout the day to keep your awareness to the fore. It doesn't have to take more than half a minute, and it can be combined with the Soul Quick Pic (tool #5) and Baby Quick Pic (tool #8).

Body Scan (tool #2)
Use this wonderful way of "climbing into your skin" every morning. Make it part of your routine, such as before you get out of bed or

after you shower, to make it easier to remember. Repeat every evening, if possible.

AS NEEDED, BUT AT LEAST ONCE DURING
PRECONCEPTION:

Dialoguing (with Your Physical Self) (tool #3)

You've probably never thought about it in this way, but you have a relationship with your reproductive system—the part of you that you'll use to conceive your baby. This encompasses your reproductive mechanics (your organs, hormones, periods, and biological clock) as well as your related emotional issues, from your feelings about children and how you view your fertility to how your period affects your moods.

What is your relationship with *your* reproductive system? Start your Preconception journey by using the Dialoguing tool to "talk" to it, as in the example in Chapter 3. Exploring this is a playful but penetrating way to gain a fuller picture of yourself as you stand on the brink of possible motherhood. It can bring up data to help you make decisions or simply bring complex feelings to the fore.

The key things to ask:

- What does your reproductive system want to say to you?
- Is there anything it needs or wants from you?
- What would you like to say to or ask your reproductive system?
- Is there anything you need or want from it?

BODY CHECKS:
WHAT MIGHT COME UP FOR YOU

OK! Let's Go!

Kara began thinking about having a baby only when she turned 35. "It just never crossed my mind in a serious way before that. But when I had a birthday, it was like, 'Whoa! Time to get going!' I wasn't sure if I was ready or not but it seemed like now-or-never timing."

Nevertheless, Kara was surprised when she did the Dialoguing exercise. She didn't expect the intensity of the all-systems-go response she felt. "The message was very clear: 'I'm healthy. I feel good. Let me do what I'm designed to do!' "

Especially in their 30s, women often report hearing their "biological clock" telling them it's time to procreate. That insistent *tick, tick, tick* is your body's way of talking to you. It's entirely possible that your body may be more ready than your soul to get pregnant. You may strongly feel the biological drive regardless of conflict or complex issues felt within your heart and mind.

There's no right or wrong answer to the question "Should I get pregnant?" These kinds of exercises are intended to heighten your awareness. It's useful to know if your body is more ready than your soul, so that you can tend to your soul and do a little more prep work in that area, like a triathlete who's not such a great swimmer might devote extra practice to that skill. Or you may decide to heed the reservations in your soul and not pursue fertility at this time, and let your body know.

Your body's messages can be reassuring in the face of other doubts, as if the body is saying, "Look, I was made to do this, we're in it together, we can work together."

I'm Not Ready.

Julia, 26, was excited about the prospect of motherhoood. She and Jake had been married for three years, earlier than most of their friends, and felt very strongly that they wanted to begin a family while they were relatively young. I saw her after she had been trying to conceive for nearly a year without success. Her regular ob had suggested she begin fertility workup and then treatment, but Julia was reluctant.

First Julia and I did a Dreamagery exercise about her fertility. I asked her to let an image come to mind representing her reproductive system and a rose came to mind. What did she have to say to it? "Hello there. What's taking you so long?" she said.

"Does your reproductive system have anything to say to you?" Julia was silent for a moment. "It doesn't feel ready."

"Can you ask it to tell you more?" I asked gently.

"It doesn't feel taken care of."

"Can it say in what way?"

A tear trickled out of the corner of her eye. "It doesn't think it can sustain the baby."

"Ask it to share why."

"Eating," Julia said. "It doesn't think I eat right."

After the exercise, she began to confide what she had been hiding: that she was struggling with bulimia. A former model who now worked for a fashion designer, Julia had been body-conscious all of her life. Her body seemed to be telling her that conditions were not ripe for pregnancy.

There are a number of different reasons that your physical self might resist the notion of pregnancy. A woman who has taken her body for granted for a while and not paid much attention to it may encounter what I call the "angry body." It's as if the body wants to know, "Where have you been? Now you're expecting me to just turn on and conceive, when I've been waiting for you all this time!" The anger usually comes from having been out of sync with one's body. Suddenly you need something from it, but it would like a little nurturing, connection, and attention first.

Or, as in Julia's case, the body may not feel ready. A woman who has eating disorders, such as anorexia or bulimia, may be drained or depleted of the nutrients her body needs to sustain a pregnancy. Any chronic illnesses, physical or psychological, can also leave the body feeling depleted and not ready to nourish another living being, as can high levels of stress.

The body can express fear: Under the current circumstances, what if I can't? I might let you down. A woman who is chronically tired may not be sick, but because she's running on empty all the time, her body might view the care and nurturing needed for nine months to be too much, one more thing than it can possibly handle. A woman who is out of shape may find a similar response.

Even when the messages your body gives are surprising or not what you had hoped or expected, I urge you to receive them as important information. It's feedback—really valuable feedback. Make the decision to conceive in conjunction with both your body and your soul.

I'm Afraid.

Joan, now 37, was raped as a freshman in college. She went through therapy and felt healed from this trauma. The rape was no longer part of her everyday consciousness. She had married relatively late, at 34, and felt too busy with her new relationship and her job, which involved a lot of travel, to start a family. Beginning to worry that she might be getting too old to conceive if she didn't do so soon, however, she began preconception planning. She decided to take a promotion that required less traveling. She and her husband made plans to convert a work room to a nursery. She felt intellectually ready to quit the Pill, although she confessed a certain ambivalence despite her preparations.

When Joan did the Dialoguing exercise and asked her body if it was ready to conceive, she got a curious answer: "I don't know."

Perplexed, Joan asked, "Can you tell me why? I'm in good shape, and I've even been working out extra hard to lose those last five pounds to get ready."

Her body told her, "I am nervous."

"Why? Tell me more," Joan asked.

"I'm just not ready," her body answered. "I'm afraid of pain."

Joan knew without further probing that her long-ago rape was at the root of her ambivalence. "It was a terrible thing but I dealt with it and considered it in the past," she said to me after her Dialoguing. "I never imagined something as wonderful as having a baby would have anything to do with the most awful thing that ever happened to me."

I urged Joan to hold off quitting the Pill until she'd explored these findings a little further. "Ask your body what it needs from you," I suggested.

Joan did Dialoguing again. "It says, 'What I need is for you to be gentle with me. To recognize that pregnancy will at times be hard for me, but if you give me the support I need, it will help me tremendously,' " she reported.

It's a surprisingly common experience for the body to express reluctance about conceiving, carrying, and delivering if you have a history of rape, sexual abuse, or other negative sexual experience. Your body holds memories even when the everyday mind has set aside or suppressed them, and being on the Fertility Pathway can activate those memories. When a woman is considering pregnancy, her body often makes the connection between prior sexual experiences— good or bad—and birth. If trauma, emotional or physical, was involved, old fears and memories of that trauma can be triggered. Exploring them now, proactively, can be extremely healing and also make a huge difference in your experience of conception, pregnancy, and birth. I believe such exploration may even make it easier to conceive.

If you don't bring your past experience into consciousness now, you can be sure it will come back later, often as issues, fears, or concerns around birth. Labor attendants are very familiar with these kinds of deliveries. A woman who has not completely processed her abuse may become overwhelmed by feelings of anxiety and fear that surface during labor. Typically, she will experience her contractions as if they were happening to her, rather than coming from within her, which can make the whole experience seem dangerously out of control. She becomes very emotional and difficult to talk to, often bewildered and scared, and she often will fight her labor. On the other hand, if you can address this and work with it, so that your heart and body acknowledge your body's memories, you will often be able to heal those wounds at a deeper level than before, allowing the body to experience pregnancy and labor as beautiful, life-giving processes coming *from* you, not happening *to* you.

You needn't have had a trauma as extreme as rape to have felt physically invaded or to have other negative body memories that surface during Dialoguing. Women who have had physical problems seemingly unrelated to reproduction might find their bodies expressing ambivalence or negativity as well. The important thing is to become aware of such feelings. I encourage women in this situation to consider putting their conception plans on hold for a little while and work through the fear and other emotions until their body feels more ready. Go *into* the discomfort. Ask your body what it needs to heal.

I advised Joan to make a commitment to check in often with her body in this structured way. I'm happy to report that, six months later, Joan was pregnant. She used the Dialoguing process throughout her pregnancy and delivered a son in an uncomplicated, normal vaginal delivery. By helping her body—which was carrying the traumatic

memories that her mind had already come to terms with—feel cared
for and comforted, she vanquished the frightening feelings that might
have surfaced during delivery—or possibly even earlier, interfering
with conception. Joan reported that she felt more whole and healthy
after these exercises than she had in a long time.

CHECK IN WITH YOUR SOUL

Before conceiving, the central question to reflect on may well be
"Why now?" Most women are not fully conscious of all of the reasons
they are choosing to enter this pathway. Because the number of candles on your last birthday cake told you it was time? Because you've
been married X number of years? Because other people in your life
(your partner, your mom, your friends) expect it? Because it's good
timing for your career? Because you want to raise a child with your
partner? Any of these reasons, however valid, are only part of your
story.

Use this opportunity to fully explore all of your feelings about your
desire to get pregnant now—the conscious ones and the unconscious
ones. And if your head has decided it's the "right" time, how does your
soul feel about this? Just as it's a little shortsighted to expect your
body to carry and deliver a baby without checking in with it, it's
equally odd to think of bringing another being into the world, one
you will likely be intimately connected to for the rest of your life, and
never see if your soul—the very essence of who you are—feels ready
for this enormous step.

See Chapter 3 for a full description of the following tools.

SUGGESTED TOOLS

DAILY:

Soul Quick Pic (tool #5)

Try doing this throughout the day at the same time you do a Body
Quick Pic. It's essentially a short pause to ask, "What's up with me
right now?" At minimum, you should run a Soul Quick Pic first thing
in the morning and again at the end of the day.

ANYTIME, AT LEAST ONCE IN PRECONCEPTION:

Journaling Your Journey (tool #6)
Explore the following in your journal:

- Write about your reasons for wanting to get pregnant now: "I want to become a mother because . . ."
- Write about the parts of you that may not want to become a mother now. Give voice to all of it: "I'm not sure whether I want to become a mother because . . ."
- Also look at the flip side. Complete the sentence "If I don't try to get pregnant now . . ." Then what? What are your concerns and fears? If you were not to enter into this path at this time, what would that be like for you?
- Explore further: What are the best and worst things about entering this pathway now? What are the easiest and hardest things? How might this impact your relationship with yourself? With your partner? With your career? When you think about entering into a relationship with another, new being, how does it make you feel? What excites you about it? What scares you?

AS NEEDED:

Dialoguing (with Your Nonphysical Self) (tool #7)
If any issue surfaces that you'd like to have a deeper understanding of, use this tool to have a conversation about it.

❧

SOUL CHECKS:
WHAT MIGHT COME UP FOR YOU

Ready? I'm Hungry for This!

When Katie's husband, Jake, whom she'd been with for six years, broached the idea of having a baby, Katie was taken aback. She was 28, and the idea of becoming a mother had always seemed off in the distant future. She wasn't sure what she thought of the idea; she worked 60-hour weeks at her public relations job and was proud of a recent series of promotions.

When she mentioned this conversation at a regular annual exam, I introduced the idea of checking in with herself just to see how her body and soul felt about the idea. She was surprised to find, when she stopped to ask, that both her body and her soul were far more psyched about the idea than her mind. Women who are very focused on their careers are often disconnected from such body- and soul-level messages because they're too distanced or preoccupied to notice. Taking the time to listen to their innermost feelings can be a true revelation to them.

For other women, an enthusiastic let's-go message is *exactly* what they were expecting to hear. Many women feel that having a baby is a central, driving part of their life that they feel wired and ready for.

I wasn't surprised to see Katie for a prenatal visit four months later. "I was ready for this," she said, "but I didn't realize it until I stopped and focused on it. Sometimes I wonder how many more years I might have plowed ahead if I hadn't stopped to ask." Sometimes the act of making conscious what you're really feeling inside can be life-altering.

Maybe, But . . .

It's also common to probe your soul and hear it give voice to one or more reservations. That was true for Amanda, 30. Her body was ready but her soul was not ready.

When Amanda got to the question in her journal, "What scares you?" she put her notebook down. "A lot of the other answers flowed at first, but not this one. . . . I had to really think about why I wasn't 100 percent psyched," she said. Eventually, she wrote: "I'm afraid of screwing up. I don't know how to be a mom and I don't have any example to follow that I remember. What do I know about taking care of a baby?"

Amanda's mother had died when she was six. Her father raised her and her two older siblings by himself. Although Amanda considers her childhood happy, she has a lot of grief around not having had a mother or even a steady mother-figure.

Her sister and brother, who are five and seven years older than Amanda, had turbulent adolescences. Her brother is not on speaking terms with their father anymore, and her sister has drifted through a series of relationships and jobs. Although Amanda herself has a good marriage and a job she likes in sales, she sees her siblings' examples as giant warning flags.

It's understandable, even expected, for events from a woman's childhood to come up and give her pause when she starts considering motherhood. You may feel unsure because of misgivings about the way you were mothered. Your intellect may dismiss such concerns as soon as they come up, but don't let it. If you feel it's an important concern, it is. Don't bury it.

Often the reservations have to do with external factors. It may emerge that your partner is more excited about having a child right now than you are. Or your mother is pressuring you to "settle down" because you've been married five years now and she'd like grandchildren. Perhaps there are such perceived roadblocks as the lack of an obvious father (no small factor), an incompatible career path, or limited resources.

None of these considerations need be the deciding factor. But it's good to be aware of them, to understand the source of your ambivalence. Some women simply don't feel wired with an inborn need to be a mother. Some of them get pregnant anyway, perhaps because they do want the life experience, or because parenthood is important to their spouse. Some decide that they'd be more fulfilled living out a destiny that does not include a child. Neither is "right" or "wrong." Be honest with yourself, as best you can, about your motivations.

Amanda decided that she did, in fact, want to have a baby. To help honor and address her concerns, she decided that she would take parenting classes and talk a lot to her husband's mother, to whom she's close. She also committed to continuing to monitor these feelings throughout her pregnancy and to Journal about them.

I Worry I Can't Get Pregnant.

Some women have a difficult time getting to the "ready or not?" question because of fears around conception itself. If the idea that there might be a problem with your conceiving has some-how been embedded, it can be hard to engage the issue of readi-ness. Examples might be the older first-time mother worried about fertility, someone who has had a previous miscarriage or who has previously lost a child, or someone with a family history of birth defects.

Laura, 32, realized while doing an imagery exercise with me that she had a great deal of anxiety about whether she could have children. Her mother had taken DES (diethylstilbestrol, a hor-mone once used to prevent preterm labor, later linked to birth de-fects that can affect fertility). Then, as an adolescent during her first gyn exam, Laura had been told she was "too small" and might need to have her exam done under general anesthesia. She didn't, and everything was fine. But a long shadow was cast over her feel-ings about her reproductive system. During Dialoguing, she asked her reproductive system, "Are you normal? Is everything all right? Will there be a problem with my fertility?"

Her system answered her, "Being a mother isn't about the physi-cal part of having a baby. You can be a mother emotionally, too."

Laura began to cry. She had never let herself think of it this way before, because she was so focused on the mechanical parts. "It's not physical, it's not physical," she repeated. Later, she re-ported a huge sense of relief, because she knew that she had what it takes to be a mother.

CHECK IN WITH (THE IDEA OF) YOUR BABY

Include this step even though your baby doesn't physically exist yet.

SUGGESTED TOOLS

DAILY:

Baby Quick Pic (tool #8)

Try doing this exercise in the morning with your other Quick Pics. It might feel especially odd at first to overcome the rational brain whispering, "A baby? You don't even have one yet!" Just notice that voice, smile, and go on with the exercise.

ANYTIME, AT LEAST ONCE IN PRECONCEPTION:

Dreamagery (tool #9)
Dreamagery can feel odd the first time you do it, so please review the directions in Chapter 3, and have fun with it!

∞

WHAT MIGHT COME UP FOR YOU

I Can't Wait, Mom!

Sometimes a woman who is ambivalent about pregnancy (her body and/or her soul have serious reservations, for example) finds that when she checks in with her baby, the baby's voice is calming: "It will be just fine. I'm ready. I'll love you no matter what." Other times the image of this future life may ask you to do a bit more inner work to get ready for motherhood. Perhaps you need to explore your relationship with your mother before becoming a mother yourself. Or it may want you to take better care of yourself physically, or address other areas of your life for it to feel fully ready to embark on this journey with you. Whatever the feedback, it's a wonderful and exciting conversation to begin now (and often enlightening).

✓ REALITY CHECK: "Yellow Lights"?
                   What to Do Next

For some women, checking in with body, soul, and baby will illuminate three green lights: all systems go. It's more common, however, for yellow caution lights to be triggered (or for one dimension, usually the body or the soul, to put out a flashing red light). This only makes sense, considering how complex the decision to become a mother is.

When a reservation surfaces, here's what to do:

1. Keep it conscious. Don't ignore or avoid any hesitation that comes up. Recognize it and acknowledge that it's a very real part of the dynamic for you. Embrace it.

2. Work with it, so it doesn't work against you later. Welcome the opportunity to go into the matter further. This can be hard, since we're so culturally conditioned to stay on the sunny side of life, especially concerning motherhood. But it's important. I call this "pay now, or pay later with interest." You need to do the hard work of facing complexities and ambivalence now, making them fully conscious, or else they will remain repressed and hidden until the day that they leap out at you—often when you least expect them, and all the more intense for being buried for so long.

3. Consider using another tool to help you understand or acknowledge a reservation. For example, if Journaling brought up a particular fear, you might want to explore it further through Dreamagery, inviting an image of something that represents your fear. All of the tools are mix-and-match, as they share the ultimate goal of making things more conscious.

4. Don't move forward until you have explored all the complexities that arose during this process, and you truly feel ready. Typically at this point, body, soul, and baby will agree that it is right to move forward, even if there are still issues you need to continue to work on throughout the pregnancy and beyond.

Chapter 7

Preconception:
The Inside Scoop

∞

What's happening biologically in order to get pregnant

The key to planning a conscious conception is understanding how your body works. While getting pregnant hinges on timing, there's more to the event than that.

YOUR MENSTRUAL CYCLE

Let's back up from the Big Moment (when egg meets sperm) to look at how your body prepares each month for possible conception. Every day, whether you're aware of it or not, hormonal shifts cause physical and psychological changes that vary throughout your cycle.

There is no single "standard" menstrual cycle. In some women, they run as short as 21 days, in others as long as 35 days. To determine the length of your cycle, count from the first day of one period to the first day of the next. Typically, cycles are shorter and more consistent from month to month when you are younger, and become longer and more variable as you age. The average cycle is 28 days, although few women fit neatly into that pattern.

The cycle is divided into four main phases, which in a 28-day cycle typically break down as follows:

- Menstrual phase: days 1 through 5
- Follicular phase: days 6 through 12
- Ovulatory phase: days 13 through 15
- Luteal phase: days 16 through 28

The first day of a cycle is the first day that bleeding begins. This is the *menstrual phase* (aka your period). Though it lasts three to five days on average, it can continue for as many as eight days. Estrogen levels are now one-tenth of what they will be at their peak.

As bleeding ends, a hormone known as FSH (follicle-stimulating hormone), secreted from the anterior pituitary of the brain, stimulates several of the egg-containing follicles in the ovary to develop, though only one of them will fully mature. The growing follicles release estrogen in increasing amounts, causing the lining of the uterus to begin to thicken again. This is the *follicular phase*. It lasts from 10 to 14 days.

As the chosen egg approaches maturity inside its follicle, it secretes progesterone in addition to the estrogen. Then FSH is joined by LH (luteinizing hormone, also from the anterior pituitary) to signal the ovarian follicle to release the egg—*ovulation*. (Rarely, two or more eggs are released, which if fertilized would result in fraternal twins or higher-order multiples.) Ovulation occurs on approximately day 14 of a 28-day cycle, midway through. Most fertilization takes place while the egg is on its several-day journey from the ovary down the fallopian tube on the way to the uterus. This is the *ovulatory phase*, when the greatest chance of conceiving occurs.

After ovulation, the uterus goes into full gear to prepare for a possible implantation of a fertilized egg in the uterine wall. This is the *luteal phase*. Once the ovarian follicle releases the egg, the follicle's structure and function are transformed and it is now called the corpus luteum, whose job is to secrete hormones, primarily progesterone, to help prepare the body for pregnancy. Estrogen, LH, and FSH decline while progesterone rises sharply. Progesterone is now 49 times higher than it was at its lowest point.

If the egg is fertilized, estrogen and progesterone continue to be produced, and the uterine lining remains full and lush, supporting the developing embryo. Soon the pregnancy itself begins producing a hormone—hCG (human chorionic gonadotropin), which is the substance a home pregnancy test detects.

If the egg is not fertilized, approximately 14 days after ovulation progesterone drops again along with the other hormones. The corpus luteum shrinks and is reabsorbed, the uterine lining breaks down and is shed through the vagina—and another period begins.

Your menstrual cycle does not function in isolation from the rest of you, however. What's going on in the rest of your body and your life plays a huge role in determining how you'll be affected by the constantly fluctuating hormonal cocktail circulating within you. The central player in this interface between your menstrual cycle and the rest of your life is an organ deep within your brain, called the hypothalamus. It regulates the entire process of hormonal secretion; for example, determining the levels of FSH and LH. The hypothalamus is influenced by stress, anxiety, poor nutrition, depression, illness, and other negative circumstances, as well as positive ones like rest, relaxation, pleasure, good nutrition, and joy.

So you can see how fertility is more than a matter of timing sex just right. The entire landscape of your life can influence whether or not you conceive in a given month, which means you can do a lot to encourage the process.

CONCEPTION

It's long been believed that when you're born, you already have in your body all of the two to three million eggs your body will ever have. New research on mice indicates that females of this species contain self-renewing ovarian stem cells that continue to produce eggs; it's not clear yet whether this is also true for humans. Be that as it may, the millions of eggs you start with are obviously far more than any woman ever needs. Each month you will typically release only one egg. If it meets up with one of the 350 million or so sperm in a typical ejaculation, as they travel up through the vagina, the cervix, and the uterus (and sometimes right out into the tube itself) toward your egg, *voilà!* Conception.

Seems simple enough. A host of factors must fall into place in order for that moment to arrive, however. That's why it takes the average healthy couple from 6 to 12 months to conceive, with only about 40 percent able to conceive in the first three months of trying. About 1 in 10 reproductive-age couples have fertility problems.

A SPECIAL TOOL FOR PRECONCEPTION:
CYCLE MONITORING

Every woman should do this kind of self-exam periodically, if for no other reason than to be intimately familiar with the particulars of her own cycle. If you do it before you conceive, you'll have an accurate baseline perception of your body. This will better enable you to know when you're ovulating and to recognize the early signs of pregnancy.

• *Keep a menstrual calendar.* If you've not been particularly mindful about your dates in the past, or if you've been using a form of contraception that caused you to not pay attention to your cycle, you should begin keeping track of the dates on which your period begins. This information will help your doctor date the onset of your pregnancy and arrive at an accurate due date. And if you are trying to get pregnant, becoming familiar with the pattern of your cycle will tell you when you are most likely to ovulate. The stereotypical 28-day cycle, with ovulation falling on day 14, is the exception, rather than the rule, for the majority of women. You need to learn what is normal for *you.*

• *Track your basal body temperature.* This is not necessary, but some women like to track their basal temperature (base body temperature, found at rest) to help them determine time of ovulation. To find this, you need to take your temperature every morning before you get out of bed with a special BBT thermometer or, if your eyes are good, with a regular thermometer. Basal temperature hits its lowest point the day before you ovulate, then "spikes" (and remains high) through the start of your period. An alternative to this rather cumbersome way of gathering information is to use a home ovulation predictor kit.

For more detailed information about your cycle and pregnancy, see pp. 93–95.

CONSCIOUS CONCEPTION

Once you're sure that you're ready to conceive, you might choose to throw caution to the wind. Or you can choose to bring a level of intention to the proceedings.

Get conscious about your "window of fertility." Your best chance of conceiving—the so-called window of fertility—occurs on the day you ovulate *or up to five days before ovulation.* The reason that intercourse on any of the several days preceding—but not following—ovulation can result in pregnancy is that active sperm can live for up to five days, while the chosen egg of the month lives just a single day. Recent research indicates that the highest odds of conception result from intercourse one or two days *before* ovulation, rather than the day of ovulation, as had long been thought.

Get conscious about your *cycle.* Relatively few women have a textbook 28-day cycle. What's more, even those who do will experience variations over time. So rather than simply counting the days on the calendar, use other clues to gauge your most fertile days. Pay attention to the nuances of your cycle across your five Centers of Wellness. How do your moods, your appetite, your levels of sociability and energy, and the feel of your body change across a cycle? Write it down. By tracking this for a few cycles, you can begin to see what the pattern looks like for you. You'll be better tuned in to the changes that transpire around ovulation.

Get conscious about detecting ovulation. More evidence that body awareness is essential: A review of fertility-detection methods reported that urine-test ovulation-detection kits identify only a part of the window of fertility (the day or two before ovulation). Taking notice of changes in vaginal discharge can be much more effective. As estrogen levels begin rising sharply during the days leading up to ovulation, your cervical mucus, which is usually scant and sticky, becomes increasingly plentiful and thick. Slick and slippery in texture, it's rather like raw egg white, with the same kind of elastic, stretchy consistency. These changes are nature's way of helping the sperm advance to the uterus, protecting them against the acidic environment of the vagina. Of those 350 million sperm racing to the egg, only one in a thousand will make it through the vagina, and only 400 or so will get as far as the fallopian tubes. Right after ovulation, the cervical mucus reverts back to its sticky, less plentiful state.

For some women, ovulation kits and basal body thermometers are a fun way to bring more awareness to the proceedings. But for many, they are an unnecessary expense and just another thing to stress out about. Cervical-mucus observation is a low-tech yet highly effective way of achieving body awareness for women who are not interested in loading up on equipment.

Get conscious about intercourse. See also the cycle monitoring tools on page 96. Many women believe that they must time intercourse to the day (or hour) of ovulation in order to conceive. Not only is this not true, it creates a lot of crazy stress in your sex life.

Of course, if you're part of a couple who has intercourse only once a month or once a week, it does make sense to have it around the two-day window when you are most fertile. On the other hand, if you're part of a couple who has sex at least every two or three days, you don't have to worry about timing, since there will always be sperm around, given that they live for up to five days.

Knowing the particulars of your body and your sex life makes conception far more natural than relying on artificial formulas. I think the best idea is to just focus on creating a steamy (or at least active) sex life. Throw out the ovulation kits and basal body thermometer if they create stress, and just have fun!

Get conscious about your relationship. If as a couple you're not feeling right and receptive together, it's going to be a lot harder for the time around ovulation to be a stress-free, loving, and *welcoming* time. Part of conscious conception is nurturing your relationship. We know that stress and tension negatively impact fertility. If you begin to become obsessed about the timing of intercourse—the "have-to-now" attitude—you risk leeching the fun, erotic spontaneity right out of the process. It's best to fuel and support your sex life, using the Fertility Pathway as an opportunity to juice up the fun rather than add artificiality to it. What's more, sperm perform better and there are higher counts when the man is more aroused. (There's reason to believe the same is true for women.)

Get conscious about your intentions. This might sound too obvious—your intention is to get pregnant, after all. But for many people, a spiritually rewarding aspect of being on the Fertility Pathway is to be really conscious of inviting this life energy, this hoped-for new being, into your relationship. For some, sex becomes a much more sacred experience when this intention is made conscious.

Chapter 8

Preconception:
Medical Care

∞

An integrative medicine perspective on preconception planning

BASIC MEDICAL ISSUES NOW

Preconception Exam

Preconception counseling has become standard care—and with good reason. The very act of making a preconception appointment brings awareness and intention to the idea of having a baby. Marking that date in your calendar creates the opportunity to focus on the transition at hand. There are practical benefits as well. In a preconception exam, your ob-gyn or midwife can review your history and your physical status and address any issues that might stand in the way of conception and/or an optimal pregnancy. For example, taking steps to alleviate depression and other psychological issues has been found to improve one's ability to conceive. You can also work with your doctor or midwife to figure out how to best prepare yourself for the experience, such as making changes in your health habits that will equip you for a healthy conception and pregnancy. Since the baby's major organ systems begin to form as early as the third week of life, which is most often before you realize that you are pregnant, what you learn during a preconception consultation can help give your baby the best possible start. This may explain the findings of a recent study which showed that birth defects occurred less often in the babies of women who got preconception counseling.

Who provides this care? Ideally, the same person whom you want to provide your prenatal care. So if your regular gynecologist does not practice obstetrics, this can be a good opportunity to look for someone you find personally and philosophically compatible. See "How to Make a Conscious Choice About . . . Your Prenatal Caregiver" in Chapter 12.

Many aspects of integrative preconception/prenatal care are exactly the same as in conventional medicine. The main difference in the kind of care I provide is wholeness—treating all of you, body and soul, which very often involves suggesting alternative options when appropriate. Because I'd like you to understand what this kind of care entails, let me describe what happens during a preconception consultation in my office:

• *A complete health history.* I include questions similar to those in the Reflective Inventory, including medical and reproductive background, lifestyle, levels of stress, and health habits. Most doctors don't go into as much detail as this, which is why I feel the Reflective Inventory is important work for you to do. Reflecting on the less typical questions helps you begin to bring relevant nonmedical or nonphysical aspects to the fore. At a minimum, however, you should discuss your basic medical history and reproductive history with your doctor.

WHY: To look for ways in which you may want to optimize your health (e.g., quitting smoking, cutting alcohol and caffeine consumption, addressing your readiness to become pregnant), and to look for any potential areas of concern (such as medicines you're taking, history of chronic diseases or depression, prior abortion or miscarriage, very high stress, and so on).

• *A physical exam, including a general physical exam as well as a pelvic exam.*

WHY: Because the best time to do a baseline assessment of the pelvis is in its nonpregnant state. Your doctor will note the size and shape of your pelvis. Gynecological conditions best treated before pregnancy include uterine polyps, cysts or fibroids, pelvic inflammatory disease, urinary tract infections, and sexually-transmitted diseases. A Pap smear is also taken in order to screen for any abnormalities that should be addressed before pregnancy.

- *Relevant prenatal tests.* These include tests for rubella, chicken pox, tuberculosis, and hepatitis B (to see if you need immunization), blood tests for anemia (iron deficiency) and toxoplasmosis (a disease cat owners, those who drink raw milk, and gardeners may be vulnerable to), and tests for sexually-transmitted diseases, including chlamydia, gonorrhea, herpes, HIV, human papillomavirus, and syphilis.

WHY: So you can detect and resolve potential problems before pregnancy. This includes bringing necessary immunizations up to date, working to restore iron levels, and treating diseases. Some results might indicate problems that could influence your decision about whether or not to become pregnant now.

- *A self-care discussion.* I go over the Centers of Wellness (Mind, Nutrition, Movement, Spirit, and Sensation) and review what patients are currently doing to support their health in these areas. Most physicians skip this step, but you can do it on your own. See the next chapter for specific suggestions, many of which might apply to you.

WHY: To begin to set the framework for optimizing self-care and to make recommendations for strengthening yourself in all domains.

At the appointment's end, I always leave time to talk. Going in to your preconception checkup with a list of questions that surfaced for you after doing the Reflective Inventory will help build the foundation of the crucial relationship between you and your care provider. If you feel you are not given enough time to discuss your concerns, this may be a problem with the system, not with your provider. If you have a good feeling about the doctor, discuss your concerns with him or her, and see how he or she suggests you both address them. If your sense is that working fast with little time for your input is his or her preferred style, this is a sign that you should look for another caregiver.

Key Preconception Issues and Why They Matter

A number of factors can influence your ability to conceive. Ideally, you and your care provider should both be aware of these before you try to get pregnant.

• *Your age.* A woman in her early 20s has a 20 percent chance of conceiving in each cycle; a woman over age 40 has just a 5 percent chance. Older mothers are also at greater risk for miscarriage, birth defects, carrying multiples, and complications during pregnancy, including preeclampsia (a syndrome that includes dangerously high blood pressure), gestational diabetes (a form of diabetes triggered by pregnancy), premature birth (before 37 weeks), placental problems (such as placenta previa, where the placenta blocks the uterine exit; or placental abruptions, where the placenta separates from the uterine wall in pregnancy). A teenage mother, on the other hand, is at lower risk physically, but often at higher risk on a soul level. Young women are extremely prone to the kind of unconscious living that can result in unwanted pregnancies and poor preconception health habits.

• *Your partner's age.* The chance of chromosomal damage is also dependent on the father's age, particularly when he is over 55. You may be referred to a geneticist for risk assessment counseling.

• *Your weight.* A woman who is very overweight or underweight may not ovulate as regularly as a woman of normal weight, or may not ovulate at all. Underweight women tend to have low birth weight babies. Overweight or obese women are at increased risk for many complications, including the development of gestational diabetes or preeclampsia. Their babies are more likely to have neural tube defects and birth trauma. Pregnancy is more challenging at every step of the way for obese women, because tests can be more difficult to administer or read, delivery is riskier (because, for example, monitoring the fetus is more difficult), even a C-section is far more complicated (because operating through fatty tissue is more challenging) and therefore dangerous. For all these reasons, if you're not within a healthy weight range for your height, it's a good idea to take extra time to achieve this or work toward it—through slow, healthy methods—before conceiving. Also, it's potentially dangerous to lose weight in pregnancy and not recommended no matter what your starting weight.

• *Your race.* If you fall into certain ethnic groups, genetic screening for disorders common to those heritages may be recommended to you. These include sickle cell disease (African Americans); Tay-Sachs disease (which can affect those of Eastern European Jewish extraction, French-Canadians, Irish-Americans, and Cajuns); Canavan's disease and cystic fibrosis (also Jewish and French Canadian); and thalassemia (Mediterranean descent). It's much easier to address these issues before conceiving.

• *Preexisting health conditions.* If you have a chronic health condition or a history of any medical or surgical disease, bring your medical records or an accurate description of the problem and treatments to your obstetrician. This is essential because the condition might place you at greater risk of complications in pregnancy, or your course of treatment may need to be revised (see the information regarding medications, below). Examples of illnesses to address and get under control before conception include diabetes, hypertension, depression, asthma, cervical dysplasia (abnormal Pap smears), and sexually transmitted diseases.

• *Medications and supplements used.* Bring a complete list of medications you regularly use to your preconception visit. Include vitamins and botanicals. Your doctor can let you know if any have been linked to birth defects and if so you can plan for safe alternatives. Depending on the medication, it's ideal to discontinue potentially harmful substances one to six months before you plan to conceive. The acne drug Accutane (isotretinoin), for example, has been linked to birth defects of the face, head, heart, and central nervous system in 25 percent to 35 percent of exposed infants, and can raise the risk of miscarriage as high as 50 percent. There are a number of classes of medications, including antihypertensives, antidepressants, and anticonvulsants, for which there are some specific drugs that are better than others to take during pregnancy. By consulting with a physician before you conceive, you give yourself ample time to switch to the drug that will work best for you. Many women assume or believe that the best thing is for them to be on no medications. This is not always the case. In many situations, the risks of the disease or disorder are far worse than the risks of the medications—including many forms of depression. However, not all drugs are created equal, and one type of antidepressant, for example, may be less risky to your pregnancy than another, so discuss ALL the options with your doctor or therapist before you become pregnant so you can make the best choice for you.

• *Type of birth control currently used.* If you are taking a hormonally active contraceptive (such as the Pill, the Patch, or Depo-Provera),

I suggest you give yourself a window of time to return to your hormonal baseline before conceiving. This makes it easier to accurately date your pregnancy, which is important because a reliable due date allows your care provider to best gauge your baby's growth. Once you have gotten your first normal period (not just spotting) after coming off hormones, you'll most likely have returned to your natural hormonal rhythm. You may revert to a normal cycle as quickly as a month after hormone use, or it may take longer. Despite the fact that some doctors recommend waiting for several months or more, there is no medical reason for waiting any longer than it takes to achieve one normal cycle.

If you have an IUD, it must be removed before you try to conceive, ideally during your menstrual period. Use the same guidelines for waiting to conceive as above; let your cycle return to normal.

If you use condoms or a diaphragm, discontinue use of spermicides for a few weeks. Use condoms without spermicides in the interim.

• *Immunization needs.* Your doctor will want to be sure your immunizations are up to date, as many diseases put your fetus at risk if contracted in pregnancy and immunization is often not recommended in pregnancy. Rubella (also known as German measles) is a contagious virus that can cause serious effects in a fetus if the mother contracts it during pregnancy. Risks include fetal blindness, deafness, and heart problems. Because the danger is greatest during the first two months of pregnancy, it's important to be sure you have had this vaccination before you conceive. Most of us received it as children. But if a rubella titer shows you to be susceptible, you can be immunized now and you can begin trying to conceive one month later. Women who have not had chicken pox should also be immunized, and wait three months to conceive.

Additionally, you should know that if you plan to travel during your pregnancy to places that require any immunizations (smallpox, cowpox, typhoid fever, or others), you will want to plan ahead and have these shots before you are pregnant.

• *History of DES*—for you or your partner. Here's a good reason for knowing a little bit about your mother's health history. A drug called diethylstilbestrol (DES), thought to prevent miscarriage, was often given to women from 1938 to 1971. Later it was found to have caused cervical, vaginal, and uterine abnormalities in many of their daughters (and have predisposed both the daughters and the mothers to reproductive cancers). The majority of DES daughters are able to carry a full-term pregnancy, but as many as 20 percent are infertile. The sons of mothers who were given DES may also have impaired fertility due to low sperm count, poor sperm motility, and genital abnormalities. The effects on women whose grandmothers had DES have not yet been well studied as sample sizes are still small; to date no increased risk for the reproductive tracts of DES granddaughters has been noted.

POSSIBLE MEDICAL ISSUES NOW

X-Rays or Other Imaging

Although you can safely receive dental care during pregnancy, it's a good idea to get routine medical care up to date before trying to conceive. That includes a dental checkup and a mammogram (if you routinely receive one or are over age 39). If you're already trying to conceive, be certain you are not pregnant before having a test involving radiation (including X-rays, mammograms, MRIs, and CT scans). Not sure? Have a pregnancy test first. Don't rely on a shield. The best time to schedule diagnostic imaging is the first week of your period, so you're sure you're not pregnant and have not yet ovulated.

HOW TO MAKE A CONSCIOUS CHOICE ABOUT . . . USING FERTILITY HELP

The medical definition of infertility is trying for a year without success. But this is a rather arbitrary amount of time; some women get help sooner and others later. How do you know when—and if— you need fertility help? Use the Feedback Loop (tool #10) to help you make a conscious choice:

First, reflection. How are *you* feeling about trying to get pregnant? Anxious? Worried? Fearful? Calm? Confident? Ambivalent? Use the information from your journal and other tools to collect your personal data on the subject.

How do you feel about the idea of beginning fertility treatment?

Does the prospect excite you or scare you? Are there some procedures you expect you would be more comfortable with than others? What does choosing to begin a fertility workup symbolize for you? Do you have a sense of what may be influencing your perspective, such as a friend who's done fertility treatments for two years without success or a friend who got pregnant on her first try at age 42? Remember at this point you're not deciding anything; you're simply gathering information that's already within you.

Second, information. How long have you been trying? What are your actual odds of conceiving based on your age? Are there other factors that might influence your conception odds (e.g., you have very irregular cycles, your mother used DES)? Use your doctor or health care provider to help obtain this perspective.

What's your doctor's advice? Depending on your situation, you may have a number of options. Be sure you have a clear understanding of what's involved. The first step is usually a fertility workup, to help identify where the problem may lie. This can include, for the woman, a laparoscopy (a surgical procedure to evaluate the pelvic organs), a hysterosalpingogram (HSG, a test where dye is injected into the reproductive tract to illuminate tubal or uterine abnormalities), and blood tests (to confirm that you're ovulating and to identify possible hormonal issues). The man will undergo semen analysis (providing a sample to be tested for sperm concentration, motility, pH level, and other factors). Depending on what's found, you may be offered additional tests, or one of many possible treatment options, from a drug to help you ovulate, to artificial insemination and in vitro fertilization (IVF), to use of a sperm donor, an egg donor, or a surrogate to carry a pregnancy. You should understand how procedures work as well as their odds of success for a couple in your situation.

I also think it is a great idea to explore complementary and alternative practices, many of which are used in concert with conventional treatments. If you are not feeling pressured about your timeline, you may want to consider taking these steps before engaging in a full conventional infertility treatment plan. While most of these approaches have not been well-studied as sole treatments, some have been studied in conjunction with conventional treatments. The approaches that I have the most enthusiasm for include Oriental-medicine and mind-body approaches (which can be used together). Infertility patients receiving acupuncture before and after embryo transfer, for example, were found to have significantly higher pregnancy rates, almost twice those of women who had conventional embryo transfer. Many women choose to work with an acupuncturist who has experience with infertility before proceeding with a medical workup. While this has not yet been studied, given the efficacy of this system in general, and also based on my clinical experience with patients, I fully support interested patients in choosing this path. As for mind-body approaches, there's no doubt that the state of our minds affects our reproductive system and our ability to conceive, so why shouldn't we use this proactively? Receiving group support and instruction in self-hypnosis during fertility treatment has been shown to as much as double the rate of achieving pregnancy. It only makes sense to engage this part of your fertility very early on. I encourage women to work with a professional one-on-one, or join support groups, meditation classes, and/or work with clinical hypnotherapists. These are very powerful approaches, with little cost, virtually no risk, and great potential benefit.

Also bring into your decision-making process whether you have any financial considerations concerning fertility evaluation. Does your insurance cover any or all expenses? Collect the information you need on these fronts as well.

It can be hard to get reliable answers. Ask a lot of questions. Learn as much as you need to feel comfortable.

Third, action. Take a step based on your reflection and information. If you decide you are ready to see a fertility specialist, make an appointment. You don't have to do anything further after this initial appointment. Alternatively, you may decide you would like to take action along a different path, such as working with a Chinese-medicine practitioner or a hypnotherapist. Or you may just want to give yourself more time.

Because you need an egg and a sperm to procreate, and because you are going to need to give one another as much support as possible, it's essential that your partner, if you have one, undergo a similar process of conscious decision-making. Share your thoughts along the way, not just your conclusions.

Then, re-reflection. Once you have taken a step, pay attention to how you are feeling about the choice. Before any next step in your fertility workup or treatments, be sure to go through the Feedback Loop again and make sure it feels right to proceed. This is not an all-or-nothing choice—try everything possible until you get pregnant, or do nothing at all. Fertility help is incremental and your approach should be, too. The worst thing you can do is climb onto a conveyor belt of no return, receiving one fertility treatment after another, without being fully conscious of what your body and your soul have to say along the way. And many, many women end up doing just that, often at great costs to themselves and their relationships. Keep checking in, deciding whether to go ahead with the next phase of treatment or not. Use the Feedback Loop every step of the way to be sure that you are making a choice that truly feels best for you at that time.

Chapter 9

Preconception:
Self-Care

∝

Centers of Wellness modifications before you get pregnant

Being in your best condition for pregnancy depends on your ability to nurture all five of the Centers of Wellness—Mind, Nutrition, Movement, Spirit, and Sensation—that comprise balanced health. The ultimate advantage to starting this process before conception is that you give yourself the gift of time to change damaging habits and bring greater balance to your life.

Follow the goals of the Basic Self-Care Plan for Pregnancy outlined in Chapter 4, with the following modifications:

THE MIND CENTER

There are growing data that the state of the mind affects ovulation and both one's ability to conceive and to carry the pregnancy to term. Pioneering research by Alice Domar, Ph.D., founder of the Mind/Body Center for Women's Health at Boston IVF, shows that women who use mind-body strategies, such as meditation, mindfulness, support groups, and tools such as those suggested in Chapter 4, have better conception rates than women who use no interventions. Women having difficulty conceiving are more depressed than those who are fertile, and alleviating depression and other mental distress appears to be correlated with increased fertility. The physiological link between depression and infertility isn't understood; it's possible that depression might reduce egg quality, delay the release of eggs, or decrease the hormonal levels necessary to allow implantation. (Stress and depression can also affect male sperm counts.) From a whole person perspective, however, it makes perfect sense. Your body is trying to choose an optimal time for pregnancy, and if you are highly stressed or depressed, your body knows it may not be in your best interest, or your baby's, to conceive now. What's clear is that a connection between mind and fertility definitely exists and therefore the better your mental health, the better your chance of becoming pregnant.

• *Know the signs of depression.* There's a link between difficulty conceiving and depression, with levels of depression peaking after two to three years of "trying," Domar reports. If you have been trying to conceive for more than a year and feel depressed, consider meeting with a fertility counselor (not necessarily a gynecologist but someone trained in fertility issues, who may be a social worker, psychiatrist, clergyman, or family counselor). Or form your own support group with women you have met along the way. The purpose is not to explore fertility workups but to help you process feelings around fertility and fertility treatment, the impact on your life, develop coping strategies, and make conscious decisions. This step alone can help lift feelings of isolation and anxiety.

Depression can also be triggered by other life events, including stress and grief, or by biochemical imbalances. Symptoms of depression include loss of interest in one's usual activities, extreme anxiety, a change in sleep patterns (such as insomnia), a change in weight or appetite, strained relationships, social isolation, and persistent feelings of pessimism, guilt, anger, or bitterness. Clearly, even if you were able to conceive while depressed, your ability to enjoy and focus on your pregnancy would be diminished, and your health compromised since even mild depression can suppress the immune system, making you more vulnerable to infection. Depression is a risk factor for increased complications related to childbearing, including prenatal depression, postpartum depression, and postpartum psychosis. If you have been struggling with depressive symptoms, mention them to your doctor. Using therapy or medication now will put you in a much better starting place for pregnancy.

• *Commit to triggering your body's relaxation response at least twice a day.* The state of deep relaxation lowers blood pressure and stress-hormone levels, slows your heart rate, and eases tension, all of which make your body more receptive to babymaking. (See Chapter 4 for examples of ways to do this.)

THE NUTRITION CENTER

Don't wait to implement the dietary changes in the Basic Self-Care Plan (Chapter 4) until after you get pregnant. Make them habits now. And because weight issues can affect the course of pregnancy, managing them now can help you avoid problems later.

• *Be aware that special diets may impact fertility.* There's preliminary evidence, for example, that consuming too much protein (more than 25 percent of total calories), as can happen on diets such as Atkins, may inhibit conception. Some researchers recommend that a woman trying to conceive should limit protein consumption to no more than 20 percent of her diet.

• *If you weigh too much or too little, seriously consider postponing conception.* I'm not saying you should not be on the Fertility Pathway. It's wonderful to focus your attention on the idea of having a baby and trying to do all you can to ensure a healthy pregnancy. But before you toss the birth control, do reflect on your weight issue and whether you are willing to take on the challenge of getting to a healthier weight range. A baby is a powerful motivator for making big health changes, so here's your chance to reframe an old problem as a new opportunity. Consult with a physician and/or a nutritionist to start a comprehensive plan to lose (or gain) weight. Be sure to use the mind-body connection to help reprogram old eating habits, through such things as mindfulness or hypnosis. Having too much body fat, or too little, can also disrupt your ability to conceive. It's not recommended that you lose any weight at all during pregnancy, so it's really now or never. Once you're pregnant, your weight will only go up.

• *If you have had a history of an eating disorder, be proactive about exploring the impact that getting pregnant can have on this.* Often these issues can be reactivated in pregnancy, so preconception is a great time to explore and get some support for these issues.

THE MOVEMENT CENTER

Exercise brings all of the same benefits now that it does in pregnancy with the advantage of there being no real limitations on what you can do. Exercise in the year before pregnancy (as well as in the first trimester) has been associated with a decreased risk of developing preeclampsia in pregnancy.

- *Get your body as fit as possible before you embark on the physically demanding journey ahead.* It doesn't matter what your starting-point condition is; anything you do to improve your overall fitness will improve your experience, allowing you to enter pregnancy physically fit. If you start before trying to conceive, you'll have your routine in place by the time you are pregnant. *If you don't have a regular exercise program, start one now.* It's best to start a new routine prior to pregnancy, when you are not dealing with the changes that come with the first trimester, such as fatigue and nausea.

- *Remember that exercise is an essential part of a weight-loss program.* If you are trying to lose weight before pregnancy, don't rely on diet alone to get to a healthy weight for pregnancy. Exercise should be a key piece of your plan.

- *Consult your doctor if you exercise intensively and have difficulty conceiving.* Although most athletic women have no trouble, athletes with very little body fat can have problems with ovulation and therefore conception. A physician can help assure that you are ovulating.

THE SPIRIT CENTER

As previously mentioned, there are well-documented links between social connectedness and fertility.

• *Find ways to connect with your spouse spiritually, not just sexually.* It's easy to let babymaking take the central role in your relationship, but even now, the focus should be on each other and the bond that you share. Nurture that, as this is the energy from which new life comes.

• *Seek out supportive relationships.* Some people don't want to tell anyone when they're trying to conceive. That's a very individual choice—and one that should be made consciously. We do know that many women who are struggling with fertility find it helpful, both emotionally and practically, to share their concerns. If pregnancy is taking a while and you are starting to feel anxious, you may want to look into fertility support groups, online or in your community. Or choose just one person to confide in, someone you can say anything to and whom you trust to keep your confidences fully. Let this potential confidant know how personal this is for you, and ask if she (or he) is willing to play this role for you. A good friend is likely to consider it an honor and can be of great support.

THE SENSATION CENTER

This center plays a starring role in preconception. Enjoy it and elevate it to the attention it deserves.

• *Tune in sexually.* Being ready to conceive and not having a worry about contraception in the back of your head can be very freeing. This is a great opportunity to explore new levels of your sexuality. Readiness can create new freedom and excitement. Go with it.

• *Make sex a priority.* Procreation should not be a chore. Make time and space to enjoy sex. Focus on pleasuring each other rather than on creating a baby. Hopefully, you'll be inspired to do it often enough that you don't have to worry about "planning" or "timing."

• *Enjoy "mindful sex."* Alice Domar recommends this to help in-fertility patients, but it's great advice for anyone. Mindful sex simply means being keenly aware of your sensations (smell, touch, taste, hearing, sight) and focusing solely on the moment at hand. It's not "I'm-ovulating-so-get-in-the-bedroom-right-now" sex. It's focusing only on each other and the potential life you are creating together.

Part Three

The First Trimester

——————— ∞ ———————

Weeks 0 to 13

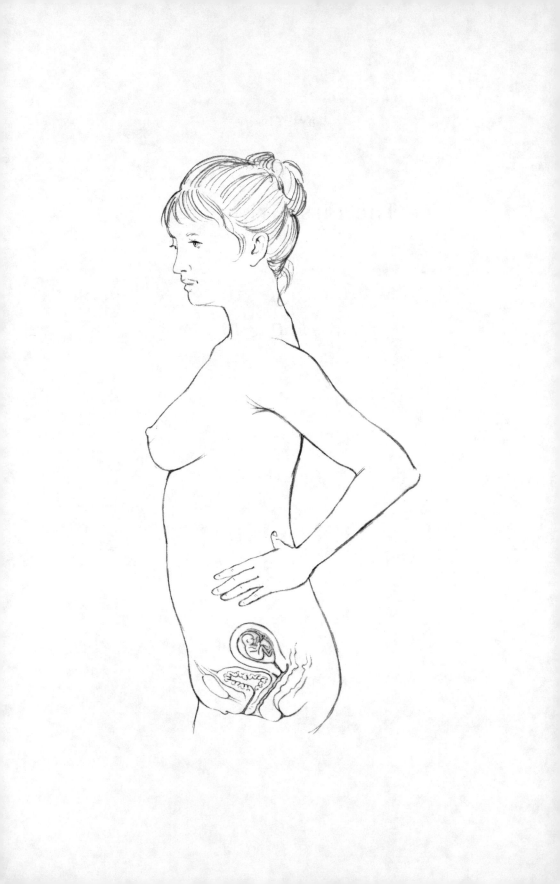

Chapter 10

First Trimester:
Reflection and Observation

∞

Checking in with body, soul, and baby, weeks 0 to 13

Pregnant? Really?!! Whether you've planned this pregnancy or been taken by surprise, being in tune with yourself is a gift to both you and your baby. Now, especially, it enables you to

- bear full witness to the miracle of pregnancy right from the start
- notice signs and symptoms that could be cause for concern and report them to your doctor
- support your daily needs in the best possible way
- take advantage of the full nine months to make the transition to motherhood
- forge a relationship with your baby from the very beginning.

CHECK IN WITH YOUR BODY

Checking in with your body is especially rewarding in the first trimester because your body has so much to say right now. You'll notice changes even on a daily basis.

Detailed instructions on how to use the following tools can be found in Chapter 3.

SUGGESTED TOOLS:

DAILY:

Body Quick Pic (tool #1)
Use this tool periodically throughout the day as a casual way of asking your changing body, "Hey, how are you doing?" It doesn't have to take more than a minute, even when combined with a Soul Quick Pic and a Baby Quick Pic (see below), and you could use it to give yourself a quick break from work.

Body Scan (tool #2)
This is really important at the start of pregnancy, so that it will become a natural habit before you are too far into the pregnancy. Do this exercise first thing in the morning and if you can, repeat it at day's end. It will be easy to remember if you incorporate it into your daily routine, such as before you get out of bed or after you shower. Make special note of new feelings you have never noticed in your body before.

WEEKLY:

Body Monitoring (tool #4)
This tool is one of the best ways to appreciate just how much your body is changing, and you will learn so much just by watching it.

AS NEEDED:

Dialoguing (with Your Physical Self) (tool #3)
Use this tool whenever something comes up in your body checks that you want to look into more deeply. Let's say, for example, that you feel the beginning of a headache. You can ask your body if there is anything that it needs, anything that might help the headache to resolve before it gets worse, anything it is trying to tell you. (You're trying to do too much, you need to eat something, you should do a quick relaxation exercise, take some Tylenol, etc.) Remember, the purpose

of Dialoguing isn't to diagnose yourself, but to make yourself more fully aware of what your body is experiencing—and what it might need to make it feel better. Then you can decide what to do next.

TELL YOUR DOCTOR IF YOU EXPERIENCE . . .

- Light bleeding that lasts for several days
- Bleeding like a period with or without cramping, with or without clotting
- Abdominal/pelvic pain
- Fever

If you have confirmed a pregnancy and have any of these symptoms, they can be signs of miscarriage or of something else amiss, and warrant further investigation. But let me reassure you that these symptoms do *not* mean you are destined to miscarry. So while your doctor should be notified and will probably want to examine you, don't leap to any conclusions. While you are waiting for more information, it's a good time to do some relaxation techniques. Keep checking in with your body as well as your soul and your baby.

BODY CHECKS:
WHAT MIGHT COME UP FOR YOU

Some of the sensations you pick up through these awareness-building exercises are specific: the beginnings of a headache, muscle tightness in your back, an overwhelming desire to nap. You can learn more about these symptoms in "Signs of Pregnancy," in the next chapter. You can then use such information to monitor the situation throughout the day, and to take an appropriate action (take a nap, take acetaminophen, and so on).

Don't assume you'll just notice things without checking in. What happens then is that you tend to notice only the very loudest shouts—a full-blown migraine or a backache—when you might have headed them off by heeding the earliest signs of something brewing.

The following are common general messages the body can send in the first trimester:

I Feel Awful. This Isn't What I Expected at All.

"I had no idea I would be this miserable," Caitlin told me. "If I had known, maybe I wouldn't have wished so hard to get pregnant." She paused a moment: "But I feel guilty for even thinking that."

Caitlin had struggled for two years to conceive before finally doing so with the help of the fertility drug Clomid. Nine weeks along, she appeared in my office pale and haggard, reporting extreme fatigue and nausea. As if the physical symptoms weren't bad enough, she was beating herself up by trying to ignore them, because she didn't feel she had a "right" to complain about anything now that she was finally pregnant.

There's no denying that for some women the early physical responses to pregnancy can be very intense. Throwing up every hour for days or weeks on end is taxing to anyone. So are extreme fatigue, breasts so tender they hurt, or a general feeling of "blahness" worse than the worst case of flu you ever had. (Although it's not always a predictor, the degree of your sensitivity to cyclical hormones—for example, whether you typically have severe PMS before your period—may be a sign of how sensitive you will be to the hormones of pregnancy.) The very real physical symptoms of the first trimester can be exacerbated when you are "supposed to be," according to the cultural dictates surrounding pregnancy, in a state of bliss. Fertility patients who have spent months or years hoping and praying to conceive sometimes feel so physically unwell in early pregnancy that they begin to wish they'd never gotten pregnant. They then feel emotionally ill, too, becoming wracked with guilt because they are having such thoughts.

Don't try to paste a smile on your face if it's green. Better to go into those feelings, and give yourself permission to accept what "is" for you—acknowledging how you are feeling, without judgment. You are then in a better position to be proactive about addressing your symptoms and working with them instead of being in battle with them. Being angry, upset, or guilty may only exacerbate them.

Remember—no feelings are bad ones. By acknowledging frankly how you feel, you're actually *less* likely to simmer in guilt. If you are having severe nausea and vomiting, then on a purely physical level, you *are* miserable. Owning up to that feeling does not negate the happiness and excitement you may also be feeling about the pregnancy.

I Don't Feel Anything Different.

At the opposite end of the spectrum from sick-as-a-dog Caitlin was April. She noticed almost no symptoms of pregnancy at all. "I feel great," she reported at her second prenatal exam, when she was 10 weeks along. "Is that bad?"

I went through a checklist of symptoms. April said she had barely a hint of nausea, no breast tenderness, no change in appetite or different sleep needs. The first thing that runs through my head in such a case is to verify the pregnancy. Although first-trimester symptoms can be annoying, they do serve to reassure you that your body *is* actually pregnant. Think of it this way— every bout of morning sickness is an affirmation!

Not all women experience this "affirmation," thankfully. Some women are less sensitive to the internal chain reaction that conception kicks off in the body. It's not unusual to go through a healthy, normal pregnancy with minimal or no nausea and not a single episode of vomiting, for example. However, if you feel absolutely no change at any time even though your pregnancy test turned positive, it's worth letting your doctor know. He or she can verify that everything is proceeding apace.

April was relieved that everything seemed all right. She then confided that she was ambivalent about this pregnancy, which was unplanned. She'd actually had a weekend of partying before she had missed her period, and had been feeling really worried and anxious. Then once she'd discovered she was pregnant, she was still unsure about how she felt. "I guess I was hesitant to really believe it or acknowledge it," she says. "And when I didn't feel anything I thought maybe it was untrue—or that I was losing the baby because I hadn't wanted it or deserved it."

I assured her that feelings don't "cause" miscarriage. I explained the basics about a conscious pregnancy and encouraged her to use tools such as Journaling and Dialoguing so that rather than denying her true feelings or blaming herself for them, she could meet them honestly and work with them. She continued to experience very few physical symptoms throughout her entire pregnancy, but spent a lot of time working on her emotional concerns. By the time her daughter, Amber, was born, April felt very excited and thankful to welcome her into the world.

CHECK IN WITH YOUR SOUL

While the most noticeable action is perhaps taking place within your newly pregnant body, your soul has a lot of adjusting to do as well. The feelings that surface at this time are not necessarily the feelings you thought you'd have when you became pregnant; they simply are what they are. Don't be surprised to discover a full spectrum of responses, with different ones coming to the fore at different times. Remember, the point is simply to acknowledge them, not to shut them away or beat yourself up over anything less than clichéd bliss. Bliss is great, and very real for many newly pregnant women—but it is only one of a huge number of emotions and reactions common at this stage.

SUGGESTED TOOLS

DAILY:

Soul Quick Pic (tool #5)
As with the Body Quick Pic, it's a brief how're-you-doing. If you don't stop to ask, you're less likely to have a sense of this part of yourself.

ANYTIME, AT LEAST ONCE IN FIRST TRIMESTER
AND PREFERABLY MORE:

Journaling Your Journey (tool #6)

Some women choose to write daily or once a week. Make the time to explore the following in your journal:

• How do you feel now that you are really pregnant? What are the best and worst things about pregnancy now that it is a reality and not an abstract notion? What are the easiest and the hardest things?

• How does being pregnant impact your relationships: With yourself? With your partner? With your friends? With your family? With your career? When you think about entering into a relationship with another, new being, how does it make you feel? What excites you about it? What scares you?

• If you did not plan this pregnancy, reflect on how this may have happened. Not in physical terms (forgot to insert diaphragm, condom broke, etc.), but on a deeper level. What do you think was going on that led you to conceive? And how are you feeling—honestly—about it now?

Whenever there is a huge disconnect between what you intended, or at least what you *thought* you intended (no pregnancy), and what actually happened (pregnancy), it's a great opportunity to explore feelings that you might not be fully conscious of. Explore them and put them on the table for acknowledgment, so that they don't cause problems during your pregnancy and beyond. Was there a subconscious part of you that had a different intention? This is not unusual at all. If so, really spend some time exploring that part of you. Get to know it in the best way you can. This is sometimes easiest to do by giving that part of you a voice. Try Dialoguing or Dreamagery with this voice to begin to develop a relationship with this part of yourself. Sometimes, however, the answer really is as simple as "The condom broke"! So if nothing is coming up for you, accept that as well.

SOUL CHECKS:
WHAT MIGHT COME UP FOR YOU

Yikes!

Tanya and her husband, Jeff, had had vague thoughts about start-ing a family for several years. But the time never seemed right—they were establishing their careers, they travel a lot—and so "it was just not something we really focused on." One night, Tanya says, she "forgot" her diaphragm and, three weeks later, realized she was late for her period.

"How are you feeling about being pregnant?" I asked at her first prenatal exam.

"Well," she said slowly, as if struggling to choose the right words, "we've talked about this for so long, so it's not really a sur-prise. It's exciting, of course, but at the same time, I lie awake in the middle of the night and think, *Oh my God, do I really want this in my life right now?*"

Second thoughts are common whether you wanted and planned a pregnancy or whether it came as an "accident." Regardless of how happy you may feel about having a baby, you may simultaneously have a strong sense of uncertainty.

The source of these reservations can be anything. Maybe you're concerned about the timing of the birth. You may be up-set that you got pregnant just when you were supposed to go on a long-planned trip. Maybe your marriage is at a rocky patch and you worry about bringing a new life into the situation. Any one of a thousand factors—physical, financial, career-related, relationship-related—can cause you concern about being preg-nant at this particular juncture in time. Your concerns don't even have to be rational. Feelings often don't make any sense to the intellect. And this quality doesn't make them any less significant or valid—even though your intellect may try to have you believe otherwise! Feelings have a wisdom of their own that deserves to be explored, and that can have practical implications. Depending on the nature of the reservations, they might lead you to look into marriage counseling, rethink your career goals, or do more self-care. If after exploring these feelings, your reservations are significant, you should explore them further, with your physician or a counselor. A trained individual can help you to understand and work with these strong feelings. For some women, exploring the full range of options means exploring adoption or abortion.

I encouraged Tanya to Journal about her mixed feelings—to give voice to both the part of her that was excited about being pregnant, and to the part that was uncertain. The next time I saw her, she shyly shared with me some of what she had written: "The idea of a baby was one thing. But now it's really happening! Jeff is excited but I am scared. Everything has been perfect with us so far and I don't know how I can handle adding a baby in the mix of our life and work, etc. Jeff says there is never a 'perfect' time and I suppose he's right. I had been forgetting my diaphragm a lot in the past year—maybe it was my way of being more ready than I thought. I couldn't make the decision to have a baby so I was hoping Fate would make it for me. Well it did—and now I am trying to get used to that idea. I think I have a hard time making changes. But here we are!"

Tanya continued to explore her feelings in the following weeks. She used some of what she uncovered during this process to sort out her ideas about how she wanted to combine career and motherhood, and to invite Jeff into the process, too, because she wanted him to understand how important it was to her that raising their child be a shared responsibility.

Unlike Tanya, who was at least aware of the fact that she was experiencing a sense of ambivalence, fertility patients often feel special pressure to be 100 percent thrilled by a positive pregnancy test and permit themselves no space at all for dealing with the shadowy feelings that are just part of the human condition. If you worked this hard to become pregnant, and now you are, you can still celebrate that fact even as you accept that pregnancy is not the sunny end point; it's merely the starting place for a different journey that, like everything in life, has both lightness and darkness.

Sometimes fertility patients who finally find themselves pregnant discover second thoughts about the pregnancy itself. It was a cherished goal three years ago when they climbed aboard the fertility-treatment conveyor belt, but now that they're actually pregnant, they're no longer so sure that this is what they want, perhaps because they hadn't done any checking-in with themselves to determine whether it was still what they wanted.

Consider all feelings, no matter how "unacceptable," to be an opening. Explore further: What part of you is feeling uneasy? What are your greatest fears?

I'm Scared.

Every time Erin stopped to check in with her soul, she got the same two responses: "I'm pregnant! This is so cool!" and "I can't believe this is happening to me. I'm scared." She wondered how she could have two such strong but opposing feelings at the same time.

"Is it common to be so nervous?" she asked.

We talked about the ways her nervousness manifested itself. Erin said she redid her home pregnancy test every couple of days for the first two weeks after she got her first confirmation. She was afraid to exercise, use the microwave, or take a bath for fear she could harm the baby. I reassured her that none of those things would place her baby at risk, but I was interested in exploring the source of her nerves.

If you are dogged by a sense of fear, ask yourself what you are afraid of. Common examples are fear of miscarriage and fear of something being wrong with the baby. When women delve deeper into the possible basis of the fear, it's often rooted in a bad outcome that they've experienced personally (for example, a prior miscarriage) or that a friend or family member has experienced or that they read or saw in a story somewhere (such as a baby born with birth defects).

"Well, I don't want to lose this baby," Erin finally said. "I can't believe I said that—I don't want to jinx anything." Upon further discussion, it emerged that Erin's sister had had a late miscarriage, at 16 weeks. The experience had been understandably traumatic. What's more, it was the only pregnancy Erin had witnessed close up.

I gave Erin information about the actual risks of loss, and we reviewed the specifics of her sister's case (she had an incompetent cervix, in which the cervix begins to dilate prematurely for unknown reasons; it does not run in families). We also talked about the importance of Erin exploring her feelings of guilt because she was now pregnant and her sister, who always did things first, was not, having had difficulty conceiving since her loss. I encouraged her to acknowledge these feelings with her sister. They were both aware of them, but they went unspoken, which created tension and discomfort between them. Over time, Erin reported feeling less worried about every little thing, which had the added benefit of allowing her to more fully relax and enjoy the experience of her pregnancy.

It sounds so simple, but it's true: Acknowledging that a particular fear is true for you is a huge step toward being able to cope with that fear.

Why Isn't My Body Cooperating?

Anika was elated to be pregnant. She and her husband, Roger, had giddily told everyone they knew as soon as the home test turned positive. Everything was just as they'd envisioned— except that Anika was very sick, nonstop sick, so sick she had to keep taking days off to lie in bed and hit the bathroom every half hour.

In Anika's case, her soul wants to celebrate and bask in maternity but her body is not cooperating.

When you get such different messages from your body and your soul, it's useful to Dialogue with both entities about the conflict and what each needs from the other. I encouraged Anika to imagine a conversation between the two.

In my experience, women who go through the process of putting their body and their soul in communication with each other tend to recover from pregnancy sickness faster than those who let the conflict and annoyance fester. This is probably because they move more quickly toward constructive steps to address the discomforts and significantly reduce stress that might otherwise aggravate the situation.

CHECK IN WITH YOUR BABY

For some women, the baby is a concrete presence right from the start, making these exercises feel natural. Others have more difficulty conceptualizing a multiplying ball of cells that's causing nausea and vomiting as an entity to be in a relationship with—though the effects it's having on you are tangible proof of a relationship! Whether you envision an actual baby or simply the idea of a new life, the following exercises can help you remain mindful of this key player in the body-soul-baby trio.

SUGGESTED TOOLS

DAILY:

Baby Quick Pic (tool #8)

Where this tool may have felt abstract before conceiving, it grows ever easier to grasp and use as your pregnancy proceeds. Even in the first trimester, before you can feel the baby moving or hear a heartbeat, you are in a relationship with this new entity, your baby-to-be. Check in with it. How is it doing? Does it have anything to say to you? You can easily run a Baby Quick Pic at the same time you do Body and Soul Quick Pics.

ANYTIME, AT LEAST ONCE IN FIRST TRIMESTER:

Dreamagery (tool #9)

Remember, Dreamagery is simply a deeper level of Dialoguing. You give yourself more time to get to a deeper state of relaxation to start, and then it's based in imagery. This gives you the opportunity to access more information because in addition to the quick conversation of Dialoguing, you have a more textured, in-depth experience.

Remember, too, that you can use Dreamagery about any topic, not just baby-related ones.

BABY CHECKS:
WHAT MIGHT COME UP FOR YOU

Hi, It's Great to Meet You!

Very often checking in with your baby in the first trimester, especially the first time you do the exercise, is like a grand opening. The baby says hello, and you say hello, and it feels like the very awesome beginning of a beautiful friendship—which it is!

I'm Here—Don't Pretend I'm Not.

Susan's first pregnancy had ended in a miscarriage at 11 weeks. That time, Susan and Dan, her husband, both 26, had told all their friends and relatives the minute they learned she was expecting. She had embraced the experience from the get-go, and was, understandably, devastated when she lost the baby.

Eight months later, Susan was pregnant again. This time, she seemed more low-key about it. At her first prenatal visit, I asked how she was feeling. "Okay," she said in a rather subdued voice. "I'm thrilled to be pregnant again, but I'm laying low about it this time. Last time, I was already trying on maternity clothes even though I didn't need them and I was thinking about the baby all the time. Now I just try not to focus on it. I'm so afraid I'll lose it, I don't want to get attached till I'm past 12 weeks."

It's not an uncommon reaction. Women who are pregnant for the first time often have it, too. In the first trimester, the odds of miscarriage are still relatively high (as high as 30 percent, according to some estimates, with 80 percent of miscarriages occurring in the first 12 weeks). Many women, whether consciously or not, avoid letting themselves become "attached" to the fetus until they're safely through the first months and can finally hear the heartbeat or see the baby on ultrasound. They may avoid thinking about the pregnancy and try to proceed as if nothing's really happening. Well-intentioned though such a wait-and-see attitude may be, it's not entirely realistic. No matter what happens, that baby is, right now, a being growing inside of you. You are already in a relationship, no matter what happens. And that's the message that often comes up in this exercise. The baby is saying, matter-of-factly, "I'm *here*."

Interestingly, my patients rarely report the baby declaring, "I'm here and I won't leave you no matter what." The reality is that nothing is certain in pregnancy, especially early on. However, it can be tremendously reassuring simply to acknowledge what *is* right now. In my experience, the women who try to avoid getting too invested in the pregnancy and do go on to miscarry have a more difficult time than those who have been conscious of the relationship from the start.

I reassured Susan that her differing reactions from one pregnancy to the next were perfectly normal. "But think about you saying you don't want to get attached," I told her gently. "You are attached already, and you should be, you can't help but be—no matter what happens this time."

I led Susan through a Dreamagery exercise. She described the image that came to her of the fetus as an iris. I asked her if it had any messages for her. She was quiet a long while. "I know you're so worried," it said to her. "But here I am, blossoming inside you."

Susan began to cry. I asked her if she had anything to share with the image. "I just don't want to be heartbroken again," she choked. "I am afraid to love you or get connected to you because, let's face it, I could lose you."

"What does the image have to say to you?" I asked.

There was a long silence. Finally Susan said, "It says, 'Whatever happens, I'll be okay, and you'll be okay.' It doesn't want to be shut out. It wants to be loved."

Chapter 11

First Trimester:
The Inside Scoop

∞

What's happening biologically, weeks 0 to 13

SIGNS OF PREGNANCY

The successful union of egg and sperm kicks off a cavalcade of events that affect you globally, not just locally. The first noticeable signs of pregnancy vary from woman to woman. You may not experience each and every one of the typical changes, but if you're checking in with your body every day in a conscious way, you'll probably notice one or more of the following as early as the first two weeks after conception (just about the time you would be expecting your next period, or about four weeks after your last period).

Some "first signs" at a glance:

• *Missed menstrual period.*

WHY: The uterine lining that builds up in anticipation of a pregnancy is shed (your period) every month when you do not conceive. If the egg you released is fertilized, however, this lush protective uterine lining has a purpose—to sustain what will become your baby—so, no period.

• *Breast tenderness.* This can range from a mild tingly sensation to a heavier, more sensitive feeling. They may be slightly full or quite painful. Often women report their breasts feel the way they do right before a period, only worse.

WHY: Hormonal changes and increased blood flow.

• *Fatigue.* You may become more winded after doing ordinary activities, and sleep more soundly.

WHY: Your body is consuming a tremendous amount of energy internally.

• *Sense of fullness and sensitivity in your pelvis and stomach.* You may feel a general (not sharp) sense of fullness, bloating, aching, or gassiness not unlike what you feel around your period, but more pronounced.

WHY: This is the area where the action's taking place inside you.

• *Frequent urination.* You may feel the need to use the bathroom as often as once an hour.

WHY: In the first trimester, hormonal changes can cause this. (It's not until later in pregnancy that your expanding uterus will push against your bladder and also create this symptom.)

• *Nausea.* "Morning sickness" can come at any time of the day or night, and in varying degrees of severity. You may have a mildly upset stomach (some women report feeling a prickly sensation, like bubbles popping), or you may feel queasy all day long, or you may be really ill, as if with the flu. Nausea may or may not be accompanied by vomiting. It usually arises about the fifth or sixth week.

WHY: It's unclear why this symptom varies so much from woman to woman—about one in four experience little to no nausea. The hormonal shifts of early pregnancy are probably the root cause of morning sickness, which means that nausea is actually a sign that things are proceeding as they should. Some evolutionary biologists suggest that nausea has a protective component,

causing a woman to avoid potentially toxic foods (such as raw
fish or smoked meats) at the very time when fetal organ systems are developing. Heredity is thought to be a factor, too.

• *Aversion to certain tastes or smells.* Although this sign is highly individualized, common instinctive dislikes that get switched on at this
time include strong tastes, such as for coffee, alcohol, tobacco, and
certain spices (such as oregano), and strong odors, including smoke,
foods being fried, and gasoline.

WHY: The same evolutionary theory behind morning sickness holds
here. These are primitive survival mechanisms that kick in to
protect the fetus from potentially dangerous substances.

• *Implantation bleeding.* You may think you are just having an unusual period because you see slight spotting or what appears to be the
equivalent of a light period, usually at around the same time your period would normally come.

WHY: Around the time the fertilized egg is implanted into the uterine cavity, some cells may be sloughed off at implantation and,
uncommonly, appear as bloody discharge. It's another reason
why it's important to pay attention to your periods, not only
their dates but also any changes from month to month in the
amount of bleeding. You'll be less likely to misinterpret this
bleeding as the start of your period if you have a good sense of
what is normal for you in a menstrual cycle.

CONFIRMING PREGNANCY

The simplest way to be sure you're pregnant is to use a home pregnancy test. You can buy a test kit over the counter at any drugstore
or grocery. Performed properly, they're 99 percent accurate—so read
the instructions carefully. Or many health clinics, such as Planned
Parenthood, will run the test for free. These tests measure a hormone
called human chorionic gonadotropin (hCG) in your urine. Produced
by the placenta, hCG doubles every two or three days for the first six
weeks of pregnancy. It's first detectable by a blood hCG test 6 to 8

days after conception (about one week before the next period is due); most women will typically show a positive blood HCG level by 11 to 12 days after conception. HCG shows up in the urine a little later—at about 10 days after ovulation by early-detection kits, or within 12 to 14 days of ovulation for standard kits, or about the time you would be having your period.

Although rare, false positives (where the test says you're pregnant, but you're not) can occur in women who are perimenopausal (nearing the start of menopause) because of naturally increasing levels of hCG, or in women who have tumors that produce hormones. False negatives (where the test says you're not pregnant but you are) can happen if you have tested too early for the hCG to be detected. Test again in two or three days if you still have not had your period and/or are having symptoms of pregnancy. Because false negatives can also occur in ectopic pregnancies (a rare event where the fertilized egg implants outside of the uterus, usually in a fallopian tube), always let your doctor know if you feel "in your gut" that you might be pregnant despite a negative test result. Listen to your body.

If you think you might be pregnant, tell your doctor so he or she can verify the pregnancy with a urine test and do your first exam. They will check to see if it is consistent with the size of your uterus and how far along you would be based on your dates. (At the time of your missed period, the uterus should be unchanged in size, which will help confirm that you are as early in the pregnancy as you thought.) An early pregnancy test and pelvic exam are among the best ways to get an accurate dating of the pregnancy.

If a urine test is inconclusive, a serum (blood) pregnancy test can also provide confirmation. Most people think blood tests are more accurate than urine tests, although this is not necessarily true. In certain individuals, it's possible to have a false positive on a blood test. (I know, because I am one of them!) This is usually because the person has a reaction to the antibody used in the test, but can also be caused by tumors, as mentioned above.

FEAR: My home pregnancy test isn't accurate.

FACT: If you follow the instructions exactly, you'll get almost certain results, so read carefully before you begin. When in doubt, try again—the tests are relatively inexpensive (or free at some clinics) and often conveniently sold in two-packs.

FEAR: I don't feel pregnant. Did I lose the baby?

FACT: Very early in pregnancy, you may not notice many symptoms of pregnancy yet. Tell your doctor and keep monitoring yourself, but give it time.

FROM CONCEPTION TO FETUS: THE INSIDE STORY

Conception

Your baby's sex is determined at the moment of conception. If a sperm bearing a Y-chromosome reaches the egg first, a male is created. If the sperm has an X-chromosome, a female is created. So the next time your partner says to you that he wants a girl or is hoping for a boy, you can let him know that that part is all up to him!

From the moment of conception, proteins are released into the maternal circulation by the fertilized egg. We believe that these proteins alter the mother's immune, metabolic, and hormonal systems—priming your body to accept and embrace the pregnancy. The production of these proteins from the embryo communicates the needs and demands of each developmental stage of pregnancy. The first proteins are released into your circulation literally at the instant the sperm penetrates the egg. The egg releases something called PAF (platelet-activating factor) when fertilized, which then releases another protein from the ovary called EPF (early pregnancy factor). The fertilized egg, known as a *zygote*, travels down the tube and into the uterus, arriving there when it's just two to eight cells big, somewhere between 90 and 150 hours after conception.

Implantation

By four and a half days after conception, the fertilized egg becomes a *blastocyst.* It begins to secrete hCG (human chorionic gonadotropin) as early as six days after conception, measurable in the mother's blood within six to eight days after conception, which is the time at which implantation into the uterine lining is complete.

Development of the Placenta

Starting at five days after conception, cells that will become the placenta are distinct from others. From the time of implantation, these cells form two layers, which have different functions and secrete ten or more different types of hormones. The placenta is an amazing structure—the unsung hero of pregnancy—that represents the physical and physiologic interface between mother and baby. After all, your baby isn't just plopped inside of you. It grows within the intricate structure of the membranes of the placenta.

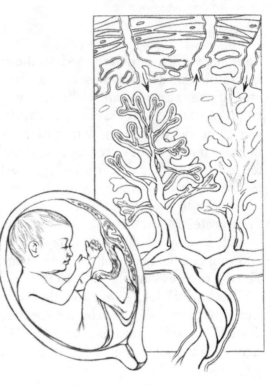

At every birth, I always make a point of holding up the placenta, its membranes, and the umbilical cord (which originates within it) to show the new parents. They can see the meaty red part that was attached to the mother, the membranes that surrounded the baby and formed the amniotic sac, and where the umbilical cord, which links the placenta and the fetus,

The amazing placenta

began. The umbilical cord has two arteries and a large vein, through which nutrients and oxygen-rich blood pass. By the time your baby is born, it can be up to four feet long. The health of the baby is completely dependent on the health of the placenta. Everything the baby needs—blood, oxygen, nutrients—is transformed within the placenta to fuel growth. That's a relationship worth being aware of! Throughout the pregnancy, the placenta adapts and alters its structure as its function changes. Early in pregnancy it's extremely active hormonally; later it becomes the organ through which oxygen and nutrients are transferred from the mother to the fetus.

Three Weeks After Conception

By five weeks after your last period, or three weeks after conception, your baby-to-be is now an *embryo*. The embryo divides into three parts: a groove called the neural tube (which will become the brain, spinal cord, and backbone), the eventual heart and circulatory system, and the foundation for bones, muscles, and the other organs. The tissue that will form the placenta also continues to develop.

Five Weeks After Conception

The embryo is now about one-third of an inch long, more than five times its size two weeks earlier. The brain is developing, the heart has begun to pump blood, and the beginnings of arms, legs, hands, feet, and facial features are forming, still in a very primitive state.

Seven Weeks After Conception

The embryo has grown to one inch long and has a recognizably human shape. Paddle-like hands and feet can be recognized and the "tail" it once had is disappearing. Internal reproductive organs are following their assigned male or female paths but external genitalia are not yet evident.

Nine to Twelve Weeks After Conception

The embryo is now known as a fetus. When the fetus is nine weeks old, it has been 11 weeks since your last menstrual period. All organ systems and limbs (including defined fingers and toes) have begun to develop. Genitalia are beginning to look male or female. The fetus is in the curled position it will mainly stay in throughout pregnancy. It can move its arms and legs, although it is still too small (barely three inches long and weighing $1^1/2$ ounces by the end of this trimester) for you to feel anything.

See how rapidly the developing embryo changes:

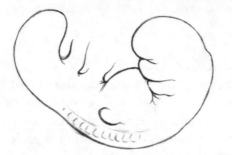

Four weeks after conception   *Actual size*

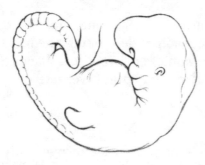

Five weeks after conception   *Actual size*

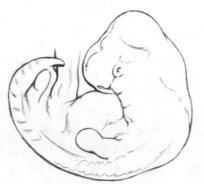

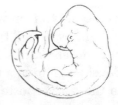

Six weeks after conception   *Actual size*

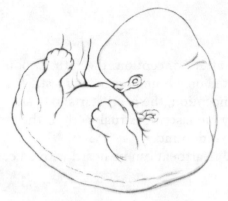

Seven weeks after conception   *Actual size*

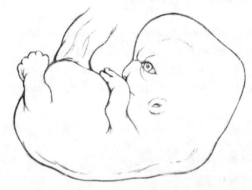

Eight weeks after conception   *Actual size*

Nine to thirteen weeks after conception   *Actual size*

Fetal Headlines

- By about 10 to 12 days after conception, the fetus produces enough hCG to be detected on a home pregnancy test.
- By 21 to 22 days after conception, the heart starts to beat.
- By 6 to 9 weeks after your last menstrual period, the fetal heartbeat can be seen on ultrasound.
- By 10 to 12 weeks, a fetal heartbeat can be heard with an electronic Doppler device.

WHAT'S HAPPENING WITH YOU: FIRST-TRIMESTER CHANGES

The physical effects are numerous as your body adjusts to the demands of being pregnant. Using your check-in tools will help you become aware of them when they first appear, allowing you to make adjustments in your care in ways that can provide comfort. Consult your doctor about other relief.

NOSE: The linings of the nose and mouth swell and secretions increase. This can translate to increased stuffiness and nosebleeds. Some women feel like they have a chronic cold. You might try sleeping with your head slightly elevated to help drain the excess fluid. A steamy shower can be comforting, as can warm liquids like herbal tea with honey. Gargling or rinsing your nostrils with salt water will also help.

EYES: By 10 weeks, the cornea increases in thickness and there is decreased intraocular pressure. This probably causes the contact-lens intolerance reported by some women. If your contact lenses are bothering you, switch to glasses and try using eye drops more regularly.

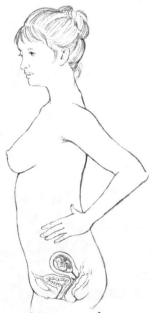

A woman in her first trimester

FACE: The "mask of pregnancy" (melasma or chloasma) is caused by hormonal changes. It's a blotchy hyperpigmentation—darkening of the pigmented cells of the skin—of the forehead, the cheeks, the bridge of the nose, and the upper lip. This occurs to some degree in nine out of ten pregnant women, especially brunettes. Melasma almost always fades gradually after delivery, though in some people it never disappears completely. Avoid the sun, which can aggravate pigment changes, and be sure to use a high-SPF sunscreen.

SKIN: High estrogen levels can cause spider veins, especially on the face, chest, and arms. They're much more common in Caucasian women. Redness of the palms—either blotchy or all over—occurs in 60 percent of pregnancies; like spider veins, they go away after delivery. Places where hyperpigmentation can occur include not just the face but the belly button, underarms, perineum, and the midline running from the lower abdomen to the pubic bone—where it's called the linea nigra.

SWEAT GLANDS: Typically you will sweat more and your skin will be oilier. Because your sweat glands control your body temperature, you may also feel overheated sometimes. Keeping your face clean and refreshed will alleviate that sweaty feeling. Try scenting your water with lemon as a natural astringent. To cool off, take a cooling shower or bath, stay hydrated, and stay out of the direct sun and heat.

BREASTS: Tenderness, tingling, heaviness, and enlargment begin within two weeks of conception, and rapid growth occurs within the first eight weeks, mostly due to increased blood flow. Breast growth after the first eight weeks is due to increased estrogen and progesterone (not fat). The nipples and areolas also enlarge, darken, and become more mobile. Sore breasts are very common in pregnancy, much like an exaggerated version of the discomfort many of us feel when we are premenstrual. If you haven't already cut out caffeine, doing so may help lessen the pain. Many women also find it helpful to change their sleeping position or switch to a less restrictive bra.

HEART: The function of your heart changes from the start. The volume of blood your heart pumps increases from about 4.5 liters per minute to 6.5 liters per minute. This rise peaks in the first trimester (or early in the second) and remains high throughout pregnancy.

Almost one-fifth of this increased output goes to the uterus, which receives only 2 percent when you're not pregnant. The kidneys also receive 50 percent more blood flow than usual, and the breasts and skin receive more as well.

Because progesterone relaxes smooth muscle, as does the heat generated by the fetus, blood vessels dilate and blood pressure is lower now, even though more blood is being pumped. Blood pressure drops progressively this trimester.

LUNGS: Increased blood flow in the upper airway often results in increased stuffiness and nasal bleeding. Breathing in pregnancy is more from the diaphragm than the rib cage. The actual shape of the rib cage changes this trimester, long before there is any physical pressure from the uterus. Even though there is a 30 to 40 percent increase in the amount of air inhaled and exhaled with normal breathing, many women experience a sense of breathlessness. The reason for this is not understood.

STOMACH: Progesterone, the same hormone that is responsible for dilation of the blood vessels, also causes the muscles of the stomach to relax, which is why your belly may be slack even before you show. This may also contribute to nausea. See pages 168–171 for tips on coping with nausea.

BOWELS AND BLADDER: More iron is absorbed because more is needed. But the digestive system slows because of smooth-muscle relaxation and water absorption, which is more than doubled. The kidneys usually grow about 1 cm in pregnancy due to increased fluids, and the right usually enlarges more than the left. The kidneys' ability to filter the blood increases significantly by five to seven weeks, and glucose excretion increases in almost everyone.

BLOOD: Plasma volume (the noncellular part of the blood) begins to increase at 10 weeks, as does production of red blood cells. Because plasma volume increases more than the red blood cells, it's normal to see anemia later in pregnancy. When you're not pregnant, anemia typically results from decreased red blood cells; in pregnancy you actually have more red blood cells but you can be anemic simply because you have more plasma volume diluting the red blood cells; this is known as "dilutional anemia" and is normal. No treatment is necessary.

Chapter 12

First Trimester:
Medical Care

∞

An integrative medicine perspective, weeks 0 to 13

BASIC MEDICAL ISSUES NOW

Choosing Your Prenatal Caregiver

The most important thing to know about this decision is that it is not irrevocable. You can change your mind. Doing so doesn't mean that you didn't do it right the first time. Often women automatically start prenatal care with the person who gives them their annual exam, whether because of convenience or a sense of obligation, only to discover that this relationship doesn't feel right during pregnancy. The earlier you act on this discovery, the better. In making your selection of obstetric caregiver, you'll want to know what choices are available and how these match up with the kind of birth experience you want.

Caregiver Options

1) *An ob-gyn.* Obstetricians (ob-gyns) are medical doctors whose specialty is women's health, including pregnancy and birth. Within this category, you can choose among obs in private practice (in solo or group settings) and those who are affiliated with teaching hospitals.

The degree to which an ob is philosophically aligned with integrative medicine can vary widely, from those who deeply embrace patient-centered care and the use of alternative therapies where appropriate, to those who strongly disapprove. If you have any factors that require care beyond routine obstetric care (conventionally referred to as low-risk obstetrics), you may be referred to or choose to seek an ob who specializes in maternal–fetal medicine (MFM). An MFM has, in addition to a four-year residency in obstetrics-gynecology after medical school, three additional years of fellowship training. Communities and physicians vary as to whom they refer to an MFM. In some places it may be as arbitrary as being over 35 at the time of delivery, a "condition" referred to as advanced maternal age, or AMA, a description that hardly cheers such moms. In addition to caring for women who do have complications with their pregnancies, MFMs often also care for women with routine pregnancies.

2) *A family practitioner (FP).* These are general medical doctors who can provide prenatal care as well as your baby's pediatric care after birth. They're trained to provide care at all points of the life cycle, which can be a useful perspective for a transition such as pregnancy. On the other hand, unlike an ob-gyn, an FP's residency after medical school is not solely in obstetrics-gynecology. It's important to get a feel for how much obstetrics the FP does (how many babies she delivers in a year on average, and how many years she has practiced ob-care). There can be a wide variation, depending on the makeup of the practice. An FP will most likely not have as much hands-on experience with pregnancy and labor and delivery as an obstetrician or MFM specialist and if you have a "high-risk" pregnancy or a chronic medical condition this difference can be quite significant. Also find out what the arrangement for "backup" is: if a situation arises in which the FP wants the opinion or involvement of an obstetrician, what happens? It will be important for you to understand this process, and be comfortable with this arrangement and with the obstetric practice that provides the backup. Many family physicians do not do obstetric care.

3) *A certified nurse-midwife (CNM).* Nurses trained in midwifery, CNMs, usually practice in birthing centers where natural delivery is the goal. Some, not all, practice with obstetricians and may deliver in the hospital setting as well. They tend to provide holistic prenatal

care and delivery. Women who are attended by CNMs tend to have lower rates of C-sections, episiotomy, and anesthesia for three reasons: 1) their philosophy; 2) their like-minded, motivated patient population; and 3) complicated or higher-risk patients who are more likely to need such interventions are not usually under their care in the first place. In my opinion, a midwife who practices within an ob-practice offers one of the best combinations of the holistic/natural and the conventional/higher-tech worlds. With this model, you have a seamless backup if your pregnancy becomes more complicated and requires ob-care. It's important to ask, however, to what degree you are exclusively the CNM's patient, both prenatally and at delivery. Some joint practices are set up so that the midwife handles the routine clinic visits but the ob handles delivery; or the midwife does part of the clinic work and the ob does part, too. In other joint practices, the CNMs function independently with their own set of patients and consult with the obstetricians as needed.

4) *A lay midwife.* Not legal in all states, these are almost always women who do not have nursing degrees but are experienced or trained in midwifery. They may or may not practice at freestanding birth centers and are seldom linked with a hospital or ob-practice. My bias is against lay midwives for two main reasons: 1) There is no standard education or credentialing body, and therefore there is no oversight to the quality of care a lay midwife offers. Anybody with or without training can claim to be one; and 2) the lack of relationship with a conventional obstetric setting is to me a potential recipe for disaster. Most deliveries are uneventful and turn out perfectly. If yours is the one that runs into difficulty, however, you'd want the best that medicine has to offer at your fingertips. Of course my opinions are in part informed by my own personal experience. I have probably seen the worst side of this care—the effects when the patient of a lay midwife and her baby have suffered because of inadequate basic care or a delay in seeking medical intervention in labor (often because of the lay midwife's and/or the patient's anti-physician or anti-hospital attitudes). I also understand that such an attitude toward the medical profession does not characterize all lay midwives. There are wonderful lay midwives, and women who have wonderful birthing experiences with them. If you choose to work with one, it's important to find someone who feels comfortable about acting in cooperation/collaboration with a conventional system if it becomes necessary, and

has a system that is happy to work with her. It is relatively easy to ignore the reality that your pregnancy may not progress perfectly, and this can result in not exploring the question of access to medical care. This is a great illustration (and one we would like to avoid) of the potential cost of not having a conscious pregnancy.

Birthplace Options

In considering caregivers, you also need to give some thought to *where* you want to give birth. Visit the options that interest you and find out as much as you can about their pros and cons relative to your situation. Your four main choices are:

1) A conventional hospital. As a hospital-based ob-gyn myself, my own bias is for a hospital delivery, because when things go wrong in birth, they tend to go wrong fast. It is potentially lifesaving to have anesthesia and an operating room close at hand. Your degree of control over your birth experience at a conventional hospital depends to some extent on the hospital's policies. Find out about standard policies such as whether you will be required to stay in bed or have an IV, who can attend the birth, the typical routines for the nursery, the visiting hours, whether your partner can stay overnight, and whether you change rooms throughout the process and how many times. Ask what standard procedures are and how much potential for variation there is within them. These questions are essentially about philosophy and will help you confirm whether you have a comfortable fit. Many, but not all, hospitals have birthing suites where you labor, deliver, and recover in the same room.

There are fundamentally two kinds of hospitals: 1) a teaching or university hospital and 2) a private hospital. At a teaching hospital, you are likely to encounter residents or medical students under supervision. Ask what this might mean for your care, such as whom you will see first and who will be present during delivery. At a private hospital, you will be dealing with your doctor or his/her associates and the hospital nursing staff. Find out how much is typically done before the physician comes in and how much is done by the nurses throughout labor. (This will vary by institution and physician, but you can get a sense of what is typical.) If it is a teaching hospital, you want to ask the same questions but with regard to the residents and their interface with your obstetrician.

Having residents involved in your care is not, in my opinion, a negative. Ob-gyn residents are physicians, and while they are still in their specialty training, they typically have a great deal of experience and are very skilled and compassionate. The advantage of this setting is that there are always physicians in the hospital—both obstetricians and anesthesiologists. In a private-hospital setting, the physicians may be primarily managing your labor from a distance, using the nurses as their hands-on providers. If the obstetrician isn't in the hospital, then the anesthesiologist may not be either. (And even if the ob is there, the anesthesiologist may not be.) Be sure to inquire about these policies as well. Either way, be aware of these distinctions so that you can make a conscious choice and not be surprised at the time of your delivery.

2) A hospital birthing center. An increasingly popular option, this is a hospital-within-a-hospital dedicated to deliveries. You labor, deliver, and recover all in the same (usually private) room, and generally find a philosophy that is patient- and family-centered. You may find this option at teaching hospitals as well as private hospitals.

3) A freestanding birthing center. These centers may or may not be affiliated with a hospital. They tend to be staffed by nurse-midwives and obs together. Studies show that about 15 to 20 percent of first-time moms who choose freestanding birth centers are transferred to a hospital (usually because they require a C-section or have other complications requiring high-tech monitoring or care). Be sure that you understand how this works and are comfortable with the hospital that is used for backup.

4) At home. Given my biases regarding lay midwives, you can probably guess my thoughts on home deliveries. Let me say up front that if I could know with certainty who would have a routine delivery, I would opt for a home birth every time. I can't imagine anything more special! The problem lies in the words "with certainty." The one thing I do know is that nothing in obstetrics can be known with certainty. Having seen what I've seen, I just wouldn't risk it. For me, *any risk* of complications that cannot be appropriately managed in a home setting is too great of a risk. If it happens to you and your baby, it doesn't matter what the odds were—it happened to *you*. Having said all of this, I know many intelligent, loving people—some of my best friends—who have chosen a home birth and had wonderful experiences culminating in a problem-

free delivery and a completely healthy baby. It's just not something I can recommend to my patients, or to you, in good conscience.

HOW TO MAKE A CONSCIOUS CHOICE ABOUT . . . YOUR PRENATAL CAREGIVER

First, reflection. What are the factors that matter to you about the person who will be your primary caregiver? Among those to consider:

- *Philosophy.* Do you want mainstream obstetric care? Do you have something different in mind? Are you not sure what you want? Your care provider's philosophy about birth and the circumstances under which interventions are used will be a huge determining factor in how your delivery goes. So spend some time thinking about what you prefer.
- *Relationship.* What is your relationship with the person who provides your gyn care, if that person is also available to provide obstetric care? What are the traits you are looking for in a caregiver? Does the size of the practice matter to you? The location of the office? The hospital that the practice is affiliated with?
- *Birth experience.* Some of the factors will relate to the way you envision your birth experience. Do you want to give birth in a hospital? At home? At a birthing center? What are the qualities or characteristics you have in mind at this point about your delivery, and how does this inform your choice of a provider?

Second, information. Once you have a sense of what you need from an obstetric caregiver, you can weigh this against the options in your area. Ask friends, especially recent mothers, for their recommendations.

Interview one or two possible choices before you commit. Ask about philosophy, office practices, how your questions will be answered between appointments, the setting for deliveries (I would recommend you visit them), the availability of anesthesia and pediatric care, payment, and insurance. Find out what the provider's experience is and about his or her rates of procedures such as C-sections, inductions, and episiotomies, as well as their percentage of vaginal deliveries. (Understand, though, that not all individual physicians keep track of these statistics, and that they may be higher than average if the physician sees a population at higher risks.) Ask about what will happen at the hospital or place of delivery once you arrive. (See these questions in the preceding section.)

Third, action. Make a choice and call to get an appointment for your first prenatal visit.

Then, re-reflection. After your appointments, reflect on the experience. If doubts or questions come up on re-reflection, remember that your first option can be to discuss your concerns with your provider. Be honest and direct, and see what comes from this kind of communication. It may resolve your doubts and deepen your relationship. Or it may confirm your doubts and cause you to end the relationship. Either way, that's good to know. You have plenty of time to change your provider if need be, and it's perfectly okay if you want to do that. Typically if you are uncomfortable and try to ignore your feelings they will surface closer to your due date, a time when there is a lot going on and making a change will be much more difficult and stressful for both you and your providers (the old one as well as the new one). Better to be conscious of it along the way, re-reflecting as you go.

Going to Your First Prenatal Appointment: What Happens and Why

Make an appointment with a caregiver as soon as you think you may be pregnant. Some issues will have been addressed already if you saw a physician before becoming pregnant. Typically, your care provider will do the following in the initial visit:

• *Confirm the pregnancy and calculate the due date.* (See "Reality Check: Due Dates," pages 152–154.)

WHY: To accurately establish the dating of the pregnancy. The earlier in the pregnancy the due date is set, the more accurate it is.

• *Take a medical history,* if this has not been done at a preconception workup, and update it if it has.

WHY: In conventional medicine, the "why" is limited to problem-finding. That's because the focus is on curing disease. Integrative medicine seeks also to optimize health in order to *prevent* any kinds of problems—a much better match for a natural, non-disease life transition such as pregnancy. This is why I believe an ideal history would be a "health history," not just a medical history, which would cover questions similar to those in the Reflective Inventory (Chapter 2), including medical and reproductive background, lifestyle, and health habits. In reality, only the biggest issues, such as smoking and drinking, may be discussed—which makes doing the Reflective Inventory on your own all the more important. But any good introductory prenatal visit should at least cover your medical, reproductive, and family histories. Certain aspects of your care may proceed differently depending on circumstances such as age or ethnicity. See "Key Preconception Issues and Why They Matter," in Chapter 8.

• *Do a physical exam and prenatal tests*, including a general physical exam and a pelvic exam.

  WHY: To confirm that you are in good health and to look for circumstances that may have an impact on your pregnancy, such as high blood pressure. (See "Prenatal Testing" on pages 155–164.)

• *Discuss self-care.* Although many doctors may give short shrift to this kind of discussion, I believe an optimal beginning to prenatal care covers all aspects of self-care. I go over the Centers of Wellness (Mind, Nutrition, Movement, Spirit, and Sensation) and review what patients are currently doing.

  WHY: So I can make recommendations for strengthening well-being in all domains, especially those that are least well tended. Since most doctors address only the most dangerous self-care issues, such as smoking and drinking, don't be afraid to ask your care provider about questions specific to your concerns. You may have questions about exercise (whether you can continue with a sport you play, for example); about sex (can you have it and what kind?); about nutrition (how can you be a vegetarian and have a healthy pregnancy?; should you get a referral to a nutritionist?). Use this time to ask about your concerns, and to assess whether or not your caregiver seems willing to address them.

• *Set up a schedule of future visits.* For a standard pregnancy, doctors typically see women every 4 weeks for the first 28 weeks of pregnancy, then every 2 weeks until 36 weeks, and weekly after that. At every visit, you'll be weighed, have your urine "dipped" (screened), and have your vital signs (blood pressure, heart rate, respiratory rate) recorded. Fundal height (the distance from the top of your pubic bone to the top of your uterus) is measured from about 20 weeks on, fetal heart tones are checked beginning in the first trimester, and in the third trimester the fetal position is noted. (Specifics beyond this depend on where you are in the pregnancy.)

WHY: To detect the beginnings of any potential problems, such as the start of a urinary tract infection or asymptomatic bacteriuria, signs of preeclampsia such as protein in the urine or abnormally rising blood pressure, abnormal weight gain (too much or too little), or any discrepancy between the size of your uterus and what we would expect for how far along you are (either smaller or larger)—just to name a few.

What You Should Do at Your First Prenatal Visit:

• *Come prepared with any questions—preferably on a written list.* If anything has come up for you in your check-ins that leaves you needing more information, bring it up with your nurse or doctor.

WHY: In order to become as fully informed as possible so that you will be able to make the decisions that are right for you.

FEAR: The doctor couldn't find a heartbeat; I'm going to miscarry.
FACT: The heartbeat of the fetus may be detectable with a Doppler applied to the surface of the belly as early as 6 weeks, but 8 to 9 weeks is more likely, and the heartbeat may not be reliably found until 12 weeks. This leaves a big window in which your doctor may be listening for heart tones (as they're called) and not finding them.

The heart is not likely to be heard if you are checked at 6 weeks unless you are very thin and your uterus is positioned optimally for this (for example, it tips toward the abdominal wall where we are listening). If it's not heard, this doesn't mean anything's wrong. If at the next visit (10 weeks, for example) the heartbeat is still not heard, chances are that your doctor will check for it with ultrasound.

Because the ultrasound can be placed vaginally right next to the cervix and uterus, and because the ultrasound is looking for cardiac movement (called "cardiac motion") rather than listening for cardiac sounds, the heart's beating can be detected much earlier and more reliably. A heartbeat can usually be seen on ultrasound by 8 weeks, and often earlier.

One very common reason for not hearing a heartbeat when we would expect to is that the pregnancy is not as far along as we thought.

✓ **REALITY CHECK:** Due Dates

At your first prenatal visit your doctor will assign your due date. There are so many misconceptions and concerns about what should be a pretty simple and important piece of information. Let me try to clear them up:

• *A due date is not a delivery date!* It's simply an educated guess as to when your baby will be born—with a two-week window on either side. Ninety-five percent of all babies are born within two weeks before or two weeks after this date. That's the most certainty we can give an expectant mom—a month-long window! And that is under the best of circumstances. Very often, because the mother-to-be has irregular periods or can't remember the date of her last period, and had late prenatal care, we are even less certain than that. Over and over, I see patients base all of their psychological prepping and pin all their expectations and plans (when to quit work, what date her mom should book a plane, when to complete preparations for the nursery) on this date without recognizing how inexact it is. If a mom-to-be delivers before her "due date," she often worries that her baby is "premature" when it's not. If she doesn't deliver by her due date, she's often in a disappointed funk, when in reality she's not "overdue" for another 14 days.

• *Here's the usual way to calculate a due date:* Start with the first day of your last menstrual period (LMP), subtract three months, and add seven days—one year from the date you end up with is your due date. Clearly, the more aware you are of your cycle, the more likely you are to know the date of your LMP. The due date you are given by your doctor is considered a "good date" if 1) you're sure of your LMP *and* 2) you have regular periods (roughly once a month) *and* 3) your last period was a normal one (extremely light flow could indicate implantation bleeding or breakthrough bleeding while you were already pregnant) *and* 4) you had early prenatal care and your earliest physical exam showed a consistency with the calculated date. Studies indicate, however, that an estimated 40 percent of women don't accurately recall their LMP—and I believe the percentage is much higher given how many women I see who are not conscious about their bodies. In general, the more aware the patient, the more accurate her date.

• *You should only be given one due date and only one at a time.* Some women think they have been given a different due date from their original one based on data generated by an ultrasound, which calculates due dates based on measurements of the fetus. They may then make the mistake of believing that this is a new official due date. But while an ultrasound-created date may occasionally lead your doctor to reevaluate your due date it does not in and of itself give you a new due date.

• *Your due date should be revised only by your care provider, and typically only if two ultrasounds indicate that the original date was wrong.* If on the basis of something an ultrasound technician or different doctor has said in passing you think your due date has been changed, be sure you get it clarified. There are a lot of reasons why the measurements on the ultrasound and your due date may not agree. Having a wrong due date is only one of the possible reasons, and not very likely if you have "good dates" (as defined above). "But how can the date shown on my ultrasound differ from my due date?" is something I hear a lot. The answer: An ultrasound is not a tool for diagnosing due dates. When an ultrasound is done, it spits out a date based only on measurements of the size of your baby. This date would be accurate only if your baby were exactly the fiftieth percentile growth-wise. But if your baby is on the small size, the ultrasound would say you were less far along than is actually the case, and if your baby is on the large size, it would say you are farther along than you actually are. Ultrasounds are most likely to be accurate when measuring a baby's size very early in pregnancy, when babies all grow at basically the same rate. By the second trimester, when growth rates begin to vary a lot, they are less reliable, and even less so in the third trimester. (Of course for seeing other things, like the structure of the heart, late ultrasounds are superior.)

An ultrasound should only be used to confirm the original due date, not to revise it, because it's only one piece of the puzzle. If your due date is January 1 and an ultrasound done in the second trimester (when most are done) indicates a due date of January 12, your due date shouldn't be moved. It's still January 1—the ultrasound essentially *confirmed* this date, because it was within two weeks of your due date based on your LMP and uterine size.

However, if a second-trimester ultrasound indicated a due date more than two weeks different from your original date, that would be a genuine inconsistency. The doctor then has to figure out if the due date is wrong, or if the baby is simply very big or very small or is not growing at a normal pace. Typically, the ultrasound is repeated several weeks later to see whether or not the baby grew at a normal rate during that interval, and the date can then be revised if necessary. If the baby did grow normally, then it is most likely simply smaller or larger than average (remember that few babies are exactly average size!). If it did not grow normally, then more tests may be needed to explore why. If your due date is changed, you should be given an explanation of what new information led to the new date.

• *Having an accurate due date is incredibly important.* Its value goes beyond helping you know roughly when to expect labor. The timing of many tests and decisions about when to intervene about certain complications such as preterm labor or preeclampsia are strongly influenced by your due date. Having "good dates" (as we say in the business) is an extremely important piece of the picture and allows your doctor to manage your pregnancy in the best interest of you and your baby.

HOW FAR ALONG ARE YOU?:
THE CASE OF THE MISSING TWO WEEKS

Throughout this book, I refer to how many weeks pregnant you are, based on how long it has been since the first day of your last menstrual period. This is indeed the convention. What this means, however, is that when you are four weeks pregnant, it has really been two weeks since conception. At 40 weeks (full term) it's been 38 weeks since conception. This may seem illogical, but it is the standard way of noting how far along a mother is.

Prenatal Testing

Prenatal care involves numerous tests, and it's important to understand what they do. A *screening test* can tell you that you or your baby may be at risk for a particular problem. A *diagnostic test* tells you that you or your baby has or does not have a particular problem. Positive results on screening tests indicate the need for diagnostic tests, but they are not themselves a diagnosis.

The Standard Tests

The laboratory tests that are most often recommended during the first prenatal visit include the following. While this list looks long, it's all obtained through a blood draw and a pelvic exam.

Hemoglobin: This test checks your blood to determine if you are anemic. Women usually become slightly anemic as the pregnancy progresses, but very low levels of iron will need to be treated with iron supplementation.

Blood type and Rh type with antibody screening: This test determines the mother's blood type, Rh status, and antibody factor. If the mother's blood type is Rh-negative and her partner's is Rh-positive, an immunization (a common brand name is RhoGAM) will be given at 28 weeks to prevent problems with future pregnancies. It will also be given if you have an amniocentesis or any other event that could expose your blood and your baby's blood to each other. You will also receive this immunization after you deliver if the baby's blood type is Rh-positive. The antibody screen done with this test is to screen for women who have been exposed to Rh-positive blood and could react against their baby's blood. (This can happen if you have not received this immunization with a previous pregnancy, for example.) If this is positive, a consultation will be done to further evaluate the situation.

Rubella titer: This test checks the level of antibodies to the German measles virus that are present in your blood to make sure that you are immune. If a woman becomes infected with German measles (rubella) during her pregnancy, her developing fetus is at risk of developing heart defects, deafness, or cataracts. If you are not immune, you will be vaccinated after you deliver. This is a great illustration of the benefit of being conscious prior to pregnancy: You can be tested for immunity prior to conceiving, and if you are not immune, you can be vaccinated before you conceive. You will need to avoid pregnancy for three months after being vaccinated, and then you will have the peace of mind of knowing you are immune.

Syphilis screen: This test checks for the presence of syphilis infection. If present, treatment can be started so that the fetus is not harmed.

Hepatitis B screen: This test checks for infection with the hepatitis B virus, which can be passed to an unborn child. If present, additional blood tests will be done to help define the state of the disease and the risk of passing it on to the baby. If indicated, the mother can then be treated during the prenatal period, and the baby can be treated at birth.

HIV screen: This test screens for the HIV virus, which causes AIDS. If the screen is positive, further blood tests will be done to determine whether the woman has the virus. If a woman is found to have the HIV virus, she can be treated during pregnancy which greatly reduces the chances of her passing the virus to her unborn child.

Pap smear: This test checks for abnormal cervical cells, which could indicate cervical cancer.

Gonorrhea and chlamydia cultures: If either of these infections is present, they must be treated, for the sake of both the mother's health and the baby's.

Urinalysis: This test examines the urine for the presence of bacteria, sugar, or protein. If present, this can be a sign of an infection or other bladder or kidney problem, or diabetes. It is usually performed at each prenatal visit.

CF screen: The American College of Obstetricians and Gynecologists (ACOG) recommends that this test be offered to all couples to screen for cystic fibrosis (CF), an inherited, incurable disease that can severely affect breathing and digestion, whether they have a personal or family history of carrying the CF gene or not.

FEAR: If I get a flu shot, I could damage the fetus.
FACT: At least part of your pregnancy is apt to fall between October and May—the flu season. The Centers for Disease Control recommends a flu immunization for all pregnant women. The vaccine is believed to be safe for fetuses, whereas flu itself presents possible dangers. Flu can increase your heart rate, decrease lung capacity, and change your immune function. Also, preliminary evidence suggests that the children of women who have influenza during the first half of pregnancy are at increased risk of developing schizophrenia. While this is not definitive, it is something to be aware of.

Prenatal Screening and Diagnostic Tests for Chromosomal Abnormalities

A key area of choice involves whether or not to undergo prenatal testing that helps detect the chromosomal abnormalities that can cause birth defects. In about 3 percent of live births, a baby will be born with a major congenital problem. About half of these are apparent at birth, and the others become evident later in childhood or sometimes in adulthood. It is estimated that about half of miscarriages are fetuses that had a major chromosomal anomaly, and about 5 percent of stillborn infants have chromosomal anomalies. While there can also be nongenetic causes for birth defects, genetic factors are most often the cause. And, most birth defects occur in families with no history of the disease (for example, about 97 percent of Down syndrome pregnancies occur in women with no family history). This obviously makes the question of genetic testing a very important one.

Although the tests done for chromosomal problems are performed at different times during the first and second trimesters, I am presenting all of them here so that you can choose consciously which tests—if any—are best for you. You will want to decide on your overall strategy for prenatal testing, which can then help you determine which tests you get when. All are optional. And now that screening methods that are far less invasive than the traditional amniocentesis are more and more effective, the decision is a very individual one.

These less invasive methods, all of which are screening tests, include two blood tests done in the first trimester (PAPP-A and BhCG), plus an ultrasound evaluation of the fetal neck called nuchal translucency. Another option is a second-trimester blood test (triple or quad screen, which includes alpha-fetoprotein or AFP, unconjugated estriol, hCG, and inhibin A). Ultrasound screening is also an important tool for finding major anatomic malformations, which can indicate chromosomal abnormalities. An ultrasound in the second trimester is now standard of care, and if abnormalities are noted, diagnostic testing will most likely be offered.

Chorionic villi sampling (CVS) is an invasive test that can be performed in the first trimester (between weeks 9 and 12), and amniocentesis is typically done later (between weeks 16 and 18). These tests are diagnostic tests rather than screening tests. The results of the screening tests can help you decide whether to have one of the more invasive, diagnostic tests done.

I sometimes see women who think that if they get *every* test done, and none indicate a sign of problems, they will know for certain that their baby does not have any abnormalities. That's an unconscious assumption. There's *no* way to rule out all abnormalities, largely due to three reasons: there is no test that screens for all chromosomal anomalies, there is no diagnostic test that tests for all abnormalities, and there are also nonchromosomal causes for birth defects.

You'll want to base your choice on many factors. (See "How to Make a Conscious Choice About...Prenatal Screening for Genetic Abnormalities," page 164.) First, let's learn about the options:

BhCG
What it is: BhCG (beta human chorionic gonadotropin) is a hormone produced by the placenta; and PAPP-A (pregnancy-associated plasma protein A) is a protein, also produced by the placenta.

When it's done: 11 to 13 weeks

What it indicates: This is a screening test for Down syndrome. (In fetuses with Down syndrome, BhCG tends to be high and PAPP-A tends to be low.) This is roughly 60 percent accurate in predicting Down syndrome, and together with the nuchal translucency, it is about 87 percent accurate.

How it's done: Blood test

Considerations: Remember this is just a screening test, and it is very dependent on doing it at the right time in the pregnancy. You may have a false-positive test, which means your baby is not affected, but you will be faced with the anxiety of an abnormal result and the choice of further testing.

Nuchal Translucency
What it is: An ultrasound measurement early in pregnancy of an area at the neck of the fetus.

When it's done: 11 to 14 weeks

What it indicates: If this area behind the neck is larger than expected, it is associated with an increased incidence of Down syndrome, congenital heart disease, and other congenital anomalies.

How it's done: Ultrasound

Considerations: This test detects Down syndrome approximately 80 percent of the time. Together with the two blood tests outlined above, it is about 87 percent accurate in predicting Down syndrome in the fetus. Because it is a screening test, you may have a false positive, or a false negative.

Chorionic Villi Sampling (CVS)

What it is: CVS involves taking a sample of the chorion frondo-sum—the part of the chorionic membrane (the outer layer of the am-niotic sac around the fetus) that contains hairlike projections called villi. The cells that make up the chorionic villi are of fetal origin so laboratory analysis can identify certain genetic, chromosomal, or bio-chemical diseases of the fetus.

When it's done: 9 to 12 weeks

What it indicates: CVS obtains cells of fetal origin (as does am-niocentesis), and therefore allows the actual chromosomes of the fe-tus to be examined. This means that the sex of the fetus is determined, along with abnormalities that are caused by an extra chromosome (trisomies) or by a missing chromosome (monosomies). These include the following: trisomy 21 (Down syndrome), which occurs in approximately 1 in 800 live births and is more common the older the mother (see table on page 168 for the risk of chromosomal abnormalities based on age); trisomy 13, which occurs in approxi-mately 1 in 20,000 live births and results in severely affected chil-dren, 50 percent of whom die in the first month, and few survive beyond three years; trisomy 18, which occurs in 1 in 8,000 live births with females three times more often affected than males, and most only survive a few months. There are other abnormalities (trisomy 8, 9, 14, 16, 22), which are far less common and present a spectrum of anomalies and disabilities.

How it's done: CVS is performed either through the vagina and the cervix (transcervically) or through the abdomen (transabdomi-nally). In some cases, the location of the placenta dictates which method the doctor uses. Both methods are effective and have similar rates of risk. Following the preparation time, both procedures take only about five minutes. Occasionally, a second sampling procedure must be performed if insufficient villus material was obtained.

For the transcervical procedure, the woman lies on an examining table on her back with her feet in stirrups. Her vaginal area is thor-oughly cleansed with an antiseptic, a sterile speculum is inserted into her vagina and opened, and the cervix is then cleansed with an anti-septic. Using ultrasound (a device that uses sound waves to produce images of internal organs) as a guide, the doctor inserts a thin plastic tube called a catheter through the cervix and into the uterus. The passage of the catheter through the cervix may cause cramping. The doctor carefully watches the image produced by the ultrasound and advances the catheter to the chorionic villi. By applying suction from the syringe attached to the other end of the catheter, a small sample of the chorionic villi is obtained. At this point a woman may feel cramping or pinching, or she may feel no sensation at all. The catheter is then withdrawn.

For the transabdominal method, the woman lies on her back on an examining table. After the abdomen is cleansed, and using ultrasound guidance, a long needle is inserted through the woman's abdominal wall, through the uterine wall, and to the chorionic villi, which is suctioned out.

At a lab, the sample is examined under the microscope. Cells with clearly separated chromosomes are photographed so that the type and number of chromosomes can be analyzed. Humans have 23 pairs of chromosomes including the sex chromosomes. Rearrangements of the chromosomes or the presence of additional or fewer chromosomes can be identified by examination of the photograph. Down syndrome, for instance, is most commonly caused by an extra chromosome 21. In addition to the chromosomal analysis, specialized tests can be performed as needed to look for specific diseases such as Tay-Sachs. Results take two to eight days.

Considerations: Because it is a newer procedure than amnio, there are fewer people trained to perform it, making it less widely available. Risks are comparable, with fetal loss occurring in approximately 1 per 200 procedures.

Amniocentesis
What it is: A needle is inserted through the abdomen and the uterus into the amniotic sac to withdraw a small amount of amniotic fluid. The fluid contains cells shed from the fetus.

When it's done: Typically 15 to 16 weeks, although it can be done earlier.

What it indicates: See the possible screening results for CVS (above).

How it's done: An ultrasound will be performed to locate the placenta and look for
the pockets of fluid. Your belly
will be washed with soap or
antiseptic and then "draped,"
meaning that sterile towels will
be placed along the perimeter of
the area that was washed. The
ultrasound will be placed on
your belly again, to locate the
best place to insert the needle.
(Some physicians give numbing
medicine before the needle is inserted; others don't, believing
that the needle with the numbing medicine causes as much dis-

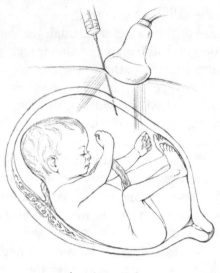

Amniocentesis

comfort as the procedure needle.) The procedure needle will then be
placed, while the doctor watches its insertion on the ultrasound. You
will feel the needle puncture your skin, and you may or may not feel
a cramping sensation when it enters your uterus. Once the needle is in
place, a small amount of fluid is drawn off (you will have no sensation
of this), and then the needle is withdrawn. The doctor will then look
at the baby again with the ultrasound.

Considerations: Because amnio is invasive, it carries up to a 1 in
200 risk of miscarriage. It's usually offered only in three instances:
1) if a mother will be over 35 at the time of delivery, because the likelihood of genetic problems rises with maternal age and at 35 the odds
of the amnio finding something are roughly 1 in 200 (equal to the risk
of the test and therefore considered reasonable); 2) if there is a personal or family history of genetic problems; and 3) if a screening test
(such as a quad test or triple screen or ultrasound) indicates a potential problem. While amniocentesis and CVS detect many of the same
abnormalities, amniocentesis does have the advantage of also detecting spina bifida, because its diagnosis is made using amniotic fluid,
which is not available from CVS.

Triple/Quad Test (Maternal Serum/Blood Screening)

What it is: This simple test, performed on a blood sample, is known as a triple screen because it screens for three substances:

1) alpha-fetoprotein (AFP), a protein produced by the liver of the fetus, which crosses the placenta to enter the mother's blood
2) hCG (human chorionic gonadotropin) a hormone produced by the placenta
3) estriol, another hormone made by the placenta, as well as by the woman and her baby

It's called a quad screen when a fourth substance, the placental hormone inhibin-A, is also screened for. As of this writing the quad-screen option is not yet widely available.

When it's done: It is most accurate when done between 16 and 18 weeks, but it can be performed anywhere between 15 and 20 weeks.

What it indicates: These markers help screen for the possibility of trisomy 21 (Down syndrome), trisomy 18, and neural tube defects. This is not a diagnostic test, but only a screening test, which, if abnormal, indicates that a problem *may* exist, and that you need to do follow-up testing.

A higher-than-normal level of AFP, for example, may indicate a neural tube defect, such as spina bifida (a gap in the bone surrounding the spinal cord) or anencephaly (a fatal brain-development disorder). Low levels of AFP, when accompanied by high hCG and high inhibin-A and low estriol, could indicate Down syndrome. These readings have been found to be more accurate when the levels of all three or four substances are factored in. Decreased hCG, AFP, and estriol are associated with trisomy 18. Serum screening does not frequently detect other chromosomal abnormalities. The ones that are likely to be missed, however, are usually lethal (such as trisomy 13) or are sex-chromosomal anomalies.

How it's done: Blood test

Considerations: Like all screening tests, the triple and quad screens are not foolproof. About 3 to 5 expectant moms per 100 who have the test will show an initial abnormal result. Compare this with the actual incidence of a defect—1 to 2 women per 100—and it is clear that there are many false positives. One common reason for inaccuracy is that the pregnancy has not been dated properly. Results are interpretted based on how far along the pregnancy is and once the correct dates are used, the results are usually found to be normal. Some physicians report that a false-positive result that is not due to the wrong dates can be associated with higher risk for preterm labor, preeclampsia, fetal distress, and intrauterine growth restriction (IUGR). Thus often these women will be monitored more closely. The presence of twins can also cause higher readings, so the lab needs to be informed when it does the blood tests in order to have accurate results.

An ultrasound can confirm or rule out multiple gestation and confirm the fetus's gestational age. If the scan disagrees with the fetal age according to your due date and your obstetrician revises or changes your estimated due date, the triple-screen results will be reinterpreted accordingly.

If your reading is low, the test is not usually repeated. An ultrasound is used to confirm gestational age and to look for the presence of possible signs of Down syndrome by looking closely at such things as the heart, the thickness of the fetal neck, and the nasal bone. To diagnose Down syndrome, however, the chromosomes of the baby must be examined, which at this time requires an amniocentesis.

HOW TO MAKE A CONSCIOUS CHOICE ABOUT . . . PRENATAL SCREENING FOR GENETIC ABNORMALITIES

Given all of the options, will you choose any of them, and if so, which? The Feedback Loop can help.

First, reflection. Consider your initial feelings about prenatal testing. There are many facets to consider, so take the time to do this work:

• How do you feel about the fact that this test has been offered or recommended? Are you worried? Confident? Ambivalent?

• How do you feel about the conditions that led to the discussion of the test (your age, family history of genetic problems, standard protocol, or the results of an earlier screen)? What is your level of concern or fear? Some women might prefer no screenings at all, for example, while others will find reassurance in knowing all they can.

• What preconceptions do you have about the test? Did you know much about it before your doctor mentioned it? Do you know anyone who had it and, if so, what was their experience like? Have you had it before? What was that like?

• What are your preconceptions of what the test will be like? Are you scared of needles (for CVS or amnio)? Worried about an invasive test and the risk of miscarriage? Eager to do everything you can to get the answers you need?

• What preconceptions do you have about birth defects? Do you know anyone who has one or has had a child with one? Have you read articles or seen stories about children with birth defects?

• What would you do if the results of the test revealed a significant problem? Would you consider terminating the pregnancy? Or do you think you would not consider termination under any circumstance? What are your thoughts and feelings about abortion?

• Are you the kind of person who would rather know about a problem ahead of time, even if it won't change what you do, so you can begin to prepare yourself? Or, if it isn't going to change what you do, would you rather not know ahead of time and avoid any potential risk?

• What does your partner think and feel? Compare your reflections.

Second, information. Understand as much about the test as you need to feel comfortable making a decision. A doctor's explanation will be sufficient for some; most people will also see a genetic counselor, who is trained to help people make these decisions. Others will also troll the Internet for other insights.

• Consider your options. There is a growing trend for women to rely on triple or quad blood screens plus ultrasound instead of amnio;

the percentage of expectant mothers undergoing amnio has dropped 50 percent in some areas. This is true even as more older women are getting pregnant. Now, with the use of first-trimester blood testing (PAPP-A and BhCG) plus the nuchal translucency ultrasound test for Down syndrome, this number will probably drop even further. When first trimester testing is combined with the quad test in the second trimester, the accuracy of detecting Down syndrome is reported to be 96 percent. We used to rely on AFP levels alone. I can imagine a day, as these tests continue to improve, when amnio and CVS will rarely be done. To some degree, using amnio as a first step, especially when recommended because of age alone, is a holdover from the days when the blood tests were not all available. The data are not yet in as to which approach is the more accurate in identifying a problem. Early evidence suggests that the new screens combined with a detailed ultrasound may catch as many or more cases of Down syndrome. On the other hand, they are still merely a screen, so if the screen indicates a possible problem, an amnio will probably be suggested. Remember, also, that there are birth defects that the amnio cannot diagnose.

• Assess the relative risks. Be sure that you understand the risks of the procedure versus the risk of having a child with birth defects. The genetic counselor is an expert in giving you this information and helping you to process it.

• Be aware of timing. Only about half of all pregnant women in the US receive prenatal diagnostic tests early enough to allow termination of an affected pregnancy. If, on the other hand, you would not terminate, the timing is less imperative, but the information is still valuable because it will give you some time to prepare for the birth of an affected child.

Third, action. If your preferred course of action is not immediately clear to you, you should take the time to imagine both having a proposed test and not having it. Sit with each hypothetical for a few hours or a few days. What do you notice about your feelings with each scenario? Notice how your body reacts to the thought of each course of action as well; is it relaxed and at ease with one and more tense with the other? Very often the choice will be clear after this exercise. Women who choose to have testing commonly do so either because they would consider terminating the pregnancy if a severe abnormality were diagnosed, or because they would want to be prepared. In my experience, the most common reason that women choose not to have prenatal testing is because they are certain they wouldn't do anything differently whatever the outcome, and they do not want to risk the stress, worry, and possible additional procedures associated with having a false-positive test.

Then, re-reflection. If you go ahead with the test, reflect afterward on how you feel about this choice. Even though you can't undo it, being conscious of how you feel is critical. The wait between the test and finding out the results can feel like an eternity. Be aware of your feelings and express them. If you do not have amnio or CVS, go through the reflection process again and see if you still come to the same conclusion.

Genetic Counseling

Based on your health history or your partner's, including your ethnic background and family history, you may be advised to consult a genetic counselor to help assess the risk of certain birth defects. In addition to those who have risk factors based on belonging to the racial groups mentioned on pages 103–104, counseling is often recommended automatically to patients who will be 35 or older at delivery. A genetic counselor's job is to help you understand your entire history in terms of genetic risk, and discuss your relative risks.

I recommend genetic counseling to anyone who is at risk *or* has a high level of concern. Even if your doctor has assured you that you're at no heightened risk, if you continue to have strong concerns, that is data that you should pay attention to. By exploring the actual risk with a counselor, you can receive factual data to help you address your concerns and decide what steps to take.

WHAT'S YOUR RISK?

This table shows your risk of having a baby with Down syndrome or any chromosomal disorder. Your risk is based on your age.

Mother's Age	Risk of Down Syndrome	Risk of Any Chromosomal Disorder
20	1/1,667	1/526
25	1/1,250	1/476
30	1/952	1/385
35	1/378	1/192
36	1/289	1/156
37	1/224	1/127
38	1/173	1/102
39	1/136	1/83
40	1/106	1/66
41	1/82	1/53
42	1/63	1/42
43	1/49	1/33
44	1/38	1/26
45	1/30	1/21

Modified from Hook, EB, Cross, PK, Schreinemachers, DM. Chromosomal abnormality rates at amniocentesis and in live-born infants. *JAMA* 1983; 249:2034–2038 (ages 33–49), copyright 1983, American Medical Association; Hook, EB. Rates of chromosome abnormalities at different maternal ages. Reprinted with permission from the American College of Obstetrics and Gynecologists (*Obstetrics and Gynecology* 1981; 58:282–285).

POSSIBLE MEDICAL ISSUES NOW

Nausea and Vomiting

Morning sickness can be felt as anything from mild queasiness to out-and-out sickness, including frequent vomiting. For some women, these symptoms can cause tremendous discomfort and disruption in everyday life. Of course, sickness is not limited to mornings; it can happen anytime. Symptoms are usually worst during the first 9 to 12 weeks. After that, you might notice a lifting of the sickness almost overnight. About 15 percent of women report no morning sickness at all. A very few women, however, remain sick throughout their pregnancy.

A minority of women, fewer than 2 percent, experience such persistent vomiting (a condition called *hyperemesis gravidarum*) that they must be periodically hospitalized in order to maintain nutrition and body fluids. Hyperemesis is the second most common reason pregnant women are hospitalized, after preterm labor.

According to the American College of Obstetricians and Gynecologists (ACOG), risk factors for hyperemesis gravidarum include carrying multiples, carrying a female fetus, being the daughter or sister of a woman who had the condition, and a history of motion sickness or migraines.

Whether your nausea is slight or severe, the good news is that this is a place where integrative approaches can have a huge impact. Mainstream ob-gyns are beginning to recognize and recommend some of these approaches, but I strongly suggest trying them right from the start. Don't wait until you are seriously ill, or until your ob might think to mention them to you. In my experience, approaching nausea from the following multiple dimensions is most likely to yield the greatest success.

- *B vitamins.* Taking vitamin B_6 (pyridoxine; start with 25 mg and you can safely increase to 50 mg) or vitamin B_6 plus doxylamine (an antihistamine) has been found to decrease the severity of symptoms by 70 percent with no effects on the baby. Prenatal vitamins can be prescribed that contain higher doses of B_6 for this purpose. If you are having a difficult time keeping the prenatal vitamins down, you may want to focus on just taking the folic acid and the B_6—both can be bought separately and are much smaller pills. Then, as soon as you are able, incorporate the complete prenatal vitamins.

- *Ginger.* This root has been shown to settle the stomach and reduce symptoms. First try increasing ginger through your diet—in foods you eat or in teas you drink. You can also get ginger gum in most drugstores. If that's not effective, one gram per day in capsule form is felt to be a safe dose.

- *Acupressure.* Based on the principles of acupuncture, acupressure has been shown in several studies to be of benefit in reducing nausea and vomiting. Antinausea wristbands, which apply constant pressure to a particular acupuncture point known as P6, are a low-tech, no-risk, low-cost method often used for other kinds of nausea such as seasickness or carsickness. You can find them in most drugstores. Stores in some states also sell electroacupressure bands (one common brand name is Relief Bands), which deliver a mild electrical stimulation to the same acupuncture point. They are also available online, and appear to be even more effective than the bands that apply pressure alone. So if the pressure bands are helping, but not giving you complete relief, I recommend trying the electroacupressure bands. Many of my patients have had great relief with this simple approach, especially when combined with B_6.

- *Acupuncture.* A National Institutes of Health consensus panel on acupuncture has found that there is sufficient evidence of safety and efficacy to support its use for treating nausea and vomiting in pregnancy. If your symptoms are not relieved by the simpler methods above, working with a licensed acupuncturist with experience in pregnancy who will individualize treatments for you is a great approach. When acupuncture is used as part of a whole-system approach, it can be far more effective than acupressure bands, which are only a tool that has been extracted from the Oriental-medicine approach.

- *Activating the relaxation response.* We all know that stress affects the digestive system—almost everyone can recall having GI symptoms, including nausea, when under great stress. So it only makes sense that stress would intensify normal morning sickness, and that any approach that reduces stress can help decrease nausea and vomiting. Low-tech, low-cost stress-reduction interventions with potentially big benefits for nausea include paced breathing, Journaling, and meditation.

- *Hypnosis.* Hypnosis is a particular kind of mind-body therapy that harnesses and focuses the power of the mind to obtain a desired outcome. It's been shown to produce measurable reductions in the amount of nausea and vomiting in pregnancy (as well as that related to surgery and anesthesia). You can buy standardized hypnosis tapes, but I find the most effective method is to work one-on-one with a clinical hypnotherapist who can develop tapes customized to your needs. You do not need to work with a hypnotherapist on an ongoing basis. Often one or two sessions will teach you what you need to know. If you ask for a tape of your hypnosis session, you can use it anytime you like. You should use the tape at least once a day, and preferably twice a day during the time you are experiencing nausea and vomiting.

• *Reframing.* No one finds nausea and vomiting pleasant, of course, but it can be helpful to understand that your body is not fighting you or letting you down; rather, it's doing exactly what it's supposed to be doing. Think of it as a normal byproduct of a pregnancy.

• *Dialoguing and Dreamagery.* As with any symptom, you can use these tools to gain insights into the symptom and what you might be able to do to help. Many women have found this to be invaluable when dealing with morning sickness and/or hyperemesis.

• *Careful scheduling of your day.* Some women feel better in the mornings, while others are sickest then. Figure out what your pattern is and try to schedule meetings or errands when you have the most energy and least nausea.

See also: "First Trimester Self-Care: Nutrition."

> **FEAR:** My nausea and vomiting are putting my fetus in jeopardy.
> **FACT:** In most cases of morning sickness and even hyperemesis, the fetus is not at any risk of ill effects. This is also true of prolonged and severe cases, although they warrant close monitoring of both you and your baby. Indeed, many studies show a lower rate of miscarriage for women with nausea and vomiting.

Urinary Tract Infections

Also called bladder infections or cystitis, UTIs tend to be more common in pregnancy. An untreated UTI can lead to a kidney infection *(pyelonephritis)*, which can be serious not only for you but for the baby, as it increases the risk of preterm labor. It can be hard to know if you have a UTI, because one of the usual symptoms—frequent urination—is a given in pregnancy. If you have a history of UTIs or kidney problems, be sure to let your provider know, because you're at increased risk for them in pregnancy. Also be sure to get checked at the first sign of burning with urination, or fever (which is a sign that the infection has probably already made its way to your kidneys). Urine is checked throughout pregnancy. This is to check for asymptomatic bacteria as well as other things. But if bothersome symptoms such as painful urination or blood in the urine show up between checkups, be sure to report them immediately. The good news is that UTIs and even pyelonephritis are most often very easily treated with a course of antibiotics—especially when diagnosed early (although pyelo will require hospitalization and intravenous antibiotics).

There is some evidence that drinking cranberry juice can prevent UTIs, so if you're susceptible, incorporating this into your daily nutrition is a good idea. Drinking a lot of other liquids is helpful, too. Although some women get so tired of going to the bathroom constantly that they start to limit their water intake (either consciously or not), you should fight this temptation. It's important to stay well-hydrated no matter what your history, but even more so if you are prone to UTIs. UTIs are also more common after intercourse, so it is a good habit to urinate relatively soon afterward. This keeps things flowing in the right direction and flushes out any bacteria that may have started up your urethra.

FEAR: I see blood; I'm miscarrying.
FACT: Most first trimester bleeding is not the result of miscarriage.

First Trimester Bleeding

Seeing a small amount of bloody discharge in your underwear or when you wipe yourself in the bathroom can be alarming—but it's not uncommon throughout pregnancy. You may also have bleeding that is heavier than just spotting. Most women panic and fear they are miscarrying, especially in the first trimester. But this is not the most likely cause. Other causes in the first trimester include:

- Implantation. As the fertilized egg attaches to the uterine wall about week four or five (when you'd normally be expecting a period), some cells slough off and can result in spotting or bleeding.

- Cervical abrasions. When you are pregnant, the blood supply to the uterus, cervix, and vagina are greater. During intercourse, the penis can rub the cervix in such a way that a slight irritation or abrasion is produced. This can cause spotting. The bleeding is not coming from within the uterus, and it does not mean that sex is unsafe.
- A cervical infection or lesion. Uncommon, but possible.
- Urinary tract infection.

Often some spotting or bleeding occurs and we don't know why. Unfortunately—in another example of medical hexing—the medical term for this is "threatened AB," which stands for threatened abortion, or miscarriage.

Always let your care provider know if you are having bleeding. She or he will typically do an exam and get an ultrasound. If your exam is normal and a heartbeat is seen on ultrasound (which is usually possible at about six to nine weeks), there's only about a 3 percent chance of miscarriage. The only "treatment" is to keep an eye on it.

If your exam reveals that your cervix is open, then you are miscarrying and this is referred to as an "inevitable or incomplete AB." This means that the miscarriage is about to happen or is in the midst of happening. A "completed AB" is when the miscarriage has happened and the cervix is again closed.

Preexisting Medical Conditions

Depending on your health history, your provider will make special recommendations for your care. There are several situations worth highlighting:

- *Anemia.* Women of childbearing age are often iron deficient. Among the factors that can cause iron-deficiency anemia: a history of heavy menstrual periods, poor nutrition (a low-iron diet or malabsorption of iron), and closely spaced pregnancies (which may not give your body enough time to rebuild your iron stores). If you have anemia, your doctor first needs to determine its cause. If it is from iron deficiency, which is the most common cause, she will prescribe an iron supplement pill. If you are prone to nausea this can be hard to keep down; try taking it at bedtime or first thing in the morning on an empty stomach. If this still doesn't work and your anemia is mild, it is best to focus first on getting folic acid in your system during the first trimester. You then can work on getting enough iron after your morning sickness has resolved in the second trimester. This still gives your body ample time to build up your iron stores and blood count prior to your delivery. Check with your care provider to make sure this is appropriate. If you can tolerate it, drinking orange juice with an iron pill enhances the mineral's absorption. Use the nutrition suggestions in Your Pregnancy Self-Care Plan (Chapter 4) for adding iron to your diet.

REALITY CHECK: "High-Risk" Pregnancy

Labels are powerful and can be self-fulfilling. We don't call underachieving students "stupid" or mentally handicapped people "retarded." I bring a similar leeriness to the term "high-risk" when applied to pregnancy. It sets the wrong tone, sends the wrong message, and, more important, it's simply inaccurate. Labeling a pregnancy "high-risk" is a terrible use of the mind-body connection. "Medical hexing" is what my colleague Andrew Weil calls it. Anything that is out of the ordinary—advanced maternal age, having a chronic disease (such as epilepsy or hypertension), or having a particular medical history (several previous miscarriages)—can get you labeled as "high-risk." That's a loosely applied category, not a diagnosis. The degree of risk of any of these conditions is highly variable and individualized.

One of my patients who had placenta previa (a placental problem putting her at higher risk for increased bleeding and making a vaginal delivery impossible) was scheduled for a C-section. Understandably disappointed by this situation, she did a lot of prep work to understand this condition and to relax about surgery. The day of her C-section, I met her in the preop holding room and we did some mind-body techniques for relaxation and some imagery. The experience was great, and she felt very relaxed, centered, and ready for the surgery. Then the anesthesiologist walked in. The first words out of his mouth: "Okay, let's understand one thing: You are a high-risk patient!" Pop! The

patient's state of mind changed just like that. It had the same effect on all of us in the room. And I'm sure if you were to have
taken her vital signs before and after his statement, you would
have seen a significant shift in them as well.

Rather than stressing about whether you are high-risk or not,
a better route is to simply be aware of your condition, and then
you and your doctor can take the appropriate steps. Often such
conditions require extra monitoring and testing, but for each
condition there are also ways of being proactive that can help
minimize your risks. Depending on the condition, there may be
nutritional strategies, exercise programs, mind-body techniques,
medications or supplements, or all of the above, that could be
useful. Being in a so-called high-risk category doesn't mean
you're a bomb waiting to go off. Refuse to "own" this character-
ization or identify yourself with this label.

• *Hypertension.* If you have been treated for high blood pressure
before you got pregnant, or if it is discovered at a preconception or
early prenatal exam, you'll be monitored especially carefully. Mild hypertension may pose no risk to the fetus, but all hypertension must be
monitored closely as it can increase your risk of complications in pregnancy, including problems with kidney and other organ functions. If
you have hypertension, the baby will also be closely monitored, because hypertension can affect the ability of the placenta to work efficiently and can result in a growth-restricted baby. It also increases
your risk for preeclampsia, a serious and complex disorder of late
pregnancy (see pages 289–293) and increase your risk for intrauterine
fetal demise, which is the death of the baby prior to labor and delivery. This is why it's essential to be closely monitored so that your
blood pressure is maintained in the normal range, which is defined as
less than 140/90. Any increase in blood pressure should cause you to
look at lifestyle issues such as diet, exercise, and stress. Blood pressures
that don't respond to lifestyle changes may need control through
medications. If you are already taking medications for hypertension,
be sure that your doctor is aware of this at your first visit, as certain
medications can be dangerous in pregnancy. If you need to switch
medications, your doctor will advise you on how and when to switch.

- *Insulin-dependent diabetes.* If you have diabetes prior to becoming pregnant (as opposed to developing gestational diabetes in mid- to late-pregnancy), managing blood sugar is incredibly important. Blood sugars that were fine for you before pregnancy can be far too high for the developing fetus, so you'll need to work closely with your health provider to achieve target blood sugar levels much lower than your nonpregnancy goals. The risk of birth defects is far greater in women who have high blood sugars very early in the pregnancy, when the fetal systems are being formed. Blood sugar levels are equally important later in pregnancy, when levels that are too high for the baby can increase the risk of many complications, including fetal death.

The good news is that insulin is not bad for the baby—as a matter of fact, insulin does not even cross the placenta to the baby, only sugar does. So it's entirely safe to use whatever amount of insulin is needed to keep your sugars in the right range for the baby. Because you'll need to achieve very tight blood sugar control, you can expect a lot more monitoring of your blood sugars—and of the pregnancy. Also be aware that as the baby grows, your insulin will need to be adjusted, because the baby's needs are changing. It is a tough and demanding disease to have in pregnancy, but with a good partnership with your health care team, and commitment from you, the baby will never know the difference!

Twins and Multiples

Multiples are usually diagnosed by ultrasound. It's a surprising, exciting moment when two (or more) fetuses show up onscreen. Other possible indications of multiples include a larger-than-expected uterus (though this can have other causes and will have to be checked by ultrasound), or hearing more than one heartbeat. Certain screening results can also be a tip-off to multiples.

Identical twins result when one fertilized egg splits into two embryos. Fairly rare, they occur in about 4 per 1,000 pregnancies. Identical twins are a quirk of nature and happen regardless of family history or other factors. Fraternal or nonidentical twins are born when two eggs are released from the ovary and fertilized at the same time. Their rate of occurrence varies worldwide. Among Caucasians, the incidence is 6 sets per 1,000 pregnancies, while among African

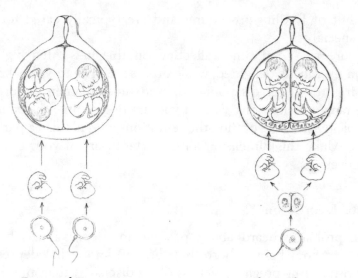

Fraternal Twins   *Identical Twins*

Americans the rate is 10 per 1,000 pregnancies. Asians have about half the rate of fraternal twins that Caucasians do.

You're not just imagining that you're seeing more double strollers these days. The overall number of twin births is on the rise, more than twice what it was in your grandmother's day. That's because multiple births are a known risk of fertility treatments. The use of fertility drugs for ovulation induction, intrauterine insemination, and in vitro fertilization all raise the odds of multiple gestation. In IVF, for example, when more than one embryo is implanted, there is a 20 to 35 percent chance of having twins, and a 1 percent chance of triplets.

Carrying twins does place you at increased risk for a number of complications, but with the quality of monitoring available today these risks are far less than in the past. If you started your pregnancy care with a midwife, you will most likely be referred to an obstetrician; consider seeing a maternal-fetal-medicine (MFM) specialist. You will most likely have more frequent checkups, and will definitely have more frequent ultrasounds, than a woman carrying a single child. Since there is more than one fetus, simply measuring the fundal height cannot reassure us that both fetuses are growing appropriately. The only way to monitor this is with ultrasound. You will also most likely be given different instructions regarding weight gain, nutrition, rest, and self-care. Most higher-order multiples (triplets or more) are the result of fertility procedures and are typically cared for by an MFM specialist.

Be sure to spend time reflecting on this news. It's big! Some women are mostly delighted, while others are primarily shocked, nervous, frightened, or disappointed. And most women experience a whole range of emotions. Even if you are predominantly excited, I'd be suspicious if some of the other emotions weren't also a part of the picture. Make this dimension an important part of your body-soul-baby check-ins.

Prenatal Depression

You've probably heard about postpartum depression, which can strike after your baby is born. But did you know that depression is also a risk *during* pregnancy? Less often discussed than the postpartum kind, depression in pregnancy is experienced by an estimated 10 to 16 percent of women. I don't mean weepiness or mood swings, which up to 70 percent of pregnant women report. Prenatal depression is a different and clinically diagnosable condition. If you experienced depression before you conceived, the condition may continue. If you wrestled with depression in the past, it can recur. And sometimes pregnancy can trigger depression for the first time.

The condition often goes undiagnosed or untreated. Symptoms include persistent feelings of worthlessness, fatigue and changes in sleep habits, decreased ability to concentrate and make decisions, changes in appetite, and thoughts of suicide. Obviously many of these symptoms overlap with common pregnancy symptoms. Often moms-to-be dismiss a blue mood as normal, or feel embarrassed to be depressed at a time when they think they "should" be ecstatic. Simply notice what you are feeling, without judgment. There is no right way to feel when you are pregnant. Depression does not mean you are unfit for motherhood; many amazing mothers have been depressed during and/or after pregnancy. But since your mental state is a critical aspect of your well-being, and you want to be as strong and healthy as you can right now, it's important to acknowledge prenatal depression and to get the necessary treatment for it.

Babies of mothers depressed in pregnancy tend to have lower birth weight and a higher incidence of preterm delivery. The impact on infant development is unclear, but worrisome, say researchers such as Diana Dell, M.D., my colleague at Duke University Medical Center, who specializes in prenatal and postpartum depression. Because depressed individuals tend to overuse alcohol, smoke, and be less vigorous about self-care including good nutrition, it's perhaps not surprising that prenatal depression predisposes you to a greater risk for obstetrical complications as well. And depression before delivery is one of the key predictors of postpartum depression, which is not likely to "go away" once you have the baby—another reason that treatment now is key.

The cause of prenatal depression is unknown. Hormones might play a role, but as with postpartum depression, the more likely culprit is a genetic predisposition that can be triggered by physiologic or life stressors. Having a history of depression before conception doubles your odds of developing it in pregnancy. Other risk factors include a history of childhood sexual abuse and a concurrent medical illness.

A self-care plan emphasizing all five Centers of Wellness can help buffer you against prenatal depression, and help you manage the condition. Of course getting yourself into a good routine when feeling depressed is a huge challenge; it can be hard enough to do this when you are not depressed! During pregnancy, however, many women find that their growing fetus provides added motivation to help them become more disciplined about taking care of themselves.

If you are taking an antidepressant, don't make the decision to taper off or quit without the participation of your psychiatrist and ob-gyn. This decision is an important one, and needs to be done very consciously. First discuss the possible effects of the particular medication you are on, and if a change is advisable. Of course, this is best done prior to conception, but if it hasn't happened yet, do have the conversation as soon as possible. If you are trying to come off antidepressants, I strongly recommend first optimizing your nonpharmaceutical approaches (a Centers of Wellness self-care plan) before attempting to wean yourself from medication.

Centers of Wellness Modifications for Prenatal Depression:

MOVEMENT: Studies have shown that regular aerobic exercise is as effective in the treatment of mild to moderate depression as antidepressant medication. Be sure that your exercise routine includes an aerobic component.

MIND: Be extravigilant about using stress-reduction tools (any of those described in this book). Take mini mental vacations often. Spend time with friends and family; reach out to the network of those who love you.

NUTRITION: Be conscious of what foods seem to trigger mood swings or emotional shifts for you. Common ones include alcohol and caffeine (both of which you should be avoiding anyway), as well as concentrated amounts of sugar. Vitamin B_6 may also be helpful; while not studied specifically for prenatal depression, it is safe in pregnancy and has been shown in some studies to be effective in treating mood changes. Be sure your prenatal vitamin contains 50 mg of B_6, but no more.

SPIRIT: Working with a counselor can be very useful throughout pregnancy, as can Journaling.

SENSATION: Touch is very important. Give yourself plenty of whatever kind of physical nurturing appeals to you—massage, lots of holding and touching with your partner, quiet evenings curled up by a fire, long walks on a beautiful beach, or whatever fulfills your sensual side.

Miscarriage

Neither our medical culture nor our society does a very good job of dealing with this difficult issue. Both tend to minimize the significance of this event and dismiss the loss, putting the grieving patient in a situation that's all the more challenging. This lack of an up-front, supportive, systematic way of dealing with miscarriage is especially curious when you consider that this is not at all a rare occurrence. By some estimates, as many as 30 to 40 percent of all pregnancies are miscarried, the vast majority in the first trimester (roughly 80 percent). Many of these, in fact, happen so early that a woman is not even aware she was pregnant. Others are more painful on every level.

The usual first signs of trouble are bleeding and cramping. It can be reassuring to remember that although bleeding is the most common sign of an impending miscarriage, most bleeding does *not* indicate miscarriage. Nonetheless, you should tell your doctor. If it is too early for the fetal heartbeat to be detected, you may be advised to do nothing and let nature take its course (a *threatened abortion* is the medical term); either the fetus will thrive and soon there will be a confirming heartbeat, or you will eventually miscarry. Similar to having a heavy period, this event is referred to, in yet another bit of unfortunate terminology, as a *spontaneous abortion*. If you have a sure due date and no heartbeat can be detected even though you are far enough along that it should be heard, an ultrasound will be done both to confirm the age of the fetus and to look for a heartbeat. If the ultrasound reveals a fetus that appears healthy, but not yet far enough along to manifest a heartbeat, you will usually have a follow-up ultrasound in a week, and/or have your beta hCG (pregnancy hormone) monitored. If the fetus is far enough along but there is no heartbeat, you will then be given the choice to wait and miscarry naturally or to schedule a D&C (dilation and curettage) to remove the pregnancy.

If you "should be" far enough along to see a heartbeat (based on your dates), but on ultrasound the fetus measures small for its estimated age and doesn't have a heartbeat, one of two things is happening— either your dates are wrong and you have a normal pregnancy that is simply not as far along as you thought, or your dates are correct and the pregnancy stopped developing. Your hCG levels will be monitored by drawing blood, and/or an ultrasound will be repeated in a week. HCG typically doubles every 48 hours in the first trimester; if after two days another blood sample does not show increased hCG levels, the pregnancy is not a normal pregnancy and you will probably go on to miscarry. If an ultrasound is done and no pregnancy is seen in the uterus, you are either very, very early, have already miscarried, or have an ectopic pregnancy.

It is also possible to have no signs of impending miscarriage until a routine checkup reveals that the fetus has no heartbeat. An ultrasound will then be done, and if it reveals the death of the fetus, the news can be absolutely devastating because it is so completely unexpected.

We rarely know exactly what caused a miscarriage. The prevailing wisdom, which I share, is that most are the result of birth defects or an abnormal pregnancy incompatible with life. It is "nature's way" (or the body's way or God's way) of taking care of pregnancies that aren't healthy. Miscarriage is not caused by intercourse, exercise, lifting something heavy, or drinking a glass of wine the night you conceived, even though most women will rack their brains to figure out if it could possibly be related to something they did or didn't do. It is essential that you understand that you did not cause this to happen. It's also important that you realize that having a miscarriage does not put you at any increased risk for having another one, or make you any less likely to conceive again and carry a completely normal pregnancy to term.

Miscarriage is a significant event in a woman's life, even when the pregnancy was not planned or desired. Aside from the tendency to feel guilty, wondering what she did (or failed to do) to trigger the loss, it is healthy for a woman to grieve for a life she had already begun to plan and dream for. She may worry that she has a physical problem that will not allow her to have a baby, or that she's disappointed her spouse or derailed their life plans. These are very real, turbulent emotions.

You may be told not to "dwell" on the loss by well-intended (but not well-informed) family or friends. It's a mistaken belief that if you put the event behind you by not thinking about it, you will recover more quickly. On the contrary, you need to turn your attention to this grieving process and give yourself the amount of time you need to come to terms with the emotions and changes you feel as the result of the loss of an unborn child. Use the tools in this book to explore how you feel, body and soul. Miscarriage can be traumatic, frightening, disappointing, depressing, painful, and, on top of all of that, misunderstood. Generally I think miscarriages are most difficult in a first pregnancy, because they give rise to doubts about whether you will ever be able to be a mother. Talking to other women who have miscarried can be tremendously helpful. You may be surprised by how many others have experienced it, and find comfort from sharing your stories. Above all, talk to your partner, who has also been affected by this miscarriage. The two of you may want to grieve together. When you feel ready, you can begin to discuss when it might feel right to try to get pregnant again.

Some women find that memorializing this pregnancy in some way helps them express grief and honor their loss. The memorializing can be as private as recording your thoughts and keepsakes in a special diary or as public as a small service for family and friends. There is no right or wrong way to do this; figure out what works for you. One woman I know found closure by writing all the names she had been considering for this baby on long strips of paper, which she then burned in a very private farewell. Another planted a tree in the baby's honor.

Medically speaking, after a miscarriage it's best to wait at least one full cycle before trying to conceive again. This will allow you to most accurately date the next pregnancy and, more important, give you some space to heal emotionally. Many women find that a month is not nearly long enough for the grieving process, however. If this pregnancy had been unplanned, you may reflect and decide that you now are ready to conceive consciously. Or you may decide to become more conscious about contraception because you are not wanting motherhood at this time.

Not everyone has a hard time with a miscarriage, but everyone does have *some* sort of response. So it's wise to spend some time listening to your feelings. Once you identify them, you can work with them.

> **FEAR:** After a miscarriage, I will have trouble getting pregnant again.
>
> **FACT:** Your odds of conceiving next time are no different than they were before you miscarried. Even after two miscarriages, your risk of a third increases only slightly. It's not until a woman has three miscarriages in a row that her odds of successfully carrying a pregnancy the next time drop significantly and usually trigger investigation and intervention.

Ectopic Pregnancy

In rare instances (less than 2 percent of all conceptions), the fertilized egg implants itself somewhere outside the uterus, most commonly in one of the fallopian tubes, and begins to grow. Implantation in the abdominal cavity or ovary is possible, though very rare. Most often, events unfold like a normal pregnancy at first: your test turns positive, you feel the usual symptoms. Within a few weeks, however, the embryo grows bigger. The fallopian tube cannot accommodate it and is at risk of bursting.

Symptoms can include abdominal pain (often on one side) or cramping, vaginal bleeding, and, if the ectopic ruptures, severe abdominal pain, and possibly feeling dizzy or faint. An ectopic (or tubal) pregnancy is usually diagnosed by eight weeks, and sometimes the painful symptoms are the first signs that the woman is even pregnant. Your doctor will use ultrasound, along with a pelvic exam and blood tests, to diagnose the ectopic pregnancy. Early diagnosis is important so that the pregnancy can be surgically or medically removed before the fallopian tube ruptures. A rupture is a surgical emergency because the woman is hemorrhaging (bleeding from the ruptured tube into the abdomen), and her life is at risk if surgery is not immediately performed to stop the bleeding. Your odds of a future normal pregnancy are only slightly less than average after one ectopic pregnancy, although they drop to half that after two successive ectopic pregnancies. As long as a woman has one normal tube, eggs released from either ovary can find their way into the uterus for possible fertilization.

Women who are at greatest risk for ectopic pregnancy include those who have had pelvic inflammatory disease (PID), sexually transmitted diseases, or endometriosis, which can damage the fallopian tube and make it easier for the embryo to lodge there; a ruptured appendix; previous tubal surgery (such as reversal of having had your tubes tied); a previous ectopic pregnancy; or those who have conceived with an IUD in place.

Chapter 13

First Trimester: Self-Care

Centers of Wellness modifications for weeks 0 to 13

What will you eat today? How will you manage stress? Will you get any exercise? The small decisions you make each day have a direct impact on your well-being. Depending on where you've started from, you can use the news of your pregnancy as an occasion to shore up existing health habits, to drop unhelpful ones, or to create some new ones in your quest to achieve greater balance in all five of the arenas that make up good health.

Work toward the goals outlined in the Centers of Wellness Basic Self-Care Plan in Chapter 4 throughout your pregnancy. The following modifications apply especially to the first trimester.

THE MIND CENTER

Your mind may be crowded with the full gamut of emotions right now, from excitement to depression. Don't neglect relaxation exercises. Do them more often than once a day if that feels useful to you.

• *Notice the state of your mind now.* It's a huge shift to go from thinking about the possibility of becoming pregnant (or not thinking about pregnancy at all) to actually being pregnant. What are you feeling now that this is a reality? Are you processing it, or pushing it aside? Does it feel real to you? What are you worried about? What are you excited about? Has this shifted now that you are actually pregnant? Remember, there are no right or wrong answers, just be honest with yourself.

• *Notice what your stressors are now.* Have they shifted since you've become pregnant? For example, discovering you are carrying twins, having a miscarriage scare, or worrying about your due date falling around the time of a big project at work can create new stresses. Because circumstances are constantly changing, it's important to revisit this. Pay attention to how the stress is manifesting itself in you now. Does your nausea get worse when you are under stress? Are you more tired, or less able to sleep?

• *Don't neglect your sleep needs.* If you feel a lot more tired than you were previously, get more sleep. The fatigue of early pregnancy is no joke; given the range of activity happening within, it's your body telling you exactly what it needs from you.

THE NUTRITION CENTER

Interest in this center often drops to an all-time low for women in the first trimester. That's not to say it ceases to be of importance. Pay close attention to what is shifting for you since becoming pregnant and how you can best address those changes.

• *Notice your relationship with food.* Has it changed since you've become pregnant? Have you lost interest? Are you turned off by certain foods? Turned on by others? Are you eating more because you feel you must "eat for two"? Eating less because of nausea? Eating about the same amount as before?

• *Pay attention to the signals your body is sending about what's not appealing right now.* Interestingly, one theory about women losing their interests in certain foods (you may, for example, notice your taste buds or your sense of smell changing) is that it is a sort of natural protection from substances that might be toxic during the critical early phases of embryonic or fetal growth. For example, fried foods and coffee are among the substances that can lose their appeal in the first trimester. You may also notice cravings for some foods. There's little evidence behind the folklore that pregnant women crave foods their bodies are lacking; rather, we tend to crave foods with which we have positive associations. In Japan, for example, MSG is a popular craving, while in the US it's chocolate, ice cream, and pizza. As long as you do it mindfully, it's certainly fine to respond to your cravings.

• *Don't beat yourself up.* A few glasses of wine before you knew you were pregnant is not going to cause fetal alcohol syndrome. Neither is that Starbucks mocha grande you had every morning until it dawned on you to take a pregnancy test. It's the continued negative habits, not the isolated event, that could place your fetus at risk.

• *Start with breakfast.* Even if you're not felled by severe nausea, you may find that having something in your stomach—even plain crackers—makes you feel less prone to bouts of queasiness.

• *If you are nauseous:* You can try several strategies (in addition to the advice in Chapter 12).

1. Graze. Although you may lose your appetite, not eating can worsen symptoms. Better to try to eat small amounts of foods you can tolerate throughout the day than to eat a perfectly balanced, nourishing diet you can't keep down in the first trimester.
2. Avoid spicy or fatty foods.
3. Eat bland or dry foods.
4. Choose high-protein snacks.

• *If you are experiencing heartburn:* Eat several smaller meals throughout the day. Don't lie down or slouch in the first few hours after eating; try sitting upright instead or walking around. Avoid eating a lot right before going to sleep. Some women report that fried foods, carbonated beverages, fatty foods, and mint aggravate this symptom. Experiment to see if any of these are offenders for you. Before taking an over-the-counter antacid or other heartburn remedy, check with your doctor. Try Dialoguing and Dreamagery to work with this problem.

• *If you are constipated:* Relieve sluggish bowels by adding fiber to your diet. Sources of fiber include whole grains, brown rice, fruits and vegetables (keep the skin on for added fiber), oatmeal, dried fruits, beans, and peas. At the same time, drink more fluids in a variety of forms, from veggie and fruit juices to water (cold or hot). Also, ground flaxseeds can be a great help. (Start slow or you may regret it!) Avoid laxatives and herbal remedies, as they can be harmful in pregnancy; seek your doctor's advice first.

✓ **REALITY CHECK:** "Eating for Two"

In pregnancy, your body needs about 300 extra calories per day, which are used to meet the physical demands pregnancy makes on your body, and to fuel the baby's growth. But the extra calories are not really needed until the second and third trimesters. A recent study by the USDA and Baylor College of Medicine put the amounts at 350 extra calories in the second trimester and 500 extra in the third, with only a slight increase in the first trimester. Ideally, the added calories should be nutritionally advantageous—for example, a cup of milk or yogurt and a piece of fruit, or an extra serving of fish, not additional orders of french fries or helpings of cake.

You *are* eating for two. But until the second trimester, the second party in that equation gets nearly all he or she needs from your normal diet.

FEAR: Artificial sweeteners can harm my baby.
FACT: Normal consumption of artificial sweeteners has not been shown to pose risk. Having said that, their use during pregnancy has not been well-studied, and whole foods and naturally occurring sweets are far better for you than unnatural chemicals. There are only 16 calories in a teaspoon of sugar, which is probably better for you than artificial

sweeteners. Craving a diet soda? Try sparkling water with lime or with a little fruit juice—or better yet, how about the fruit itself?

FEAR: Microwave ovens are dangerous to the fetus.
FACT: There is no evidence that using a microwave poses any risk to a fetus.

✓ REALITY CHECK: Weight Gain

I'm going to give you some numbers—but with the caution that there are a lot of "ifs" and "buts" attached to them. Statistics and numbers are meaningless without an awareness of your unique situation and history.

First, how you think about weight gain in pregnancy depends on where you're starting from. And like everything else in a conscious pregnancy, that starts by being fully aware of "what is." Weight is a place where many of us go unconscious. We'd just rather not think about it or look too closely. Many of my patients believe that they are starting pregnancy at a "normal" weight when they aren't. The way to do this consciously is to start by calculating your nonpregnant Body Mass Index (BMI). To do this, see the charts below ("What Is Your Body Mass Index (BMI)?" and "What Does Your BMI Mean?"). If you're beginning pregnancy at a normal weight for your frame, you should gain 25 to 35 pounds over the nine months. If you are underweight, you should gain 28 to 40 pounds. If overweight, add 15 to 25 pounds and if obese, 15 pounds or whatever your doctor advises. Why should a woman who is overweight to begin with add pounds in pregnancy? Because most of these pounds are not gained as body fat, but rather as important elements needed to sustain the demands of pregnancy and avoid intrauterine growth retardation (IUGR), a syndrome of poor growth that puts a fetus at risk. (See "How Weight Gain Adds Up" chart.)

In general, the 25-to-35-pound average weight gain should consist of a total of three to six pounds during the first trimester, and one-half pound to one pound per week during the last two trimesters. Your actual gain may vary from these recommendations, but this gives you a general sense of whether you're on track. Women who are very sick in the first trimester often worry that they're not gaining enough weight. It's reassuring to know that you have to be extremely calorie-deprived before your baby is deprived. Only in very severe cases of hyperemesis is hospitalization warranted in order to protect those fetal needs. However, gaining fewer than 10 pounds by midpregnancy (when morning sickness has lifted) is a red flag.

Here's where awareness of your own body and soul come in.

Women who feel the most uncomfortable and unhappy about the necessary weight gain and bodily changes of pregnancy tend to be those who have some history of anorexia or bulimia. These women and others with food issues may be acutely reluctant to add pounds, but the problem may not become apparent to the physician until the third trimester. If this is an issue for you, it's important to be conscious of these feelings right from the start. If your disorder is active, your fear of a big belly and other bodily changes may cause you to do anything to prevent that from happening, which could be harmful to your baby. If you are in a later stage of recovery, the reality of pregnancy can trigger a relapse of old tendencies.

At the same time, for those with food and body image issues, this can be an opportunity to heal. If you can come to embrace and love the reasons you are getting bigger, great things can come from that. Respect the reality that this is a hard issue for you, then work with it. This is a great time to get professional support to help you optimize your health in this important life transition. Better to be proactive with it rather than struggling alone or just hoping everything goes okay.

I'm increasingly worried about a new phenomenon: moms who purposely try to gain a bare minimum of weight in order to preserve a "sexy" profile in pregnancy. These women stop short of having a true eating disorder, but put their fetuses at risk by skirting the very edge of acceptable weight gain. Instead of tuning in to their bodies and souls to find out what they really need, they subscribe to an external dictate about what's chic or acceptable. This is a real sign of unconsciousness. If you find yourself being pulled in this direction, take note of it, and make some time to further explore these feelings. Explore them in your journal or with a trusted friend. What are the fears underlying these tendencies? What are your concerns? What are your needs? A quick look at the chart below will clarify why a certain amount of weight gain is absolutely vital to the health of the baby, and may be of help as you address these concerns.

Women who tend to gain the most weight in pregnancy are those who have some history of an underlying issue with overeating, such as binge eating or yo-yo dieting. Food issues are tough in pregnancy because food, unlike tobacco or alcohol, can't simply be forsworn. We have to eat! And now, with a new life growing inside you, the prevailing cultural mandate tells you to eat for two—a real switch in the message! If you have a tendency to overeat, this can be an invitation to go wild. Pregnancy can be a great opportunity to mindfully work with overeating or binge eating. The voice to be wary of is the one telling you that now you can eat whatever you want, and at long last no one will criticize you for it. Be conscious of that voice and bring it to the forefront. Bring mindfulness to what you're eating, when you're eating, and why you're eating. As with many lifestyle issues, if you recognize this and choose to address it head-on, your pregnancy can often help motivate you to new levels of health. Additionally, you'll be less apt to wind up with a large number of postpartum pounds to drop, and you may well have a healthier relationship with food than ever before in your life.

WHAT IS YOUR BODY MASS INDEX (BMI)?

Body mass index, or BMI, uses a mathematical formula that takes into account both a person's height and weight. BMI equals a person's weight in kilograms divided by height in meters squared ($BMI=kg/m^2$). Doctors and health professionals can use this to correlate a risk of associated diseases like heart ailments, diabetes, and others. First locate your height in the far left column. Then find your prepregnancy weight in one of the columns on the same line as your height. The number in bold at the top of that column is your prepregnancy BMI. (Note: Do not use this chart to evaluate your BMI as your pregnancy progresses.)

Risk of Associated Disease According to BMI and Waist Size

BMI Height	19	20	21	22	23	24	25	26	27	28	29	30	35	40
	Weight (lb.)													
4'10"	91	96	100	105	110	115	119	124	129	134	138	143	167	191
4'11"	94	99	104	109	114	119	124	128	133	138	143	148	173	198
5'	97	102	107	112	118	123	128	133	138	143	148	153	179	204
5'1"	100	106	111	116	122	127	132	137	143	148	153	158	185	211
5'2"	104	109	115	120	126	131	136	142	147	153	158	164	191	218
5'3"	107	113	118	124	130	135	141	146	152	158	163	169	197	225
5'4"	110	116	122	128	134	140	145	151	157	163	169	174	204	232
5'5"	114	120	126	132	138	144	150	156	162	168	174	180	210	240
5'6"	118	124	130	136	142	148	155	161	167	173	179	186	216	247
5'7"	121	127	134	140	146	153	159	166	172	178	185	191	223	255
5'8"	125	131	138	144	151	158	164	171	177	184	190	197	230	262
5'9"	128	135	142	149	155	162	169	176	182	189	196	203	236	270
5'10"	132	139	146	153	160	167	174	181	188	195	202	207	243	278
5'11"	136	143	150	157	165	172	179	186	193	200	208	215	250	286
6'	140	147	154	162	169	177	184	191	199	206	213	221	258	294
6'1"	144	151	159	166	174	182	189	197	204	212	219	227	265	302
6'2"	148	155	163	171	179	186	194	202	210	218	225	233	272	311
6'3"	152	160	168	176	184	192	200	208	216	224	232	240	279	319
6'4"	156	164	172	180	189	197	205	213	221	230	238	246	287	328

WHAT DOES YOUR BMI MEAN?

18.5 or less	Underweight
18.5–24.9	Normal
25.0–29.9	Overweight
30.0–34.9	Obese
35.0–39.9	Obese
40 or greater	Extremely Obese

HOW WEIGHT GAIN ADDS UP

In a typical pregnancy, here's how the necessary weight gain adds up.

2–3 pounds	increased fluid volume
3–4 pounds	increased blood volume
1–2 pounds	breast enlargement
2 pounds	uterine enlargement
2 pounds	amniotic fluid
1–2 pounds	the placenta
4–6 pounds	maternal stores (fat and protein needed for breastfeeding)
6–8 pounds	the baby
Any extra pounds	basically, fat that you will need to lose at the end of pregnancy

THE MOVEMENT CENTER

Regular exercise in the year before pregnancy as well as in the first trimester has been found to decrease the risk of preeclampsia. And the mood-enhancing effects can give you an added boost now if you're struggling with ambivalence, nausea, fatigue, or stress. But your body is not the same as it was a few weeks ago—so be aware of changes you will need to make to fulfill your movement needs as you progress through pregnancy.

• *Notice how your body feels throughout the day.* Do your muscles and joints feel any different? What is your energy level? Do you feel like you want to move, or not? How is it different from day to day? Adjust what you do accordingly.

• *Be flexible.* Don't, for example, force yourself to tough it out through your usual workout if you don't feel up to it. Especially now, energy may be at a low ebb, or vary by the time of day. You'll feel stronger some days than others. Honor that.

• *Take it slow.* Guidelines from the Canadian Academy of Sports Medicine advise that women who have been inactive and are in low-risk pregnancies wait to start a program of mild or moderate exercise until the second trimester. Already active women can continue as usual with the caveat that they should tune in to their bodies with extra care. Many athletes are all too good at overriding their bodies, playing in spite of pain and "powering through." This is not a good idea if you're pregnant.

• *Find a comfortable balance between movement and rest.* This balance point is highly individualized, as pointed out by exercise experts Carol Krucoff and Mitchell Krucoff, M.D., authors of *Healing Moves:* "An athletic woman accustomed to running 20 miles a week is likely to feel unbalanced and frustrated if forced to stop exercising vigorously when she becomes pregnant. Likewise, a totally sedentary woman would probably become upset and injured if she were instructed to begin intense activity during pregnancy."

• *Consider yoga.* Yoga means "union." Based on ancient Hindu philosophy, yoga uses physical postures, relaxation, and movements to reach a state of physical and spiritual unification. This central concept, combined with yoga's gentle movements and relaxing effects, make it an ideal exercise for pregnancy. Do not, however, take just *any* yoga class. There are many different approaches to yoga, and some poses that you should not do during pregnancy. A class especially designed for pregnant women is ideal. Failing this, seek out an instructor who has worked with pregnant women before, and always let your instructor know that you are pregnant. Avoid any type of yoga, or any fitness approach for that matter, that involves extremes—including those that are done in high temperatures, as elevated body temperatures are unsafe for your fetus. Even if you are experienced with yoga, pay attention to your body's signals and do not push it beyond its current abilities. Stop if any pose causes pain or discomfort.

• *Consider a prenatal exercise class.* Many fitness centers, gyms, YMCAs, YWCAs, pools, dance studios, and hospitals offer classes tailored to pregnant women. Even in such a program, know your limits and adhere to them.

• *Consider being "moved."* Therapies such as massage or Watsu (shiatsu done in water) can be very relaxing and nurturing, especially now when you may be feeling particularly lethargic or drained and your body may not feel up to moving itself. Find a massage therapist who has experience with pregnant clients.

• *Don't forget walking.* A great, gentle way to move your body through space, it's sometimes the best option for days in the first trimester when you may feel fatigued yet still feel the desire to move.

FEAR: Swimming is dangerous to the fetus.
FACT: Your baby is already swimming—safely in the amniotic fluid of your womb. Swimming is ideal exercise in pregnancy because it uses your arms and legs, makes you feel weightless and cool, and puts you at little risk of injury.

THE SPIRIT CENTER

In the first trimester, when you are really integrating the concept and the reality of this new life within you, some women find they are naturally drawn to more spiritual aspects of life. They report being drawn to spiritual readings and books (poetry, the Bible and other religious texts, existential explorations, reflections on life, philosophy, and so

on). Or they may find a renewed interest in classes, religious participation, or other activities that help them explore their relationship to
God or spirituality. Other women find that their focus and energy in
this domain is low. Or they find their spirit inclinations primarily focused on the self, which makes them feel much more reflective and
inwardly focused. Neither is wrong or right. But it's interesting to be
aware of your spiritual side, and gratifying to support this aspect of
yourself.

The first trimester is also when you begin to see everyone around
you in a new light (as they in turn are seeing you, once they know the
news). It's a time of beginning to marshal the support network that
will see you through the coming months.

• *Notice your tendencies regarding spirituality now.* Have they
shifted since you've gotten pregnant? If your inclinations have
shifted, have your actions shifted, too? Or are you still in your old patterns, even though they're not what you are really drawn to now?
Give yourself permission to follow your spiritual tendencies where
they take you, regardless of how much of a departure they might be
from your norms.

• *Do what's right for you in sharing the news.* Don't feel pressured
to tell the world right away—or to keep it a secret until you're safely
past the first trimester—if either course makes you uncomfortable.
Everybody's different. If you and your partner disagree about when to
spread the word, talk about it so that you appreciate each other's perspectives. Also realize that you are the one who is carrying the baby,
which means that your own feelings merit an added dollop of respect.
Be clear about who you want to know. You may, for example, decide
to tell your immediate families right away, but not your boss. Or your
best friend but not your parents. Revisit the issue; how you feel the
day you discover you're pregnant may be different from how you feel
at 8 weeks, or 12 weeks. Just make it conscious.

• *Pay attention to how pregnancy has impacted your relationship.* It's
a big development for you and your partner. Do you feel closer? More
distant? A little of both? Pay attention to how this unfolds. Talk about
it. Your partner has his own set of doubts, worries, insecurities, and
fantasies for the pregnancy and the birth and your future as a family.

- *Begin building your emotional support network.* This can include:

  Other pregnant women. Women in the same situation can be an unexpected source of support. If you don't have any friends, neighbors, or family members who are also pregnant, or whose support would feel right at this time, consider turning to the Internet. You'll find many sites where pregnant women can chat, some of them organized by due date so that you'll be sharing many of the same questions and concerns. You can also read and sometimes comment on the blogs of other moms-to-be (or perhaps start one yourself).

  Friends. Now that you're pregnant, you may find that some friends eagerly embrace the news while others, often those without children, are less interested. Friends with fertility problems or a history of miscarriage or loss might find it difficult to hear your good news, even if they are thrilled for you. Recognize this and consider sharing the conflict you feel between your excitement for yourself and your sensitivity to their sorrow with them.

  Your mother and mother-in-law. These relationships often come into particular focus now, given that you are about to become a mother yourself. If it feels right to share experiences with these two important women in your life, this can be a special time for deepening your relationships and helping you to see them in a new, more nuanced light. If your mother is no longer alive, consider using Dialoguing or Dreamagery to have a conversation (or many) with her. You'd be surprised how rewarding this can be.

THE SENSATION CENTER

The start of pregnancy is a great time to elevate this center in your life and keep it a priority for the next nine months (and beyond). It's the center of pleasure, a dimension of life that a pregnant woman needs and deserves as much or more than anybody! Make it a habit now, while pregnancy is new, and you'll be more likely to view it as absolutely essential by the time you're on your way to the delivery room.

• *Notice whether your levels of sensuality and sexuality have changed.* Some women feel incredibly sexual, as well as sensual, knowing that they're pregnant. Others feel the opposite, especially if they are struggling with morning sickness and other physical symptoms. Feelings may fluctuate dramatically across these first three months. Toss aside expectations about how you're "supposed to feel" right now, and honor how you're really feeling.

• *Nurture your altered sense of smell.* If you experience this, go out of your way to avoid unpleasant odors (leave the room when your partner's frying the onions or better still, keep the malodorous foods out of the house for a few weeks). Also important: find ways to indulge scents that you find pleasing now. Keep fresh flowers on your desk (but sniff 'em first . . . some women find all flowers too strong). Wear your favorite perfume, or skip it altogether. Be sensitive to what works for you right now. Your usual nose usually returns by week 12 or 13.

• *Nurture your altered sense of taste.* Indulge cravings, within reason. Find foods whose textures appeal to you when nauseous. Eat what makes you feel happy, mindfully and in moderate amounts. Although there's a great deal of pressure to make food choices that are nutritious and supportive of physical needs, remember that food has a psychological component. Find ways to use it to make you feel good, such as experimenting with different flavors of herbal tea or switching from cold cereal to a favorite comfort food, like oatmeal.

• *Fuel your changing sense of touch.* While you may not be feeling particularly sexual, remember that the body loves to be touched. Notice what your body loves—and provide it. This may range from a full massage weekly, to daily foot and hand massage by you or your partner, to wearing something that is particularly soft and appealing to you right now.

FEAR: It's best not to have too much sex in pregnancy, to keep the baby safe.

FACT: This is a very common misconception, not true at all if you're in a low-risk, normal pregnancy. On the contrary, a healthy sex life can be a great stress reliever and a way to remain connected to your partner during this potentially stressful time of life. And if you don't feel well and don't desire sex right now, honor that. Chances are good that this will change next trimester.

OVER 40? IN YOUR TEENS?

People often think that teenagers are at greater risk in pregnancy than adult women. The opposite is actually true. From a purely physical level, your teens are a great time to be pregnant and give birth. I used to work with and do research on the pregnancy outcomes and complications of teenage mothers-to-be. It was remarkable how they had overall fewer complications and bounced back quickly.

When you are 40, strictly from the "body" standpoint of the physical demands of pregnancy, you are past your peak. From a "soul" perspective, though, your experience, wisdom, maturity, intellect, emotional preparedness, and other traits tend to provide far greater advantages.

For any woman, young or old, what's most important is to be proactive about being in the best possible condition, across all five Centers of Wellness. If you are older, this is essential. Your body needs your active partnership to optimize your health.

Part Four

The Second Trimester

Weeks 14 to 28

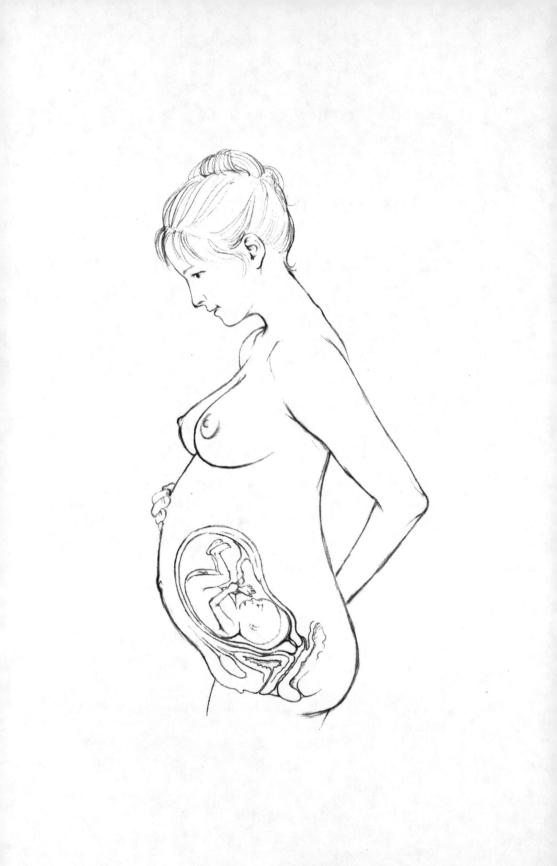

Chapter 14

Second Trimester:
Reflection and Observation

∾

Checking in with body, soul, and baby, weeks 14 to 28

I call this trimester "the calm." Not because there isn't anything happening—plenty of change goes on. But these mid-pregnancy months are bracketed by the highs and lows of the first trimester, when pregnancy is new, and the last trimester, when the fetus becomes viable and labor is around the corner. Months four, five, and six tend to be a time when the body and soul have adjusted to the reality of being pregnant while not yet engaged in the drama of imminent labor and motherhood. Checking in every day remains an important way for you to:

- Fully embrace the life experience of being pregnant, and enjoy this often wonderful "in between" stage
- Be aware of the ways in which your body and soul are evolving
- Detect worrisome changes promptly
- Begin to sort through the many different ways your life will change when you become a mother
- Forge an ongoing relationship with your baby-to-be.

Detailed instructions on how to use the following tools can be found in Chapter 3.

CHECK IN WITH YOUR BODY

In general, this is a peaceful and happy time physically, with a low incidence of worrisome complications or uncomfortable changes. The biggest physical changes are that you begin to "show," if you haven't already, and you feel the baby move for the first time, a wondrous event known as *quickening*. The fetus has been moving for weeks, but it's now grown large enough that you can feel its movements. Some women feel these movements as early as 16 or 18 weeks, while others don't feel anything until 21 or 22 weeks, or even later. If you haven't felt anything by the 22nd week, mention it to your doctor.

What does the movement feel like? It's not painful, but it does vary a lot from woman to woman. Moms report everything from very subtle "flutters" to "bubbles" to "thumps." Many women at first mistake it for gas! You may gradually realize that you've been feeling the same unfamiliar but unmistakable sensation, usually very low in your midsection, below the navel, for days or even weeks. Or you may suddenly one day feel something and realize, "This must be it!" The movement is not constant; your baby stretches and kicks, stops, naps. Before long, you will realize that you are feeling the baby's movements every day. You'll feel them at night, too. The baby doesn't follow the same sleep-wake cycle you do, so as it grows and its movements are more easily felt, you may be awakened by fetal acrobatics in the middle of the night. Eventually, it will be hard to remember there was a time when you didn't feel them. As your baby grows, you will even be able to see the ripples of movement across your belly.

Feeling your baby move is exciting and, once it can be felt externally, makes pregnancy seem all the more "real" to your partner, too. It not only presents another way to bond with your baby, it's also a terrific indicator that things are going well, since a lack of fetal movement can be a sign that the baby is not getting adequate oxygen for some reason. Once you begin to feel kicking regularly and clearly, usually late in this trimester, you should make an awareness of fetal movement part of your daily check-ins. By week 28 you will want to do this in a more systematic way and to do it without fail every single day. See "The Kick Count" in Chapter 18 for directions.

SUGGESTED TOOLS:

DAILY:

Body Scan (tool #2)
Hopefully this has become part of your regular routine. Resist the temptation to drop it once the wild ride of first-trimester changes has ended.

Body Quick Pic (tool #1)

WEEKLY:

Body Monitoring (tool #4)

AS NEEDED:

Dialoguing (with Your Physical Self) (tool #3)

WHAT MIGHT COME UP FOR YOU

I Feel Fantastic!

For many women, the first trimester is plagued by tentativeness. The specter of miscarriage hangs over every long week until the heartbeat is heard. Often the parents-to-be tell no one the news yet. And then there are the physical discomforts that get in the way of fully enjoying the experience of being pregnant.

The second trimester is a time when the pregnancy seems more "real," and much more pleasurable, too. Sickness subsides, energy increases. As you begin to show, you share the news, or people guess. Best of all is feeling the baby move—a constant daily reminder of what pregnancy is all about.

Meg, 28, had a rough beginning. Almost from the time her pregnancy test turned positive, she vomited nearly every day and felt leveled by exhaustion. "I was completely taken off guard," she says. "I had expected to get a little sick in the mornings, but this was virtually constant." She lost four pounds, and all her plans for healthful eating and exercise went out the window. (Or as she put it, "down the toilet—pun intended.")

"Everybody around me was so psyched about my being pregnant but as time went on, I couldn't find any joy in it. I mean, I wanted this baby, but day to day it was a struggle to remember that," she says.

Around week 10, however, Meg's worst symptoms began to subside. She went a week, then two, without getting sick. By week 14, her energy had returned, and with it a sense of pleasure and pride in being pregnant. "My favorite exercise now is Body Monitoring," Meg says. "I love noticing the changes—it's as if I'm a flower coming into bloom after being in the desert." Her skin went from sallow to pink. Her breasts no longer ached. Best of all was her growing belly.

My Sex Drive Has Gone Through the Roof.

For weeks, the only context in which Lucia had thought about bed was sleep—she couldn't get enough of it in the early stages of pregnancy. In her fourth and fifth months, she was surprised to discover something different that she couldn't get enough of in bed—sex. "Whenever I paused to check in with my body, it seemed, I was hot to trot," she marvels.

The same hormonal changes that fuel pregnancy may stoke sexual arousal. As much estrogen is now produced in a day, for example, as a nonpregnant woman's ovaries produce in three years. In the second trimester, when the fatigue and nausea lift, this turbocharged libido often becomes more apparent. With the genitals already engorged and nerve endings growing more sensitive as they stretch, many women achieve orgasm more quickly or intensely now, or have multiple orgasms easily. Some women have orgasms for the first time in their lives. Feeling aroused several times a day is common. If it happens to you, enjoy it! Sex can't harm the fetus.

Not all women experience this sexual bounty, however. Some report no interest in sex at all. This is not a sign of anything amiss, simply that every woman is different. You may want to take the initiative and do more sexual exploration to see if your body responds differently during this time, even if your libido has not shifted significantly.

Still Sick!

Natasha's morning sickness was so severe that it was diagnosed as hyperemesis, and she twice came close to being admitted to the hospital because she was so severely dehydrated. Her doctor told her not to be too discouraged, that she would most likely feel better by weeks 10 to 12. She didn't. This is a hard situation, because no one knows why morning sickness sometimes persists. It can be almost as frustrating for doctors as it is for patients.

Natasha found it difficult to move on to the stage of reveling in pregnancy because she still felt so sick. Her anger with her body began to build. "I was like, 'What's the matter with you? We're supposed to be happily pregnant and instead of buying baby clothes, I'm still hanging over a toilet every day,' " she said. "I knew intellectually I was supposed to be taking care of my body and getting excited about the baby, but frankly I had a hard time doing much more than feeling sorry for myself."

I suggested Natasha try Dialoguing with her body to explore these feelings further. Asking her body, "What's up with all this sickness?" helped her to get that anger out in the open. This was the beginning of a conversation that helped Natasha see in depth what she was dealing with. The message she received from her body was: "I'm not the enemy here. This is hard on me, too." This helped Natasha see that the morning sickness wasn't "me versus my body." Instead, they were in it together. Bringing this awareness to the fore didn't make her symptoms go away but it did help her to become more nurturing to her body, and thus to enjoy her pregnancy more. By tuning in, she became better aware of the first symptoms of nausea. This enabled her to eat some crackers to settle her stomach. She also realized that for her, nausea and vomiting were worse when she was exhausted, so she made an effort to rest more. She became more self-nurturing, too, incorporating the integrative approaches of hypnosis tapes and acupressure bands. As it happened, Natasha continued to feel occasional nausea and vomiting throughout her pregnancy. But by continuing the dialogue with her body, she found ways to give it relief. Natasha absolutely believed that her symptoms would have been much worse had she not been directly in touch with her body's needs.

CHECK IN WITH YOUR SOUL

You're now at a place where you can really relax into the reality that you *are* pregnant. What are the implications of that for you? How do you feel about it? Dive in and help those responses surface.

Suggested Tools

DAILY:

Soul Quick Pic (tool #5)

ANYTIME, AT LEAST ONCE IN THE SECOND TRIMESTER:

Journaling Your Journey (tool #6)
As you continue your exploration of how pregnancy is affecting you, ask yourself the following:

How has the change in your physical symptoms changed your experience? How do you feel now about having this baby?
What was it like to feel the baby move for the first time? What emotions did it evoke? How do you feel about your baby?
What are your greatest fears at this point in pregnancy?
What are your greatest hopes and joys?

AS NEEDED:

Dialoguing (with Your Nonphysical Self) (tool #7)

∞

SOUL CHECKS:
WHAT MIGHT COME UP FOR YOU

Shouldn't I Be Happier?

"I'm sick and tired of everybody congratulating me and giving me booties and making googly eyes at me just because I'm pregnant!" Wendi declared emphatically at our first visit. She had recently moved, and when I first saw her she was already 16 weeks pregnant.

"How are you feeling about being pregnant?" I asked.

Wendi slumped. "It was an accident," she whispered. "I thought things would be okay, but they seem to get worse as the weeks go on. I'm not physically tired like I was at first, but I keep telling my husband that I am, just so I can stay in bed and be left alone." She began to cry. "I'm sorry!" she said, dabbing at her eyes. "I can't help it. I cry all the time."

When a woman in her second trimester tells me she's having the blues or just feels generally "blah," I consider it a warning sign. Because this is a time when most women are really "up"—feeling great physically, and on an emotional high because they can now feel the baby moving inside—being depressed can indicate something amiss that is worth exploring more deeply. If you are ambivalent about being pregnant in the first place (and there are any number of reasons why this may be the case) and don't come face-to-face with these feelings, they aren't likely to just go away. They worsen. Often women don't feel well enough in the first trimester to address these feelings, or they think they feel them *because* they don't feel well, and are surprised to feel that way even once they are doing better physically. If you continue to ignore such mixed feelings about the pregnancy, they will continue to haunt you right through to your labor, and possibly on into the postpartum phase, putting you at a very real risk for postpartum depression. It's important to be aware and honest about your emotional state, both to yourself and to your care provider.

I encouraged Wendi to use tools such as Journaling and Dialoguing to explore her depression. I also referred her to a psychiatrist who works with pregnant women, using both therapy and medication, as indicated. I knew counseling would help her to go more deeply into her feelings, and also allow for her situation to be adequately evaluated and followed. In this situation it's also critical to focus on your health plan and optimize all five Centers of Wellness. Mind-body strategies, exercise, better nutrition steps in the Sensation center, and social support can all lift mood and provide needed support. (See "Prenatal Depression," in Chapter 12, pages 178–180.)

Wendi spent a lot of time exploring her feelings toward this pregnancy, addressed some of her concerns with her partner, and enrolled in a parenting class to help calm some of her fears about her ability to be a good mom, which stemmed in part from her feeling that her own parents had not been good models. These steps, along with her Centers of Wellness plan and continued counseling, resulted in her beginning to feel like she understood where her negative feelings were coming from and how to listen to them. As she grew in confidence about her ability to be a mom, she found herself becoming more and more excited about the pregnancy and her transition to motherhood—authentically!

CHECK IN WITH YOUR BABY

In the second trimester, the baby within you moves from being a concept to being a reality, a tangible presence that you can feel and even see moving across your skin. Many women have ultrasounds this trimester as well, which provide a first "portrait" of their child. Most women find it a unique joy to be in a relationship with this being. Even if you were having trouble with this step earlier, checking in with your baby is likely to become easier and more natural now.

Suggested Tools:

Baby Quick Pic (tool #8)

Dreamagery (tool #9)
Remember, Dreamagery is simply a deeper level of Dialoguing. First get centered and deeply relaxed, and then invite an image of your baby to join you. Take your time and notice every detail about this image. Feel free to let the conversation with this image representing your baby go wherever it wants to. Have fun with this great and precious opportunity.

BABY CHECKS:
WHAT MIGHT COME UP FOR YOU

A Deepening Bond

Like many women, Jane looked forward to doing the Dreamagery exercise with her baby. She always saw the same image: her plastic childhood baby doll, only in a full-motion, come-to-life representation. (More often when you are inviting an image of the same thing across different sessions, what you "see" changes over time.) Remember to accept the first thing that comes to mind—whether it makes sense to your logical brain or not, whether it is the same or different from previous times.

The way Jane used Dreamagery is worth sharing: "About once a week I have what I call 'Me Time,'" she explains. "I take about an hour on Friday night, after work, to have a nice long shower and do a full Body Monitoring, write down in my journal what I've found, and then write about a different Journaling exercise question each week. After that I do a little Dreamagery with an image of the baby—I think of that part as the 'dessert' to the whole indulgence because I like it so much.

"As my pregnancy has gone on, the baby and I 'talk' about all kinds of things. Usually it just says that it's happy and growing well, and that it can't wait to be held in my arms, and that's reassuring," she adds. "I think of each kick as kind of a 'hi Mom!' message. Then we just let the conversations evolve however they want—and it is so much fun, and always full of surprises!"

Remember, too, that you can use Dreamagery about any topic, not just baby-related ones. Below is the account of a woman who used it to explore a problem with her placenta.

The Placenta Is My Baby's Best Friend.

Sara used Dreamagery to help her cope with a second diagnosis of placenta previa, a condition where the placenta is partially or completely (as in her case) covering the cervix. In many cases, previas that are seen on second-trimester ultrasounds resolve themselves before delivery. If they do not, however, they put the mother and baby at increased risk for sudden bleeding during the pregnancy, and the baby ultimately must be delivered by C-section because the placenta is literally blocking the baby's exit from the womb. Sara was upset about this development. Her first child had been delivered by C-section because of a placenta previa, and she'd had her heart set on a smooth second pregnancy and a vaginal delivery. Even worse, there was a small risk that because of her prior C-section, the placenta had implanted improperly into the scar tissue (a placenta accreta) rather than along the uterine wall, a rare development that can't be seen on ultrasound and requires a hysterectomy at delivery.

The first time Sara used Dreamagery, inviting an image of the placenta, the image that came to her was of her baby in a life raft, bobbing on the water. "What are you doing? I don't understand why you are making this pregnancy so difficult," Sara inquired.

The image responded, "Actually, I am here supporting our baby, and you."

Sara: "But how can that be? You're not even in the right place!"

The image: "I didn't have any control over my position. I am disappointed in that, too, but even though it's not ideal, I'm still able to keep you and our baby alive and well."

After the exercise, Sara realized that she had been so focused on what was *wrong* with her placenta, she had never considered what it was doing *right*. This new insight helped diminish her feelings of anger and frustration.

The next time Sara did Dreamagery, the image that came to her was of a scene: she, her baby, and the placenta all in the water together, swimming and playing. She was amazed at the shift. This was a joyous image of interconnectedness. "Is there anything I can do to help you?" she asked.

The image: "Just take it easy, listen to your doctor, and we'll be all right."

Over time, as she continued to use Dreamagery weekly, she was able to reframe her perception of the placenta from "My Big Problem" to "A Slight Problem with My Baby's Best Friend." "The placenta is keeping the baby alive," she noted. "And I feel grateful to it for that."

She continued to do this imagery work with both the placenta and the baby throughout pregnancy. It was heartwarming to see the very significant change in her experience.

In the end, Sara *did* have placenta accreta and needed a hysterectomy following her C-section. It turned out to be a difficult surgery, as such cases can be, involving a lot of blood loss. So I was surprised when she asked, in the middle of all this, to see the placenta when it was removed. Later she said, "Of course this was not the outcome that I wanted. But I still feel great about it because my baby is fine. The placenta allowed my baby to thrive, and I survived. That's a great ending."

Chapter 15

Second Trimester:
The Inside Scoop

∞

What's happening biologically, weeks 14 to 28

WHAT'S HAPPENING WITH YOU:
SECOND-TRIMESTER CHANGES

Using your check-in tools will help you to become aware of the physical effects that take place as your body accommodates your growing baby, and to make adjustments in your self-care.

TEETH AND GUMS: Like the membranes of the nasal area, your gums can be swollen and prone to irritation. Ordinary brushing of your teeth or flossing can cause bleeding—but it is important to continue, because the gums are more susceptible to plaque and cavity-causing bacteria, which can lead to dangerous infections. Be sure to drink plenty of water after eating or drinking anything sweet, and don't forget to use a good natural mouthwash to keep bacteria at bay.

BREASTS: They may continue to increase in size; soreness and tenderness should decrease. Periodically check that your bra is not digging into your skin. You may need to go up in bra size several times during your nine months.

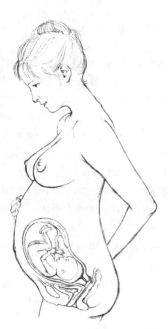

A woman in her second trimester

LUNGS: A sensation of shortness of breath affects 60 to 70 percent of all women beginning early this trimester. It's a normal result of changes happening within the respiratory system, but it can be unnerving.

HEART: Blood pressure continues to decrease from prepregnancy norms during the second trimester, with the systolic pressure falling 5 to 10 points and the diastolic decreasing 10 to 15 points. If, for example, your blood pressure before pregnancy was 110/65, at 24 weeks it may be 100/50.

STOMACH: Appetite continues to increase as the body needs more energy and nausea subsides.

BOWELS: As your gastrointestinal system slows, it can take six hours for food to move through the small bowel now. The volume of the gallbladder is twice that of prepregnancy, and it empties much more slowly. These changes can lead to feelings of indigestion, constipation, or bloating.

URINARY TRACT: The dilation of the ureters (the tubes that carry urine from the kidney into the bladder) is greatest in the second trimester. Each ureter can be 2 cm in diameter, up from a few millimeters, and hold 20 to 55 ccs of liquid—which means you can have almost half a cup of urine just sitting in the ureters!

SKIN: Stretch marks are said to occur in half of all pregnancies—although from what I see, it seems like the actual total is higher. Common sites for these silvery lines include breasts, lower abdomen, and upper thighs. They're actually tiny tears in the elastic tissue of the skin that allow it to stretch normally. Some women have a genetic predisposition to developing more marks; a large weight gain (as when carrying multiples) can also increase stretch marks. Moisturizers and other creams may make your skin feel better, but there's little that can be done to prevent the marks.

Tiny loose growths of skin on your breasts and upper arm called skin tags may also appear. They sometimes disappear after delivery. If not, they can be easily removed by a dermatologist.

UTERUS: It's growing! By 20 weeks, the top of the uterus is typically at the level of the belly button. (Check—you can feel it.) This stage of growth, when the uterus is growing and moves up and out of the pelvis into the abdominal cavity, is when many women complain of pain in the lower abdomen. This is called *round ligament pain*. The round ligaments are at the top of the uterus, and the theory is that they are stretching a great deal during this phase of uterine growth. Many physicians say there is no such thing, although enough women disagree to convince me. These pains tend to feel sore, dull, or aching, but can sometimes be sharp, and are normal. If you do feel sharp or excruciating pain, you should report it to your doctor.

VAGINA: *Leukorrhea*, a constant, thin, whitish discharge, is normal and tends to increase each month. Leukorrhea is *not* bloody, mucusy, brownish or greenish, thick and cheesy, watery, or especially malodorous, and it does not burn, itch, or make the perineum feel sore. Any of these symptoms may be signs of a vaginal infection or other problem and should be reported to your doctor. Use pantyliners or change underwear as needed during the day to feel fresher. (Cotton underwear is preferable, because it helps the area breathe better.) Don't use tampons, vaginal sprays, or douches.

LEGS: Cramping is common, possibly due to the uterus pressing on nerves. Try to walk regularly, and if needed wear support hose. Yoga can help, too.

FEET: Water retention can cause swelling, which is normal. The loosening of ligaments (a by-product of the same hormones that allow your hip bones to separate and widen for birth) may also cause the feet to get bigger, sometimes by as much as a whole shoe size. These changes are temporary for some women, although others report them to be permanent.

WHAT'S HAPPENING WITH YOUR BABY NOW

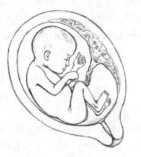

Fetus at 14 to 18 weeks

19 to 22 weeks

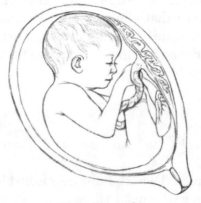

23 to 27 weeks

MONTH 4 (14 to 18 weeks)

The details of your baby's features are starting to become more defined, including ears, eyes, and fingerprints. The fetus can now suck its thumb and swallow amniotic fluid. Where the head was once much larger than the body, now the body is catching up. Limbs are lengthening and bones are getting stronger.

MONTH 5 (19 to 22 weeks)

Your baby looks more like a "real" baby. By 17 to 20 weeks, it weighs just one pound and is seven or eight inches long from head to rump.

The skin is coated with vernix, a waxy protective substance, and lanugo, downy-fine hair.

It moves a lot and can even react to sounds heard outside the uterus. As the arms and legs grow, the muscles get stronger, and the skeletal system hardens, the fetus practices flexing and moving these limbs. This increased movement plus bigger size account for your finally being able to feel the movements.

MONTH 6 (23 to 27 weeks)

Your fetus is now like a cake that's half-baked. It resembles what it's going to become, but is not quite "done" yet. By the end of the trimester, a fetus may weigh between 2 and 3 pounds and be 12 to 16 inches long. There is very little body fat, and the skin is very thin and translucent, almost like Saran wrap. The lungs are developing surfactant, a substance that allows them to expand more easily on their own. (The lack of surfactant used to be a major reason that babies seldom survived if born during the second trimester. Now we can provide this to babies born prematurely.)

Fetal Headlines

- Around 16 weeks, the fetus's gender can usually be determined on ultrasound.
- Between 18 and 20 weeks, most moms first feel the baby move (quickening; see Chapter 14).
- By 24 weeks, half of babies who are born prematurely will be able to survive outside the womb.

✓ REALITY CHECK: Viability

Incredible things are being done to save babies who are born earlier and earlier. But this trimester is where you see how every single extra week and every single extra *day* in the uterus is of tremendous benefit. Babies born at 23 weeks (gestational age) rarely survive. By 24 weeks, about half survive, although usually with very serious complications. By 25 weeks and beyond, survival rates go up and complication rates slowly go down.

If something unexpected arises such as the premature rupture of your membranes and you face a possible delivery at a very early stage, spend extra time really exploring this. The tendency is to just hope it doesn't happen and to try to "not dwell on it." This is actually the very time to fully turn your attention to this possibility. Focus on your feelings, on your own, with your partner, and with your health provider. This is very often the most complex of situations for all involved because being on the border of viability creates very difficult choices. Many women reflexively say to their doctor: "Do everything you can to save my baby." That's an entirely understandable first reaction, but very often a mom says this without a full understanding of what "saving" a baby at the very limits of viability means. As painful as it is to contemplate, I believe there are some extremely premature infants who would be better off not surviving. Risks for an extremely preterm infant include brain damage, cerebral palsy, lung disease, blindness, and deafness. About 70 percent of infants who survive when delivered at 23 to 25 weeks are disabled. There may be no more important time to be conscious, and let this awareness be the basis of your choices. If you request that your baby be saved at all costs, the medical team will most likely follow your wishes, and you need to be aware of the potential consequences for the baby—and for you and your family.

Whether you choose to "do everything" or "let nature take its course," the decision is a very difficult one, and has significant ramifications. You will be the one guiding this course of action because there is no "right" or clear choice in such a situation. If there were, the medical team would offer more direction in the decision. The Feedback Loop can be invaluable in helping you to make these choices consciously.

Chapter 16

Second Trimester: Medical Care

∞

An integrative medicine perspective, weeks 14 to 28

BASIC MEDICAL ISSUES NOW

Checkups and Tests

If your pregnancy doesn't turn up any red flags, you'll see your care provider once a month this trimester. Here's what's done at each checkup, and why:

- *Urine dip.*

  WHY: To screen for signs of infection. Moms-to-be are at an increased risk of urinary tract infections and you may have no symptoms but still have bacteria in the urine. We also screen for protein in the urine, a possible sign of preeclampsia. Protein can come from many sources, including normal vaginal secretions. This is why a "clean catch" is so important. To get this, your provider will ask you to swab an antiseptic pad over the vulva before you provide the sample; you should also capture the middle of your flow, not the first part that comes out. (If protein in the urine is still detected and there is reason for concern, you may be catheterized in order to get the cleanest possible sample.)

- *Blood pressure.*

WHY: We want to see that blood pressure is following normal patterns. As in the first trimester, blood pressure normally continues to drop from its prepregnancy baseline because of the effects of progesterone and some heat from the fetus, both of which cause blood vessels to dilate. Blood pressure typically drops to its lowest point in the second trimester, and slowly returns to baseline in the third trimester. It should not trend higher. Increasing blood pressure is a possible sign of preeclampsia.

- *Weight check.*

WHY: To ensure you're on track. If you haven't gained much weight by midpregnancy, this could cause a problem with fetal growth. Gaining too rapidly can also be a concern, or can be a sign of fluid retention.

- *Fundal height.* Starting at about 20 weeks, the growth of your uterus is tracked through external abdominal measurements called fundal height. The distance from the top of your pubic bone to the top of your uterus (the *fundus*) is the fundal height. Each week beginning at week 20, the fundal height should increase by 1 cm, with the measurement correlating roughly to how many weeks along you are. So in the 24th week, a typical fundal height is 24 cm, and would be expected to reach 28 cm by your monthly checkup four weeks later. More important than the actual numbers is the growth curve; we want to see a steady increase in fundal height from month to month.

WHY: To help gauge your baby's size and growth pattern. If the size and growth rate are less than what we expect given how far along you are in your pregnancy, this *may* indicate a possible problem with the baby's growth. The fundal height can also exceed what we expect, called "size greater than dates."

The most common reason for a discrepancy, however, is human error. This measurement must be done very precisely and consistently each time, but often individuals do the measurement differently or inconsistently or one or more of them does it inaccurately. There are two common errors. One is that the provider does not press deeply enough to clearly identify the top of the pubic bone, where the measurement starts. Perhaps because this pressure can be a bit uncomfortable, or because it is in an intimate part of the body, many people will just place the tape measure in the region, which can change the measurement by a centimeter or two. The second common error is that the tape measure is carried too far down the belly. This is not the accurate way to measure and can add several centimeters (see illustration). When you're counting in centimeters, it doesn't take much imprecision to appear as a significant discrepancy from what was expected.

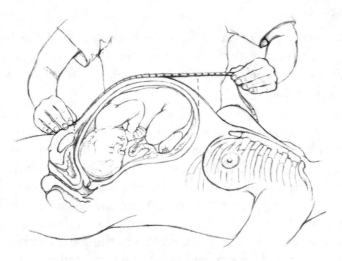

Measuring Fundal Height
The tape measure should begin at the top of the pubic bone (dotted line on the left) and end at the top of the uterus, which is the fundus (dotted line on the right). For an accurate measurement, the tape measure should not be draped down the belly but extended into the air at the fundus.

Whenever there is a real or suspected fundal height lag, the possibility that the baby is not growing normally needs to be investigated. An ultrasound can be done to more accurately assess the size of the fetus, rather than just measuring the uterus. The length of a femur (the leg bone), the circumference of the abdomen, and the diameter of the head, will all be measured, and together they are used to predict the baby's approximate weight. If the measurements are within a normal range, then as long as the fundal height continues to follow the expected growth curve, all is well. If the baby does indeed measure small, then your doctor may recommend other tests or monitoring to determine if you just happen to have a small baby that is growing normally or a growth-restricted baby, which can be a sign of something wrong. Too little amniotic fluid is another possible culprit for fundal height lag that requires further investigation. Fundal height measurements can also be affected by something as benign as the baby's position.

A baby who measures larger than dates indicate is also reevaluated with ultrasound. A similar range of possible explanations exists, which includes poor measuring, a baby who is simply very large, or too much amniotic fluid.

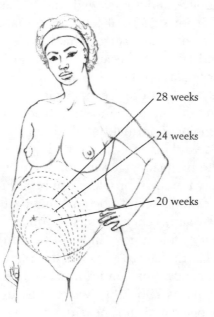

28 weeks

24 weeks

20 weeks

Fundal height

- *Verify fetal heart tones.* At each visit a care provider will check for the presence of fetal heart tone and rate.

WHY: To verify the baby's well-being.

- *Ultrasound* (optional). In routine obstetric care, you typically receive one ultrasound (sonogram), which is done during the second trimester around 18 to 20 weeks. (Others may be ordered earlier or later if you have one of many different situations that warrant more frequent observation.) The kind of ultrasound performed in the second trimester is abdominal. A device called a transducer is moved across your abdomen, causing sound waves that bounce off internal structures to create an image on a screen.

WHY: A basic ultrasound study documents fetal life, the number of fetuses, the presentation, and estimated fetal size and age. The placenta's location and maturity are checked, as is the amount of amniotic fluid. A basic ultrasound study also looks at fetal anatomy, including the heart, skull and brain structure, bladder, stomach, kidneys, abdominal wall, and hip and leg bones. Most but not all major structural fetal abnormalities in these areas can be detected at this stage. This kind of study is generally timed around 18 weeks because the fetus is developed enough to see major organs (you can see all four chambers of the heart, for example), and yet the pregnancy is not too far along to preclude making decisions about what to do if problems are discovered. If major abnormalities are found, there is still time to do more of a workup and consider all options, including termination of the pregnancy. It's important to remember, though, that not every potential problem can be seen on ultrasound.

If the placenta is seen to be covering part of the cervix, this will be noted and rechecked in the third trimester. It doesn't pose any real problem now and will hopefully be lifted into a safe position as the uterus expands. If it remains in this position later in pregnancy, this condition, called placenta previa (see Chapter 20, pages 296–299), will be discussed in detail with you. If your placenta is not near the cervix now, you're fine; it won't migrate downward later.

An ultrasound at 18 weeks can also be useful in confirming your due date.

Your doctor may want to do repeated ultrasounds to check the progress of certain situations, such as a baby who is measuring large or small, or a possible problem with the placenta or amount of amniotic fluid. A detailed or comprehensive ultrasound is a more in-depth exam used to look at specific areas when there is concern, such as the baby's heart or spinal cord.

HOW TO MAKE A CONSCIOUS CHOICE
ABOUT . . . FINDING OUT YOUR BABY'S SEX

Often the baby's genitalia can be seen on ultrasound, which means you can find out the baby's gender. Nowadays, in fact, finding out has become the default scenario. The person doing the scan says, "Do you want me to tell you?" and the patient says, "Um, sure"—often without having thought much about it.

It's not a huge issue, but worth mentioning because you should realize that receiving this information is a choice. So before you go for your ultrasound, give some thought as to whether you really want to find out.

First, reflection. How do you feel about knowing the baby's sex before it's born? (It's a pretty basic question but many people never stop to consider it.) How does your partner feel?

What are the reasons that you might want to find out? To narrow the name-selection process? To choose the color of your nursery or layette? Because your family or friends want to know? Because you have your heart set on one sex and want time to adjust in case the baby is the opposite sex? Just because you can? Because it seems weird to you that someone else will know but you won't?

What are the reasons you might not want to find out? Do you like the old-fashioned element of mystery and surprise of hearing "It's a boy!" or "It's a girl!" in the delivery room? Because either gender is fine with you? Or you don't want the baby to seem too "real" yet? Because knowing would be like peeking ahead to the last page of a novel?

Second, information. The most pertinent piece of medical info to know is that ultrasounds can be wrong. Although this becomes less and less of a possibility as technology advances and ultrasound images become sharper, I've seen it happen. Only an amniocentesis can definitively determine gender.

Third, action. If you decide you don't want to know, you can always change your mind later. Even if you don't have another ultrasound, the gender will probably be noted in your records—so the trick is to make sure that it is clearly written that you do *not* want to know!

✓ **REALITY CHECK:** Souvenir Ultrasounds

Go to the mall, pay some money out of pocket, and get a 3-D snapshot of your fetus to send to Grandma. Sound good? Walk-in ultrasound businesses are multiplying, often offering imaging in 3-D and 4-D (3-D plus movement, the fourth dimension being time).

I can appreciate the appeal: human curiosity and excitement. I've even seen pregnant ob-gyn residents scan themselves every other day at the hospital in order to watch their babies grow. But since my overall medical philosophy is "less is more," even though I understand the temptation, I have reservations about it. While we have not seen problems with 2-D scans, which are the standard for medical ultrasounds, the long-term risks of long, high-powered scans or frequent scans, especially in 3-D and 4-D, are not known. In 2004 the US Food and Drug Administration issued a statement that ultrasound should not be used solely for entertainment. Also, these ultrasounds are often not done by trained medical personnel and can be misleading in terms of your care. I sometimes see patients who insist their due date must be different based on a walk-in ultrasound finding, or who want to skip an ultrasound altogether because "I just had one at the mall and everything was fine." Your doctor does ultrasound as part of your complete medical evaluation. A walk-in ultrasound in no way replaces the medical ultrasound.

But once you find out, there's no taking the knowledge back. Imagine choosing one way or the other, and live with that choice for a day. Then reverse your decision and live with that. Notice how you feel living with each choice.

Then, re-reflection. Whatever you decide, revisit how you feel about it.

- *Glucose screen*
  Between 24 and 28 weeks, your blood sugar will be tested with a glucose screen, also called a one-hour postprandial glucose test. It involves drinking a glucose solution, usually like a thick,

flat, flavored soda, and having your blood drawn one hour later. Some doctors ask you to fast the night before this test, but it's technically not necessary.

WHY: This is a screening test for gestational diabetes, a pregnancy-induced resistance to insulin found in 1 to 2 percent of all pregnant women. In general, pregnancy creates some degree of insulin resistance in most women. If it causes too *much* insulin resistance, the result is gestational diabetes. Although we aren't sure why some women get it and others don't, those who are older, overweight, or have a family history of diabetes are at heightened risk. These women are also at greater risk for developing diabetes later in life. If untreated, this disease can lead to serious complications for your baby. Treated and managed well, virtually all of the risk can be eliminated.

About 15 percent of women have an abnormal result in their one-hour screening test; this only means that the *possibility* exists that you have gestational diabetes. If your results are abnormal, you will have a diagnostic test as soon as possible. This second test is a three-hour glucose-tolerance test, which does require fasting beforehand. You'll drink a much more concentrated glucose solution, and have your blood-sugar levels checked prior to taking the glucose, and at one-, two-, and three-hour intervals afterward.

(See "Gestational Diabetes" in "Possible Medical Issues Now.")

BLOOD SCREENS, AMNIOCENTESIS, AND SCREENING FOR FETAL ABNORMALITIES

Because two common tests you may be offered fall in the second trimester, please refer back to the discussion of prenatal tests for genetic abnormalities (pages 157–164) and information on how to make a conscious choice about them (pages 164–167).

POSSIBLE MEDICAL ISSUES NOW

Gestational Diabetes

Gestational (pregnancy-induced) diabetes is one of the most common complications of pregnancy, and its management requires a lot of effort on your part. That's the downside. The upside—and it's a big one—is that most cases of gestational diabetes can be managed very effectively, giving you a great deal of control over how well the baby does.

One of the more common risks of gestational diabetes is *macrosomia*, a condition in which the fetus is of excessive size and is built like a sumo wrestler, with more weight distributed across the chest and shoulders. This condition predisposes you to a difficult delivery or an inability to deliver vaginally, because of the possible risk of *shoulder dystocia*—a situation in which the head is delivered but the body cannot follow because the chest and shoulders are so outsized. The baby can be trapped in the birth canal, suffer complications such as nerve damage from a very difficult delivery, or even die. (Babies of nondiabetic mothers can also have shoulder dystocia, just not at the same incidence.) Gestational diabetes also causes an increased risk of intrauterine fetal demise, or fetal death. The risks don't end at birth. Immediately following delivery, the baby's body may have difficulty adjusting blood sugar levels because it has been exposed to the mother's sugar levels. This does not mean the baby will be diabetic.

The key to controlling the risks of gestational or any other kind of diabetes is controlling your blood sugar levels. As long as you keep them within a normal range—which can often be done through just diet and exercise—your baby grows normally and everything's typically fine. You may be referred to a nutritionist to plan appropriate meals, and should eat multiple small meals throughout the day to keep your blood sugar stable. Depending on the degree of insulin resistance, some patients may also require insulin. This is given with injection, and can be given in a variety of regimens. A typical one requires injections three or four times a day. Some studies are now investigating oral agents that could negate the need for insulin in some gestational diabetics.

You'll be responsible for monitoring your blood sugar, just as insulin-dependent diabetics do. The monitoring may be as intensive as seven times a day (before and after each meal and at bedtime).

Though most doctors do not suggest that many checks, you should do whatever your doctor advises. Monitoring your blood sugar is a job you do for your baby's well-being and your own. Take it seriously. Too few people do. A study at the University of Texas at San Antonio gave patients glucose monitors that had a secret memory chip embedded in them that recorded each check. Patients were asked to keep a log of their readings. It was incredible to find that two-thirds of the patients lied about how often they were checking blood sugar and lied about what the values were, making up entries in the logs that didn't match the monitor—just to placate their doctors! That was a scary discovery, because the management of diabetes (for example, the decision of how and when to start someone on insulin) is based on patients' own blood checks. Falsifying these values could really place a woman's baby at risk. Obviously, being conscious about these numbers and sharing them honestly is crucial. If your sugars are high, it does not necessarily mean you are doing anything wrong; it most often means that your insulin resistance is increasing, and your treatment needs to be adjusted accordingly, which often naturally occurs as the pregnancy progresses.

About half of the women who develop gestational diabetes will have abnormal glucose tolerance later in life. Therefore, the American Diabetes Association recommends follow-up testing at the first postpartum checkup, with annual retests from then on even if the first test is normal. The best thing to do, in addition to screening, is to make the recommended lifestyle changes now (or better still, at preconception) and continue them postpartum and beyond. This is the best way to prevent the disease from ever recurring.

Rh-Incompatibility

When a mother's blood type is Rh-negative and a father's blood type is Rh-positive, the possibility of Rh-incompatibility arises. This can occur if the baby's blood is also Rh-positive. If some of the baby's blood intermingles with yours during pregnancy and delivery, amniocentesis, a miscarriage, an abortion, or an ectopic pregnancy, your blood will produce protective Rh-antibodies. This is not a problem in a first pregnancy. But if you have a second pregnancy carrying a baby with Rh-positive blood, these antibodies can cross the placenta and attack the baby's red blood cells. To prevent this, a mom-to-be with Rh-negative blood is given a shot of Rh-immune globulin (RhoGAM) with each pregnancy at 28 weeks, as well as following amniocentesis. RhoGAM is also given following a miscarriage, abortion, or ectopic pregnancy, and after delivery if the baby's blood type is Rh-positive. If this is done, there is no chance for antibodies to form and no risk to future pregnancies. If it is known with 100 percent certainty that the father of the baby is also Rh-negative, however, RhoGAM is not necessary.

Second-Trimester Bleeding

If bleeding occurs in the second trimester it can be worrisome for the mom-to-be, although it doesn't always indicate a serious problem. As in the first trimester, report any spotting, clots, or bleeding to your doctor. Bleeding is of particular concern now because if it is caused by one of the usual suspects behind late-pregnancy bleeding, such as a placental problem or the onset of labor, it can put you at risk for hemorrhage and premature delivery. This is much more problematic in mid-pregnancy, because the baby would be very premature.

(For a complete discussion of possible causes of bleeding, see Chapter 20, "Third Trimester: Medical Care.")

Spotting is sometimes also associated with incompetent cervix (see below).

Incompetent Cervix

Let's set aside for a moment the rude and discouraging name for this rare but difficult problem. ("Incompetent" is strong language for any part of your body.) Cervical incompetence refers to a cervix that is unable to stay closed under the physical pressure of a pregnancy. It thins ("effaces") and opens ("dilates") without contractions and for no apparent reason. This is of course a problem, as you do not want the cervix to open until uterine contractions cause it to open as part of the normal process of labor at term. Cervical incompetence is not common (less than 2 percent of all pregnancies), but it's thought to account for as many as a quarter of all miscarriages in the second trimester.

The cause of this condition is most often unknown. Risk factors that we do know about include: a previous operation on the cervix (such as a large cervical biopsy or conization), cervical damage from a previous delivery, a birth defect (such as from DES exposure), previous second-trimester miscarriage, or carrying multiples.

This premature and covert dilation is usually a slow process. Since there are no contractions to feel and therefore no pain, the mother often notices nothing amiss. But body check-ins can be useful, especially if you are at risk, because even though there are no contractions there may be other signs. These include spotting, a thick vaginal discharge (bloody or mucusy), and a sensation of heaviness or pressure in the lower abdomen or back.

Because checking the cervix (by inserting two fingers in the vagina) is not a particularly pleasant procedure and can introduce problems such as infection, the cervix is not checked routinely at prenatal visits. A somewhat controversial new approach is to measure the cervix during the routine second-trimester ultrasound as a noninvasive way to check its length. The downside is that the results may be unclear or misleading, causing unnecessary worry or even risky intervention.

If a prematurely thinning (effacing) or opening (dilating) cervix is noticed early (for example, you're found to be 2 cm dilated at 22 weeks), the area above the cervix can be sutured closed until delivery. This can help prevent miscarriage or preterm birth and is a surgical procedure known as a *cerclage*. Cerclage is most successful when done early to mid second trimester. This is an invasive procedure, however, and the risk of preterm birth remains high. If you have a cerclage placed, you will be watched carefully immediately following the procedure and for the rest of the pregnancy. Sutures are removed when you approach your due date. A woman who has had incompetent cervix in a prior pregnancy may have a cerclage placed early in the second trimester to hopefully prevent the cervix from dilating prematurely in this pregnancy. Anyone with a history of second-trimester loss may want to discuss cervical measurement by ultrasound with her doctor.

Undergoing a cerclage is bound to create a great deal of anxiety in your life. Since we know that the physiologic response to stress is a factor in contractions and labor, it is important to be proactive about stress-reduction techniques at this time—both prior to the procedure as well as during the entire period when you are facing the possibility of a miscarriage or premature birth. I recommend hypnosis for the procedure itself and suggest to these patients that they consider a wide variety of mind-body strategies for their daily lives.

Preterm Labor (PTL, Also Called Premature Labor)

Many women are more familiar with the image of a preemie—a smaller-than-average baby born before 37 weeks gestation—than they are with premature labor. Preterm labor means having uterine contractions that lead to cervical dilation and effacement before 37 weeks. (Deliveries between 37 and 42 weeks are considered full term.) PTL is more common in the third trimester, but you should be aware of its possibility now because some cases occur late in the second trimester.

PTL does not necessarily mean that the baby will actually be born prematurely. Many women who have preterm labor go on to have a full-term or near-term delivery.

Interestingly, obstetricians have still not figured out an effective way of preventing preterm labor or preterm deliveries. More than one in eight deliveries in the US is preterm, a rate some are calling an epidemic. The amazing science of neonatology is able to save more and more of these premature infants. They are at immediate risk for respiratory illness and other problems. Some, especially those born before 32 weeks, may suffer lifelong complications. And prematurity is still the leading cause of death in newborns without birth defects. On the brighter side, many babies born prematurely catch up to their full-term peers in growth and development by two years of age.

We can't predict who will develop preterm labor. Usually those who do have no known risk factor; anyone can develop it. We do know, though, that women who make certain lifestyle choices experience PTL more often. These include poor nutrition, poor weight gain, smoking, use of drugs or alcohol, and long hours of standing. Other known risk factors include a previous preterm delivery, DES exposure, certain uterine abnormalities, excess amniotic fluid, carrying twins (or more), and obesity. African Americans, those under 17, and those over 35 also have higher rates of PTL. Some PTL is triggered by an underlying cause that can be treated, such as infection.

There's also an established link between prenatal stress and preterm labor. Bizarrely, there has never been research into stress reduction as an intervention to decrease the risk of preterm labor or deliveries! For me, this is one of the most unfortunate examples of the way that modern medicine discounts the mind-body connection. Unlike the drugs commonly used to treat PTL, (none of which have proven to be effective), stress-reduction techniques have no side effects and I believe can have potentially great benefits. At a minimum, stress-reduction techniques can help you cope better and reduce anxiety. Given that the diagnosis of PTL is itself a stress-inducing factor, these approaches are even more critical. It is also possible that by using these techniques, you may have a very real impact on your outcome. (See "Centers of Wellness Strategies for Preterm Labor," box on pages 234 and 235.)

It's not always easy to know if you're in preterm labor. Rather than the strong, rhythmic contractions of full-term labor, you may feel back pain, cramping, pressure, or a sensation that the baby is balled up inside. Diarrhea can also occur. So this is another extremely important reason to stay attuned to what's happening in your body and report anything that seems different or makes you uneasy.

If you do have symptoms, the first thing that will be done is to evaluate you to see if you are actually in preterm labor. If you are, an underlying cause must be sought. While it's true that the cause is often unknown, if PTL has been triggered by a diagnosable condition such as a kidney infection or even a bad UTI, treating the underlying problem is usually easy and will almost always stop the labor. Even something as basic as increasing hydration can sometimes stop contractions. In other cases, preterm labor without a known cause stops on its own and the woman goes on to deliver a healthy full-term baby.

Many times, however, labor progresses. Bed rest or hospitalization with monitoring and sometimes medication are usually advised to try to forestall labor as long as possible. The hope is to create a window of at least 48 hours, so that steroids can be given to the mother in order to speed the maturation of the baby's lungs. The use of steroids has helped to dramatically reduce the complications of premature lungs.

Most people are surprised to learn that there is no proven therapy to postpone preterm labor by more than a couple of days, if that. The drugs often used have varying side effects or risks for the mother, and some for the baby as well. Beta sympathomimetics (such as ritodrine and terbutaline), for example, can cause an increase in fetal heart rate and temporary side effects in the mother such as low potassium and high glucose. Magnesium sulfate appears safe for the fetus but has some side effects for the mother, most often nausea, vomiting, headache, weakness, and shortness of breath.

The bottom line: if you are at risk, be very disciplined about a stress-reduction program, in addition to using the daily and weekly tools recommended. Many pregnant women coping with stress find it useful to work with a psychologist, perhaps one who also does imagery and hypnosis or runs group therapy for women. If your doctor is recommending the use of drugs, be sure to understand the effectiveness of the drug as well as the potential side effects, and make a conscious decision together with your doctor.

CENTERS OF WELLNESS STRATEGIES FOR PRETERM LABOR

Preterm labor patients face a stressful diagnosis and then more stress if they are on hospital bed rest. Try techniques that will help you buffer stress and use the mind to work toward your desired outcome: a healthy delivery.

Here are my recommendations for a woman in such a situation:

Every day:

• Do paced breathing twice daily as well as at any other time you feel stressed or feel contractions or pressure. Follow this with a mental vacation, which is explained in Chapter 4 (page 42).

• Journal. Use a journal to vent all of your emotions, the full spectrum. Often this is the only place where women can truly express all of the feelings they are having, and express just how difficult this situation is for them. What are you feeling—anger, sorrow, frustration, fear? And to whom are your emotions directed—your baby, your body, your partner, God? Describe it all. What you write down does not have to be rational or defensible; it actually helps to start with your least rational feelings and go from there. You want to access the whole range of your feelings, and if you don't start with the scariest ones you run the risk of repressing them and never off-loading them.

• Incorporate movement in some way into your day even if you are on complete bed rest. Examples: body massage, stretching, or progressive muscle relaxation. All of these can be terrific in helping to relieve stress.

• Do Dreamagery or hypnosis. If you work with a professional, he or she can create a tape for you that you can then listen to daily, preferably twice a day.

Every week:
• Tap in to other expressive therapies beyond Journaling that may work well for you. For example, does it help you to pray? To meditate? Just to talk to someone to whom you feel you can say anything? If so, reach out to them on a regular basis.

Before a procedure:
• No procedure is simple when you are anxious and worried about your baby. Even something as "simple" as a nonstress test can create more stress. Do paced breathing and take a mini mental vacation beforehand to help you relax.

Preterm Premature Rupture of Membranes (PPROM)

The breaking of your amniotic sac before the 37th week is a serious matter. The loss of fluid can feel insignificant, almost like the trickle of liquid that's sometimes released when you cough or sneeze. Preterm premature rupture of membranes can also be experienced as a large initial gush with continued leakage afterward, since the fluid is continuously produced. PPROM occurs in about 2 percent of pregnancies.

When this happens, the goal is to give the baby as much chance to mature in the uterus as possible, which means avoiding both labor and infection. It becomes a wait-and-see situation, with mother and baby monitored closely in the hospital. Seventy to 80 percent of women who experience PPROM between weeks 28 and 36 deliver within the first week after it happens, with more than half of those within the first four days.

The earlier PPROM happens, the more agonizing the situation. About 20 percent of those who experience PPROM before 26 weeks' gestation can, however, gain as much as four weeks, which greatly improves their baby's chances of survival. Hospitalization is required, to help prevent infection and to watch for other complications, which can include prolapse of the umbilical cord. This is when the cord slips out of the cervix, which puts it at very high risk for cord compression and can cut off the blood supply to the baby. It requires emergency C-section. Medications given include antibiotics and steroids to help the baby's lungs mature. Daily nonstress tests and weekly fluid checks (using ultrasound to evaluate the amount of amniotic fluid around the baby) are also important aspects of care.

PPROM is a condition of particular interest to me. Much research has demonstrated a link between stress and the onset of labor. A patient with PPROM is in an extremely stressful situation. She knows she's at high risk of delivering prematurely or developing complications such as an infection that again result in a premature delivery. What's more she has suddenly and unexpectedly been hospitalized, requiring her to leave her home, family, and work until she delivers. This could be a matter of weeks or, in some cases, months. And then what? She's told there is nothing she can do except lie there and hope that nothing bad happens (like labor, infection, or fetal distress to name just a few of the little things she should try not to stress about!). And we give her no tools to cope.

At Duke, we're studying the use of mind-body techniques to help reduce stress and prolong such pregnancies. Our thinking is that since approaches such as visualization and meditation have been found to reduce stress outside of pregnancy (in conditions such as hypertension and diabetes), similar results could be achieved during a stressful situation in pregnancy. Given that we know stress increases the risks of preterm labor and weakens the body's ability to fight infection, our hope is to help delay the delivery and allow the baby more time to mature. We teach PPROM patients a variety of the same approaches described in this book, such as checking in with their body, soul, and baby; paced breathing; Journaling as a process to bring their stressors to consciousness and unload them; Dreamagery; and guided imagery and mindful meditation. We also support the woman in transforming a sterile hospital room into a more nurturing environment. (See page 239, "Savannah's Story.") What we're finding anecdotally is that such strategies do seem to alleviate stress and may help delay delivery. More research is needed to understand the real benefits. In the meantime, there is no risk to these approaches and they definitely help the mom. Many of my patients say they would never have been able to stay in the hospital and do what they knew was best for their baby without these stress-relieving strategies.

The example of Jill is typical: At 28 weeks her membranes ruptured and she was hospitalized. Quite knowledgeable and insightful, Jill noted that her body had tried to tell her to take it easy and that she had ignored all of its messages. So now she was in the hospital until she would deliver, which of course we hoped would not be for quite some time. Initially, she was quite chipper. She utilized the tools I've described and was quite receptive to them, especially breathing and Journaling.

Two weeks later, though, Jill hit bottom. "I can't take it anymore," she declared to the nurses. She demanded to go home, even though this was against medical advice. On top of worrying about her baby, she had an 11-year-old son at home who was having a hard time with her being away and she felt her husband, Jim, was unsupportive of her plight. Her family lived several hours from the hospital, which of course made the situation all the harder on everybody.

As she packed, she began to experience some vaginal bleeding. Her body was "screaming" to get her attention, to say that this was not in its best interest. I came in to see her. She herself said that she felt the bleeding, which she had never had before, was her body trying to get her attention. We talked about how the approaches had helped her thus far and I encouraged her to use them more intensively. I asked her about her journal and it turned out she had been writing in it but was using it to give herself the same very upbeat pep talks she gave her husband and her son. I asked her to use it to candidly express what was really in her heart, to say to it what she wouldn't allow herself to say to her family. We talked about how miserable and frightened she was. "I am really scared," she admitted. "I have been trying to hold it together for everyone but it's so hard." After she had shared a lot of her feelings with me, I led her through some guided imagery.

✓ REALITY CHECK: When the Order Is Bed Rest

Bed rest has traditionally been recommended for a host of conditions. It's always necessary with PPROM, because of the risk of cord prolapse, and often recommended for preterm labor (the most common reason), and preeclampsia. It may also be prescribed for women who have incompetent cervix, unexplained bleeding, or who are carrying multiples. And sometimes bed rest is thrown into a list of recommendations as a good thing that "can't hurt," more so that the doctor can feel that all bases have been covered than because of clear medical necessity. Despite its prevalence, surprisingly little hard data have been collected about the usefulness of bed rest. Most existing bed-rest studies have been done on women who were carrying twins—and have yielded mixed results about whether the practice can actually prevent preterm deliveries.

Bed rest may be broadly (and sometimes even cavalierly) prescribed, but for the woman in the bed, it's a hugely significant life event. And it is stressful—the very thing you want to avoid, since it's well-documented that the onset of labor is affected by stress.

If you receive this recommendation, I strongly recommend that you push your care provider to make very clear what is being recommended and why. Ask for specifics. "Bed rest" can mean many different things. It's one thing to have a history of preterm delivery and be told to "try to take it easy" in your last trimester. It's quite another to have preterm premature rupture of membranes at 27 weeks and need to be on bed rest to decrease your risk of cord prolapse and labor. In many of the situations in between, you probably have more choice in the matter than you may think.

Some questions to ask:
What is the rationale for the bed rest?
What is the evidence that it may help? What is the evidence that it may not?
How strongly are you recommending it? (You can even ask on a scale of 1 to 10!)
Exactly what is meant by bed rest—what can you do and what can't you do?
How much bed rest?
What activities are permitted? (Can you get out of bed at all? Have intercourse? Take a shower?)
For how long?

Bed rest is a serious prescription. If it is really necessary, and sometimes it is, you need to know why and understand exactly what is being prescribed so that you can be sure you are doing what is best for you and your baby.

If indeed you are placed on bed rest, there are many steps you can and should take to make this time happier and healthier. My plan for this is outlined in "Centers of Wellness Strategies for Preterm Labor," on pages 234–235.

The bed rest continued to be very difficult for her, but she agreed that it was crucial and went back to the practices that had helped her before. She also began writing what she felt rather than what she thought she should feel, and the journal played an important role in keeping her sane and determined. Two weeks later she delivered a premature but otherwise healthy son. She also had a smooth postpartum transition and both mom and baby are now doing well. She feels that the tools she used during her four weeks of bed rest gave her a more intimate relationship with her body, her soul, and her baby than she would ever have had without them. And while it was hard, she is very grateful for the experience.

Our hope is that as we research the impact of these approaches in PPROM patients, we will prove that such therapies can not only help the mother to cope better, but may also significantly improve outcomes. If this is the case, these approaches could be applied to the broader population of women at risk for preterm labor and delivery. I love to think of the day when every pregnant woman receives instruction in these techniques as standard medical practice, and is offered more intensive approaches if she develops any of these complications.

Savannah's Story: Surroundings Matter

After two years of fertility treatments, Savannah was pregnant for the first time, with twins. She had been on hospital bed rest for three weeks already because her membranes ruptured and her water started leaking. I was brought in to consult with her because she was demanding to be discharged. "I feel fine," she insisted. "I'm tired of just sitting here. I want to go home and wait for labor." She was now 30 weeks pregnant, and as with any woman with premature preterm ruptured membranes there's a risk of infection and other complications, so she needed to stay in the hospital. I asked her to talk to me about *why* she was wanting to leave. On probing, she told me that she didn't feel that the doctors (or anyone else) understood how hard it was to be on strict bed rest.

I looked around the room. It was so stark you would have thought she had just been admitted. There were no personal items, no photos, no blanket or pillow from home, no music, no flowers, no appealing scents such as those from aromatherapy, nothing at all to reduce the clinical atmosphere and make it a place remotely appealing to live in day after day. As I discussed the power of the mind-body connection with her, and why changes in her environment could make a significant difference in how she felt about being there, she shared more of her feelings of isolation and distress. Her mother visited whenever her partner could not, but she didn't feel comfortable talking to either of them about her distress. I talked to her about using a journal to express the feelings that she was reluctant to share, so that she had an outlet for them whenever she needed it.

Savannah was frustrated because she felt helpless. Understandably, she wasn't aware of how much influence she could have over this situation and how many ways there were to make it more bearable. Her favorite parts of the treatment plan I outlined included the Journaling, which allowed her to express her anxieties to a nonjudgmental party (the paper), and bringing CDs and items from home to make her space more inviting. She agreed to remain in the hospital until her babies were born, and she delivered three weeks later. Both mother and babies did well.

Preeclampsia (Toxemia, or Pregnancy-Induced Hypertension)

Preeclampsia is most common in the third trimester, but can develop in the second. A kind of hypertension that affects all the body's organs, this serious complication is being seen more and more often, and we don't know why or what causes it. The earlier in pregnancy it occurs, the more severe form it tends to take. That's why you should be alert for changes that may be symptoms of preeclampsia.

Signs of preeclampsia include headache, swelling of the face or hands, sudden rapid weight gain, visual disturbances, and pain in the right upper part of your abdomen. Tell your doctor if you experience these symptoms. If you do have this disease, close monitoring is required, including bed rest and possibly hospitalization. There is no "cure" for preeclampsia other than the delivery of the baby, but in many cases it remains mild for weeks, enabling the fetus to grow and mature.

(See "Preeclampsia," pages 289–293.)

CENTERS OF WELLNESS STRATEGIES FOR BED REST

In addition to the preterm labor measures listed earlier, it's important to intentionally send signals of comfort and safety to your body, soul, and baby. There's probably no more important time to create and achieve a very clear self-care plan across all your basic Centers of Wellness.

• Mind: The Mind tools described in the daily plan can go a long way toward easing your stress and therefore improving your baby's odds of a safe delivery and good health. Use them often.

• Nutrition: Get clear about what you enjoy and need, and communicate this to those who are taking care of your food. Look into grocery delivery services or restaurants and supermarkets with delicious premade meals-to-go to help make food preparation easier for your caregivers. Indulge yourself with modest treats as a pick-me-up.

• Movement: Don't overlook this center simply because you are lying in bed. Find out exactly what limitations you have. Most women can still do stretching. Even repetitive isometric contractions of muscle groups can make your body feel more alive and grounded.

- Spirit: Make sure that the people who visit you are those to whom you have a real connection. Perhaps you can arrange for distant friends or relatives who fall into this category to visit you now, rather than waiting until the baby is born. To find a community of women in similar situations to yours, look into online chat groups for women on bed rest. (One to try: sidelines.org.) Get books or poetry or tapes that nurture your spiritual life, have a Bible or other spiritual or religious writings on hand if appropriate to you.

- Sensation: Create an environment that feeds all of your senses. If you will be on bed rest for a prolonged length of time, change the ways you stimulate and soothe your senses from time to time. Vary the scents and music to which you are exposed. Change the fabrics on your bed (new sheets, a different blanket) and on your body (pajamas, bed jacket, shawl) periodically. This creates a healing environment that helps decrease that cabin-fever feeling.

Chapter 17

Second Trimester: Self-Care

∞

Centers of Wellness modifications for weeks 14 to 28

You may find yourself especially energized, motivated, and involved about self-care this trimester. If this is true for you, use this time to review what's worked well for you so far and whether there are new things you'd like to try.

Continue to aim for the goals in the Basic Self-Care Plan in Chapter 4, with the following modifications:

THE MIND CENTER

In addition to continuing to incorporate mind-body approaches into your day, you may discover new ways to apply breathing and other centering techniques, such as the following:

- *During your daily relaxation breaks, do your kick counts.* Focus on the presence of your baby and its movements. That way, the important work of monitoring your baby's movement becomes part of your routine.

- *Use breathing exercises before tests or procedures (or anytime you're feeling anxious).* You can mentally prepare yourself for the sometimes unnerving prospect of having a prenatal test or a procedure, whether it's amniocentesis, the glucose tolerance test, having blood drawn, or even an ultrasound. Do some of the breathing exercises or another mind-body approach you've found helpful both before and after the experience.

✓REALITY CHECK: Childbirth Education

I think childbirth preparation is a great idea. Knowledge really is power when it comes to labor and delivery. Childbirth preparation classes generally cover the mechanics of labor and delivery and how to use your mind, your body, and labor supports to ease pain, optimize your experience, and participate fully in labor. Women who have taken childbirth courses tend to have slightly shorter and less painful labors, perhaps because they have a better idea about what to expect. Their training gives them great confidence and helps them to work with their bodies better during contractions. Your partner will also learn what to expect and practical ways to play a supportive role in labor.

I don't have a particular preference whether my patients take Lamaze, Bradley, or the generic course offered at the hospital that covers basics. Classes reflect different birth philosophies, formats, and teaching styles, which suit people differently. What's important is simply to take a course which you are drawn to that familiarizes you with the basics of childbirth and offers a few tools for helping to work with your body.

Start exploring your options now. Ideally you should start the class in your seventh or eighth month, depending on its duration. Some classes meet weekly over the course of a couple of months, and you want to wind up your sessions several weeks before your due date. (Remember that you may go into full-term labor two or three weeks before your due date.)

To find a course that's right for you, ask around. Get recommendations from friends who have recently given birth, from your care provider, or from the hospital where you plan to deliver. Your doctor or midwife may have suggestions, or you can ask at your local hospital or contact the International Childbirth

Educators Association (ICEA), which certifies instructors and can identify those in your area (see www.icea.org).

In making a choice, you will want to consider the course schedule, class size (five to seven couples is ideal), and the instructor's personality and philosophy on childbirth. Some classes (and individual teachers) are more oriented toward natural drug-free delivery than others.

The most common types of childbirth preparation are:

• Lamaze. This method portrays birth as a natural process and emphasizes breathing exercises and relaxation for pain management. The most common medical interventions and medical forms of pain relief are also usually covered in Lamaze classes. There's no single Lamaze class format, so the individual teacher sets the tone.

• Bradley. This method prepares women for the goal of natural childbirth through emphasis on nutrition and exercise during pregnancy and deep-breathing work as well as the active participation of the partner as an integral player during labor. (Bradley used to be known as "husband-coached delivery.") Reportedly 90 percent of Bradley trainees go on to have drug-free deliveries.

• Other methods. Hypnosis can be used to reduce pain in childbirth and speed labor; some hypnotherapists teach courses focused on labor and delivery. You can also find hospital-based hypnosis programs or those sponsored by health organizations or other groups.

As you check out the various class offerings in your area, run the other way if you come across someone touting their particular philosophy of childbirth with near-religious zeal. This is a red flag, even if the teacher is credible and the curriculum valid. When the message is delivered with that kind of you-must-do-it-this-way urgency, there's no room to make the process your own—which is what being truly conscious during labor is all about. A rigid program (requiring you to breathe an exact way, refuse all drugs, and so on) is a prescription for unconscious be-havior, because it doesn't take *you* into account.

The whole point of childbirth preparation should be to em-power you, not to intimidate you.

Once you choose a class, keep checking in with yourself about it. Is it working for you? If so, great. If not, explore why. Sometimes people stick with something that's not right for them because they think that changing midcourse suggests in-stability or a failure to commit themselves wholeheartedly to the well-being of the baby. My take is that you can learn from lots of different approaches—so if you don't like the class you're enrolled in, look for something else. For example, some Lamaze-style classes, which teach relaxation and breathing, may be too elementary for a woman who has meditated her entire life; yet other Lamaze classes might be a blast and a boon to that same woman, depending on the instructor, the other students in the class, and her alignment with the group. That's another reason to start checking out options now—to give yourself plenty of time to find a course you click with.

Rarely, a woman may find that childbirth classes add to her stress rather than relieve it. If this is true for you, ask yourself why, and give yourself permission to leave if you are comfort-able.

THE NUTRITION CENTER

Nutrition is one of the most changeable centers in pregnancy. As you approach the halfway point (week 20), it's a good time to take stock of how things are working for you and what kind of fine-tuning is in order.

• *Notice your food and eating preferences now and how they have changed from the first trimester.* Are you better able to tolerate certain flavors or smells that were previously difficult? Do you crave any-thing? How has your appetite changed?

• *Switch to multiple smaller meals.* As your stomach begins to be compressed by the growing fetus, it can't hold as much food as previously. Rather than eating three main meals each day, try dividing them into four to six mini-meals. Digestion also takes longer now.

• *Drink water throughout the day.* Some women like to fill a two-and-a-half-quart pitcher in the morning and drink from it throughout the day. If it's empty by the end of the day, they know they're drinking enough. Others carry portable sports bottles or bottled waters (flavored or plain) with them wherever they go.

• *Be conscious of your weight gain and adjust your food intake accordingly.* If nausea and vomiting were a problem for you, you may not have gained much weight in the first trimester (or you may even have lost a few pounds); pay careful attention to sticking with desirable gains now. If, on the other hand, you gained too much during the first trimester, don't diet your way back to a normal curve, but do pay attention to how this happened. Have you unconsciously been "eating for two"? Noshing nervously? Think about how you can make better food choices so that you don't continue to overgain the rest of pregnancy. Use the mindful-eating tools described on pages 43–55.

> FEAR: I look so fat!
> FACT: Your shape is changing, but it's not flab. Reframe the way you see yourself by banishing this kind of false labeling from your mental vocabulary. The pregnant shape is beautiful: Your body is gearing up for a remarkable thing—a new life! Celebrate your body for its bounty.

THE MOVEMENT CENTER

Take advantage of the wonderful energy and "bloom" you're likely to feel during these three months. But don't overdo it. Your body, even if it's feeling great, is undergoing enormous changes that you need to respect.

• *Avoid lying on your back.* After the fourth month of pregnancy, when you lie on your back you will be putting the entire weight of your growing uterus on the vein that returns blood from the lower body to the heart, thus decreasing the flow of blood back out to the body, including the uterus, to the heart and possibly lowering your blood pressure.

• *Listen to your body.* Do a Body Scan before you exercise. How does your changing body feel right now? Are there any places that need extra TLC? Your body will tell you how far you can go; take care not to override its message.

• *Listen to your doctor's recommendations about limits on your physical activity.* These restrictions may be related to problems such as incompetent cervix, placenta previa, pregnancy-induced hypertension, or sometimes to a multiple-birth situation. Or they may simply be restrictions that your doctor feels are appropriate to this stage of pregnancy.

• *Avoid high-risk sports.* Even if you're a longtime participant, now's the time to find replacements for recreational sports that put you at risk for: falls or abdominal kicks (soccer, gymnastics, basketball, downhill skiing, vigorous tennis or racquetball); for accidents due to a shifting center of balance (gymnastics); or for changes in air pressure (scuba diving, mountaineering).

• *Avoid extreme movements.* As your pregnancy progresses, ligaments loosen and stretch, placing your joints at risk of injury. To prepare to lift something heavy, plant your feet apart and lower your body by bending at the knees rather than the waist. Push from your thigh muscles, not your back, as you lift. Never twist your body while lifting. And don't overdo it.

• *Watch your weights.* If you do strength training switch to lighter weights, because the hormone relaxin makes your ligaments looser and places joints at greater risk of injury. Weight machines are generally safer than free weights, because they make it easier to maintain proper balance and posture.

• *Watch your balance.* As your center of gravity shifts, you may find it difficult or impossible to safely maintain certain yoga poses, to ride a bicycle, or to walk in very high-heeled shoes, among other activities. Take precautions and lower your heel height by an inch or two.

• *Stretch your legs to avoid muscle cramps.* Pay attention to your calves and feet. Take breaks so that you're not sitting or standing in one position for a long time. To relieve a cramp, straighten your leg and flex your foot upward, then pull your toes toward your head. Report persistent painful leg cramps to your doctor; rarely, they can be a sign of a clot.

• *Realize that you may feel more clumsy and drop things more often.* Loosened joints and water retention can affect your grasp and make you feel all thumbs.

WARNING SIGNS

Stop exercising and get medical attention if you experience any of the following:

- vaginal bleeding
- shortness of breath before exercise begins
- dizziness
- headache
- chest pain
- muscle weakness
- calf pain or swelling
- contractions
- decreased fetal movement
- leaking vaginal fluid

THE SPIRIT CENTER

Use this quiet time of pregnancy to lay groundwork for the future.

• *Reflect on the meaning of this transition in your life.* Explore what it may mean in your life to go from woman to mother, wife to mother, professional to mother. Explore how stepping into that identity will feel and how it may reshape the other roles you play. You can write about it, use Dreamagery (invite an image that represents you as

"Mommy"), or ask other women who have children to reflect honestly on these transitions with you. How does being pregnant shift your perception of yourself and your place in the world?

• *Set boundaries to protect yourself.* Pregnancy is a time that invites a lot of unwelcome conversations and unwanted advice. That's why it's wise to be conscious of who you spend time with. Notice who fuels you, and who drags you down. I believe that being around negative energy—people who drain you or conversations that make you anxious—can have a very real impact on your well-being. Give yourself permission to make conscious choices about those relationships that sap your energy. Do you still want to maintain them? If not, have the courage to drop them. If you decide to continue them, then be sure to set boundaries around the interchanges with them. Choose when and how much time you want to spend with someone who "pushes your buttons." Use a mind-body technique such as paced breathing before the interchange, and after. This simple act can help isolate the energy and emotions that may be stirred, so you don't carry them around within you. Setting boundaries doesn't make you rude; it makes you strong and proactive about your health. As life coach Cheryl Richardson says, practice saying "no" with grace and love.

THE SENSATION CENTER

Notice what is shifting for you now. Are you finding different smells and textures appealing? What about your sexual side?

• *Acquire some maternity clothes that you love.* Out of necessity, pulling together a maternity wardrobe usually involves borrowing or buying basics to see you through the coming months. There are so many great choices available today that you needn't sacrifice style for maternity. If you feel like hiding your condition under sacks for the next six months; explore why that is and experiment with clothes that reveal it proudly. Splurge on a gorgeous pair of shoes a half size larger to accommodate your swollen or spreading feet. Accessorize with shawls or scarves you really love. Make one of your maternity tops something lively and outrageous—leopard print, shocking

pink—so you can reach for it to perk you up when you're feeling
blah.

• *Notice if you are feeling an increase in your libido, and if so, fuel it!*
Since many women feel hypersexual in the second trimester, and
more easily orgasmic, this is a great time to have fun and share increased intimacy with your partner. Plan a bed day, where you and
your partner block out everything else for 24 hours alone together,
and fill it with all of the things you love. Get movies, music, foods,
all the things you like, and then enjoy: It's like having a mini-
"babymoon" (a second honeymoon before the baby) without leaving
home.

• *Try different intercourse positions to accommodate your belly.* For
most women, being on top provides both comfort and the ability to
control the depth of penetration. Rear-entry positions (with the
woman on all fours, or lying side-by-side in a spooning position) also
avoid placing any pressure on the abdomen. Remember you can't
hurt the baby; it's a question of what's comfortable for you.

• *Whatever your sexual inclinations, don't neglect sexual time.* Sex is
part of the glue of a relationship, and if that relationship is strained
during pregnancy (as many are), sexual time can help you and your
partner stay close. Build "skin time" into your week, whether or not
your activities include intercourse. Many pregnant women find that
they like to be touched and held now, and many men find their partner's swelling breasts and belly, as well as other skin and hair changes,
to be incredibly sexy. Enjoy this.

FEAR: Orgasm can trigger miscarriage or labor.
FACT: The uterine contractions that occur in orgasm are different
       from those that trigger labor. Even an intense orgasm isn't
       going to start labor in a body not otherwise ready for it (i.e.,
       a normal pregnancy).

Part Five

The Third Trimester

Weeks 29 to 40

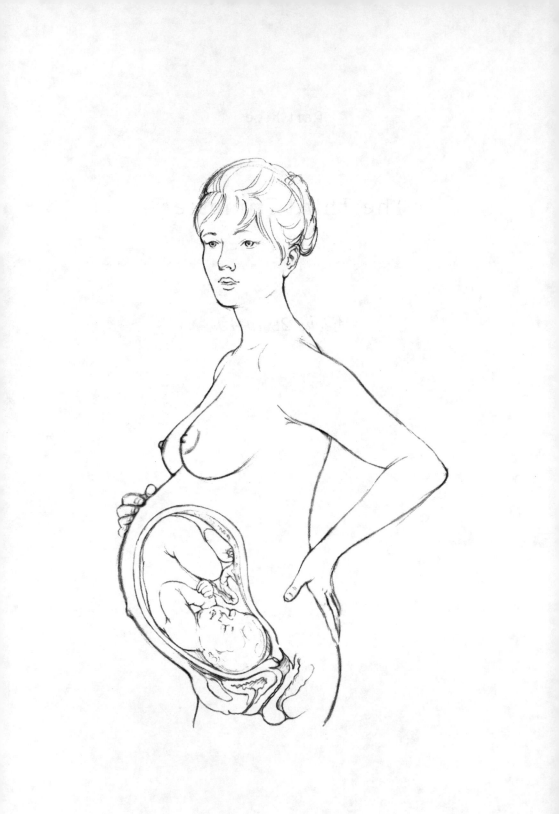

Chapter 18

Third Trimester: Reflection and Observation

∞

Checking in with body, soul, and baby, weeks 29 to 40

Developing the practice of paying attention during the first parts of pregnancy really pays off in the home stretch. If you are in tune with yourself now, it will help you to:

- be on "first alert" for physical changes that could signal problems
- prepare mentally and physically for labor
- identify signs of labor
- prepare for the imminent transition to motherhood
- bond with your soon-to-be-born baby.

Often the physical and emotional changes of this stage are written off as "just part of being pregnant." Feeling crampy? "Oh, that's just part of being pregnant," you might be told. Feeling weepy? "That's just part of being pregnant," you think. A conscious approach, in contrast, recognizes that these experiences aren't insignificant things to be ignored. Pregnancy consists of many, many incremental changes that reflect the incredibly dynamic process of reproduction. Recognizing them and paying attention to them, rather than dismissing them, allows you to reap some benefit from their presence. Cramps become not an annoyance, but a possible sign of labor, for example. An increased puffiness in your face could be the first signal of preeclampsia. Noticing changes in the way your baby moves can help you know when labor is near, or whether your baby needs to be evaluated. Resting when you feel fatigued can play a role in lowering your risk of preterm labor.

Paying attention allows you to influence the outcome—a healthy baby, a healthy you, a labor experience you feel great about, a joyful and rewarding transition to motherhood. If those aren't great reasons to pay attention, I don't know what is. Turning your attention to the things that cause you to weep can help you reveal underlying concerns or fears you may not have been aware of.

A SPECIAL KIND OF AWARENESS: FETAL MOVEMENT

Now that your baby takes up most of the available space in your uterus, its movements begin to change. In mid-pregnancy you probably noticed flutters, dramatic flips, and rapid movements. Now the movements feel more restricted—a poke or kick, for example. These sensations are the result of wriggling and stretching as opposed to the earlier out-and-out somersaulting, because the more the baby grows, the less space there is for doing the big flips! You may even be able to feel with your hand or see the contour of a rump or a foot. The frequency of movements is unchanged from the second trimester. By the very end of pregnancy, when the fetus assumes the usual delivery-ready head-down position and the head engages in the pelvis, there is still another change in movement. It becomes more localized and less varied (you might feel the same foot in the same place every time, for example), but you will still feel the movements. It's a myth that babies "stop moving" when they're ready to be born. The movements do become smaller, but they are still easy to detect.

Your baby won't move all the time, however. Fetuses sleep. They also have periods of lower activity and higher activity. A fetus is typically more active when blood sugar is low—that is, right before you eat. You may notice more movement in the evening simply because this is when you are still and less distracted by other things.

Studies show that in the third trimester, the fetus spends 10 percent of its time making large body movements (kicks, rolls, big stretches)—up to 30 an hour! By late pregnancy, you can feel about three-fourths of these large movements. Your baby is also flexing muscles, grasping, suckling, and making many other smaller motions that you cannot feel. Periods of fetal activity last about 40 minutes and quiet periods generally last about 20 minutes, but can stretch as long as 75 minutes. Unfortunately for your sleep, this inner action tends to peak between 9 PM and 1 AM. Fetal hiccups are another baby-related event you may notice. They feel like a persistent, rhythmic, slight sensation—like you're hiccuping on the inside. They are not a cause for concern.

Remember, good fetal movement is the sign of a healthy baby, and changes in fetal movement can be the first sign that a baby is not doing well.

THE KICK COUNT

Beginning in your 28th week, monitoring your baby's movement is one of the most valuable things you can do. There are many different ways to do kick counts; one way is not more right than another. Here is my recommendation for how to do it:

- Sit still and free from distractions.
- Count every movement you feel your baby make until you reach 10, which usually happens pretty quickly, though it can take up to an hour.
- Call your care provider if you feel fewer than 10 movements per hour, or no movement at all during any 12-hour period. Your doctor may want to do some tests, such as fetal monitoring, to confirm fetal well-being.
- Do your kick count three times a day. Just before each meal is a good time to do it, because fetal movements tend to increase when blood sugars are low. Once you are familiar with your own baby's rhythms, feel free to do kick counts whenever you know the baby is most likely to be active. Check with your care provider to see what kick-count method she prefers.

CHECK IN WITH YOUR BODY

Especially on a physical level this trimester, problems can be caught early and disasters avoided when a woman is paying attention. In fact, since you're with yourself 24/7, you are in a better position than your doctor to monitor such key aspects of late pregnancy as fetal movement (an assurance that everything is okay); swelling of your hands and face, headaches, or visual changes (all possible danger signs of preeclampsia); contractions (possible sign of preterm labor or labor); and leaking fluid (possible sign of preterm premature rupture of membranes, or PPROM, if it happens before week 37 and prior to labor); as well as backache, shifts in your energy level, and changes in vaginal discharge.

To be sure, cultivating awareness can't prevent problems from occurring. But because it enables you to detect the earliest signs of a possible problem, you can enlist help swiftly, if needed, and possibly prevent a small or controllable event from escalating into something dangerous. By the very end of pregnancy, of course, paying attention also helps you recognize labor. Throughout this trimester, listening to your body can help you be more responsive to its day-to-day needs.

Detailed descriptions of how to use these tools can be found in Chapter 3.

SUGGESTED TOOLS:

DAILY:

Kick Counts (see box above)

Body Quick Pic (tool #1)
Continue to use this tool together with the Soul Quick Pic and the Baby Quick Pic, periodically throughout the day to keep the incredible dynamism of your state at the front of your consciousness.

Body Monitoring/Body Scan combination (tools #4 and #2)
These tools can be a lifesaver in the third trimester—literally. That's why it should now be used every day. Start with the Body Scan to get a snapshot of any physical sensations, then follow with the

Body Monitoring tool. Together they provide a solid, intimate picture of your physical state.

In addition to what you usually cover during Body Monitoring, pay particular attention to:

- *Your face and hands.* Do they seem puffier than usual? If yes, make your doctor aware of this. You know what's normal for you better than your doctor, who sees you only periodically. Monitor changes from week to week and day to day. Also smart: Get the opinion of someone who knows you well, like a family member or trusted coworker. Have they noticed any significant changes in your face recently?

WHY PAY ATTENTION: While some swelling in pregnancy is normal—especially "dependent edema" or puffiness in the feet and ankles, which happens because gravity causes the additional fluid in your system to pool down below—nondependent edema, as in the face, can be a sign of preeclampsia.

- *Any involuntary leaking of fluid.*

WHY PAY ATTENTION: When your membranes rupture, or your "bag of water breaks," fluid doesn't necessarily come out in a flood. You may notice only a slight trickling that can be mistaken for urine or discharge—and there is no way you can tell the difference. Let your doctor know so that you can get a professional assessment of what's going on. Don't wait, because a rupture or even a leak in the membranes of the amniotic sac sets up the possibility of infection, which can be perilous to the fetus.

- *Your belly, uterus, and fetus.* In addition to monitoring your baby's movements, pay attention to your midsection more generally. Notice the shape of your abdomen and how the baby feels inside your uterus. How are you carrying it—does it feel lower than before?

WHY PAY ATTENTION: Can you feel or see your belly becoming intermittently taut? Known as Braxton-Hicks contractions, this sensation reflects your uterus having "practice contractions." The uterus tightens and then relaxes, which you feel as a temporary hardness across your belly. They can last from 30 seconds to two minutes and are the body's way of rehearsing for labor. But they are not a sign that you are *in* labor. Braxton-Hicks contractions are usually painless and disappear when you shift position, and they lack a rhythmic pattern. (See "True or False Labor?" on page 369 in Chapter 24.) Braxton-Hicks contractions help the cervix thin and prepare for labor but are not strong enough to trigger labor. Some women notice them for weeks, some only right before labor, others not at all. If Braxton-Hicks contractions develop into a regular pattern, even if they remain painless, they may signal the beginning of preterm labor and will need to be evaluated immediately. Paying attention to your abdomen can also provide a snapshot of fetal movement throughout the day, and prompt you to do kick counts if you feel you haven't noticed movement.

- *Your back—and backaches.*

WHY PAY ATTENTION: If you have persistent lower-back pain, tell your doctor. It's probably just the normal but uncomfortable result of the loosening of the musculature that supports a straight back, which occurs so that the weight of the growing belly can be counterbalanced by a sway-backed posture. But if the back pain comes and goes in a rhythmic pattern, report this immediately. Your doctor can then evaluate you for preterm labor. This involves monitoring the uterus to determine whether your back pain is in fact originating in the subtle contractions of your uterus rather than in your back. Sometimes the only symptom of preterm labor is lower-back pain.

- *Headaches or visual disturbances.*

WHY PAY ATTENTION: Severe headaches, or those that don't get better with Tylenol, should be evaluated as they can be associated with preeclampsia. The same is true of migraine-like auras or other visual disturbances.

- *Pelvic sensations.*

WHY PAY ATTENTION: Any significant change, such as an increase in pelvic pressure or mild cramping before your due-date window, can be a sign of labor, including premature labor. This is an especially dynamic area now.

AS NEEDED:

Dialoguing (with Your Physical Self) (tool #3)

Use this tool whenever something comes up in your body checks that you want to go into further, as in the stories that follow.

***

FEAR: My puffy feet and ankles are a sign of preeclampsia.

FACT: Swollen feet are common in pregnancy because gravity causes the added fluids in your system to accumulate there, especially after you've been standing or walking awhile. They're little cause for alarm unless accompanied by swelling in your face and hands, or if the swelling doesn't start to go down after putting your feet up for an hour.

BODY CHECKS:
WHAT MIGHT COME UP FOR YOU

Enough Already! When Will This Be Over?

Some time toward the middle or end of the last trimester, most women experience a shift from the vitality of mid-pregnancy to the unmistakable bigness and slowness of late pregnancy. Even the most upbeat and reveling-in-my-condition woman can have moments of thinking, "Enough, already!"

A sense of impatience for delivery day rises pretty naturally from the cumulative effects of carrying extra weight, having difficulty bending over or rising from a chair, and being awakened by frequent bathroom runs and an inability to get comfortable—as well as your desire to hold this baby in your arms and begin the next phase of motherhood!

My Baby's Not Moving!

This is the kind of distress call that always puts a doctor on high alert. Mia, 31, in her ninth month, called my office to report that she had not felt the baby move in the past 24 hours. As worrisome as such a message is, and as much as I would have preferred she called much sooner, I was glad that she hadn't waited any longer. The alternative scenario is all too common: a patient comes in for a routine weekly checkup and during a check of the baby's heartbeat, there is nothing. "When did you last feel the baby move?" I'll ask such a patient.

"I'm not sure," comes the answer.

"Did you feel it in the last 24 hours?"

"I'm not sure."

"Did you feel it yesterday?"

"Gee, I don't know."

I told Mia to come to my office immediately. By the time she arrived, I could tell from the look on her face and the way her arms caressed her belly that she had begun detecting movement again. "I was so worried this morning when I realized I had gone all day yesterday without noticing anything," she confessed. "It was a really busy day at work and I sort of skipped my kick counts. When I didn't feel anything the first time, I just put it off until later. But that evening I didn't feel anything. Jim said not to worry and I was so tired, I didn't. Then I slept unusually soundly and when I woke up, I realized I couldn't even remember when the last big kick had been. That's when I called.

"But while I was getting dressed, I felt strong kicking, like a leg reaching out and stretching down my side. I felt better but I still wanted to come in and be sure."

I could hear the heart beating at a normal rate. We did a non-stress test on Mia just to be sure the baby was doing well, and it was. I reassured her she had been right to come in, and emphasized that next time—though hopefully there wouldn't be a next time—she should not wait 24 hours.

A third-trimester fetal death is one of the most awful events in obstetrics. Although we don't know the reason for every case, sometimes it can be what's referred to as a "cord accident." Cord accidents include situations where the umbilical cord either wraps around the baby's neck (a nuchal cord), or forms a knot that isn't a problem in earlier pregnancy when there's still plenty of room for the baby to move around, but then later can tighten and cut the blood supply to the baby. Neither condition is necessarily fatal to the fetus. I have delivered innumerable healthy babies with a nuchal cord or a true knot. Other potentially serious complications that can arise in the third trimester include problems with the placenta and certain genetic disorders.

The earlier we get an indication of a possible problem the better. And your own ability to tune in is the best possible early-warning system. If you begin to notice decreased movements, it's extremely important to let your caregiver know. Though the chances are good that nothing is wrong, if the baby does appear to be compromised, labor can be induced; if the baby is in distress and needs to be delivered immediately, an emergency C-section can be performed. Mia's story illustrates why kick counts are so valuable. If you do them often and regularly, you'll be quick to notice if there is a decrease in movement or no movement at all.

If the baby seems abnormally still, shift your activity (if you're seated, stand up and walk around) or eat something and see whether the baby responds. These actions sometimes make a difference. If you still feel no response, let your doctor monitor the baby to confirm that all is well.

CHECKING IN WITH YOUR SOUL

SUGGESTED TOOLS

DAILY:

Soul Quick Pic (tool #5)
Don't be surprised if you pick up very different readings from day to day, or even within a day, when you do this exercise. There is a lot going on in the third trimester, not just in your growing body but within you—who you are, how you see yourself, and how others see you. Explore the things that come up on a Soul Quick Pic more deeply in your journal or through Dialoguing.

ANYTIME, AT LEAST ONCE IN THIRD TRIMESTER:

Journaling Your Journey (tool #6)

Labor and parenthood—two incredible experiences—are right around the corner. Take some time to contemplate them as they approach. In your journal, explore the following:

- What do you most look forward to as labor approaches?
- What are your greatest fears about labor?
- What brings you the greatest joy as you think about becoming a mother?
- What are your greatest fears about motherhood?
- Reflect on your partner as a father. What hopes and expectations come to mind about his new role and your relationship as parents?
- What are your greatest fears about your partner as a father and the impact that having a child may have on your relationship?

These are deceptively simple questions. Because they get at the heart of a truly huge and magical life transition, they're a great way to bring to the surface feelings that can easily be repressed. If the feelings aren't acknowledged, they will often find other ways to express themselves. For example, fears about the kind of father your partner will be can result in "unexplained" irritation with him. Or unaddressed fear around labor or your own transition to motherhood can surface as the blues, as generalized anxiety, or as increased physical symptoms (heartburn, back pain, headaches, and so on).

Dialoguing (with Your Nonphysical Self) (tool #7)

Because Dialoguing is a wonderful way to explore a symptom or problem more deeply, and because fears can be rife in the third trimester, pick one of your fears to Dialogue with. Examples: fear of labor pain, fear you won't know how to take care of your baby, fear of being a bad mother, or fear of not bonding with your baby.

SOUL CHECKS:
WHAT MIGHT COME UP FOR YOU

I'm Not Just Having a Baby—I'm Becoming a Mother!

Chloe is excited, involved, and *aware*. For her, pregnancy has been everything she'd dreamed, and more. "She even liked morning sickness," her partner, Stephen, says good-naturedly. Indeed, Chloe has really blossomed across all eight months of pregnancy. She kicked a sporadic smoking habit six months before she conceived. She's made small diet and exercise changes to further support the baby's health, taken up yoga as a way to unwind and relax, and joined an online support group of other women slated to deliver in the same month. She even has her nursery fully furnished and decorated, right down to a stack of pastel onesies in the bureau drawers.

Lately, though, Chloe has become aware of a subtle change in the focus of her preparations. "For a whole year before I got pregnant and all through it so far, all my focus has been on one thing—bringing home a healthy little baby," she explains. "And of course that's still Priority Number One. But lately I've been thinking that if I have an actual baby in my arms then I am a mother. Me!"

How can this be such a startling realization this late in the game? Intellectually, of course, we understand that giving birth to a child makes us mothers. But "mother" is a huge concept. It represents a dramatic change in our place in the universe, our day-to-day life, our self-image, and in the way others view us. Pregnancy is such an all-enveloping experience for a woman that it's not surprising that it leaves little space for focusing on the life change that awaits us at the end of it. Adjusting to the reality of oneself as a pregnant woman is such a big shift in and of itself that reflecting on actually becoming a mother takes a backseat.

Frequently the mental transition to motherhood is expressed as a fear: *How will I know what to do? How will I know how to hold it or feed it or stop its crying?* These can be very real worries if you, like millions of today's moms, live far from extended families and have children later in life and don't have much experience around babies. There you are, soon to deliver, with no turning back. The baby is less a figment of your imagination and more a very real creature who will depend on you for everything. That's big!

Chloe's dawning awareness of the momentousness of this change is natural and very healthy. As you prepare for delivery and begin to integrate this shift from pregnant woman to mother into your identity, how does your soul redefine itself? How will the essence of who you are change when it goes through the crucible of one of the most significant, life-altering experiences that will ever happen to you?

Chloe spent time Journaling about her concerns as well as her fantasies about what motherhood would be like. She also began asking her friends who had children how this transition had felt for them. She was thrilled to discover that most of them had plenty to say about the fears they too had felt during pregnancy and the surprising confidence they soon felt as new moms. Simply by diving into these fears, rather than running from them, Chloe was able to feel much less anxiety and much more excitement.

Will I Be Able to Love My Baby My Way?

A different sort of fear may arise concerning your emotions toward this future baby, specifically, the key parental emotion of unconditional love. Tai, 28, expressed this fear as "Will I be able to love my baby the way I want to?"

"Can you say more about what you mean?" I asked. She said she couldn't put it into words. I asked her to Journal about her concern and reflect on all the emotions that surfaced.

For many women, their fears are rooted in their relationship to their own mother. Beginning usually in the third trimester, and intensifying after delivery, such issues often become magnified. You may find yourself feeling unreasonably irritated with your parents or agitated by thoughts of events from the past, even if your parents are no longer living. If you feel that they made mistakes with you, then you may be wondering: *Will I make those same mistakes?*

Alternately, if you have mainly positive feelings about your parents, you may have a different kind of fear: *My parents were so great with me; will I be able to be that great with my child?*

Tai felt that she had always had a difficult relationship with her mother, a prominent physician. "I did not feel that she was really there for me when I was younger. My siblings and I were cared for by a string of nannies," she reflected. "I am a lot more creative than my mom and she always discounted my artistic endeavors. My having a painting in a national show when I was 16 was not as important to her as acing my math courses. And when I dropped out of college to paint, that was a really hard time." While she had never really processed how painful this was, she always felt that her mother's love for her was conditional. Now that she was approaching motherhood herself, she wanted nothing more than to make sure that her child always felt loved, with no strings attached. And she was a little scared about that—how would she know how to give unconditional love, not having received it herself.

Just making these questions conscious in her journal and through talking to me helped her feel better. She had the same concerns as before, but now she had a sense of why. She also began to understand that her mother had probably done the best she knew how. She knew that her mother's family had not been very loving, which helped her to view her mother in a much more compassionate light. With this new awareness, Tai felt ready to change this pattern. While she was still a little scared, she was also excited. We also talked about where she could get further support in counseling if she needed it, and resources for developing the parenting style she wanted (such as websites, local educators, and organizations offering classes).

From Partners to Parents—What Will That Be Like?

Along with questions and concerns you feel about becoming a mother, you may also quite naturally be having thoughts about what your mate will be like as a father. He is probably facing many of the same questions himself.

Is he more psyched than you? Is he going along with the

whole "baby thing" because of your wishes? Is he right there experiencing every symptom and checkup with you? (Some dads-to-be even gain weight and experience symptoms such as backache, insomnia, and morning sickness right alongside their wives, a condition known as *couvade syndrome* or sympathy pains.) Is he supportive and happy, but a little worried about finances and a little freaked out every time you're spooning in bed and he can feel your surfing fetus kick him in the back?

Two very common scenarios: You think he'll be a great parent because he has a great family, while yours is all screwed up. Or vice versa.

Whatever your expectations—about either yourself as a mother or your mate as a father—use these perceptions as a starting place for a conversation about what you're each thinking and feeling. Just as you have a mental story about him, he will have one about you, and it's likely that both of you will be surprised by some aspects of what the other is thinking. This is a great time to build a foundation for communicating and sharing—which is always better than worrying alone in the dark or being surprised. And it can be fun and enlightening, too.

How Will a Baby Change How I Feel about My Work? Or How My Work Feels about Me?

"The baby shower they gave me at the office was excruciating!" Sofia confessed. "That morning, I felt physically ill. When I ran through my Quick Pic checks, my soul was on red-alert: '*Whoop! Whoop! Whoop! Baby shower day! Bad!*'"

At 39, Sofia had been thrilled by how easily she had conceived. A single mother, she had planned her pregnancy carefully, even timing her delivery to coincide with a less busy time at work. Still, she worried throughout her first trimester and much of the second as well, not telling a soul until around 20 weeks when her expanding middle was becoming more and more visible. Even then, she told only one of her colleagues. "I kept buying larger navy blazers and it worked pretty well to hide things."

The head of human resources for a Fortune 100 company, Sofia had worked hard to get to the top post. Although she reveled in being pregnant, she was anxious about being perceived differently at work. By the third trimester, when her condition was unmistakable to even the most casual observer, she was finding it harder and harder to keep up the ruse of "business as usual."

By the time her department threw her a luncheon shower—her best work friend having insisted on it, over Sofia's protests—she was in full-scale panic over this collision between the efficient, successful business Sofia and what she perceived as the frivolous, distracted mommy Sofia.

I see this impulse all the time, especially in "older" moms-to-be. With 10 or even 20 more years in the workforce than a young mother right out of high school or college, older first-time moms often have a huge amount of themselves invested in their professional lives. This can be true of any woman who works. It's only natural that your concerns about how motherhood will affect your life would focus on work. These feelings will intensify, and perhaps change, after the baby is born. For now, it is important to embrace and accept them, no matter how turbulent they may be—and to continue checking in with them throughout the third trimester and after delivery.

HOW TO MAKE A CONSCIOUS CHOICE ABOUT . . . YOUR POSTPARTUM WORK PLANS

Will you go back to work after you have your baby? Will you become an at-home mom? Work part-time? If you take maternity leave, for how long? Will your partner take a leave, and for how long? Before you can negotiate the details of your post-baby work life with your boss, you have to negotiate them with yourself and your mate. It is impossible to know now, during pregnancy, how you will feel about these questions after giving birth. I have seen many flip-flops (in both directions), so do this process along the way, *and* recognize that a lot might change when the baby is actually in your arms.

First, reflection. Start by reflecting on what your "story" is about being a mother and having a career. Is there a part of you that feels that "good" moms are those who choose to stay at home full-time? Or have you always had deep respect for women who appear to "do it all"—have a job and a family, and never miss a beat? Consider also your idea of what it means to be a "good" father. What does that involve from day to day? What role do you hope your partner will play in childrearing? Look honestly at your feelings, and try not to be influenced by the feelings and values of those around you. This is about *you* and how *you* feel.

Then give some thought to the practical issues. What is your economic situation? How critical is your income to the well-being of your household? What is important to you in terms of lifestyle? In terms of childrearing?

What are your feelings about your job? Does it fuel you? Drain you? Do you feel fulfilled? Like you're just marking time? Do you have a career plan?

What are your feelings about being a working mother? How do you feel about child care? Did your mom work when you were a child? Did your dad leave most of the parenting to your mom? What was that like for you?

How do you envision daily life as a working mom? As an at-home mom?

What do you think others in your life would do or think? Your partner? Your mother? Your boss? Your colleagues? Are their feelings influencing you, and if so, how and why?

Second, information. Explore your feelings with your partner and ask him about his thoughts, feelings, and preferences at this stage. Both of you may find that your preferences change throughout this process, and again once the baby is a reality.

Investigate child care. Familiarize yourself with the range of options: in-home care, such as a nanny; family day care in someone else's home, day-care centers—at churches, schools, or in independent facilities—or the care of a family member (such as your mother or your partner). Visit some choices. Ask friends what they use. Look into cost, credentials, experience, admittance policies, and atmosphere. Get a sense of what you prefer and can afford.

Explore career trajectories. You can't be sure what will be true for your working life once you have a child, but you can get some sense by looking at others in similar situations. What happens to your prospects for career advancement if you quit this job? If you become a working mom? If you switch to part-time? What about the possibility of your mate being the stay-at-home caretaker?

Explore the policies of your employer and your mate's. How

much maternity leave are you entitled to (paid and unpaid)? What are your partner's family- or paternity-leave options? Is there a part-time work option? A job-sharing option? You should be able to have this conversation with your human resources representative in confidence.

Economically, what are your options? Are there places you can cut your budget to accommodate staying home if that's what you want to do? Would working part-time give you enough money? Is it feasible for you and your partner to split child care? How much money do you need? Factor in everything, including the cost of child care, commuting, dry cleaning, and so on, whether you are considering returning to work either part- or full-time.

Third, action. Make a plan, remembering that you will not have a complete picture until your baby is born and you are actually a mother. If you aren't sure, you can always take your entitled maternity leave and make a final decision when you come close to the end of it. While this may not be the most ideal solution for your employer, it is an option if you are really uncertain about what is best for you.

Then, re-reflection. This is essential! Nothing you choose is carved in stone. Once you make a plan it's ideal to let it sit for a while. In a week or so, go back to it and review it. How does it feel? Right for a starting place? In need of a few minor adjustments? In need of rethinking altogether?

After you give birth, you can continue to re-reflect on your choice and see if you still feel the same way. Whether you will or not is totally unpredictable; I have seen women who were sure they would continue working suddenly decide to quit, and those who swore they'd stay at home with their babies decide that they preferred to balance work and motherhood.

CHECK IN WITH YOUR BABY

SUGGESTED TOOLS:

DAILY:

Baby Quick Pic (tool #8)

It's probable that you'll naturally find yourself doing more baby checks this trimester, as what's going on inside your belly becomes harder to ignore. Building a Baby Quick Pic into your daily routine helps you to keep your awareness at the forefront, even when a busy day or week might otherwise lull you into paying attention to everything *but* your baby.

ANYTIME, AT LEAST ONCE IN THE THIRD TRIMESTER:

Dreamagery (tool #9)

After you are in a relaxed state, invite an image of your baby to join you, and have a conversation about the upcoming labor and delivery. Ask the baby how it's feeling about getting close to leaving your body and entering the outside world. Ask how it's feeling about the labor and delivery process. Is there anything the baby needs or wants?

Take this time to share your thoughts and feelings with the baby. Is there anything you want or need from the baby? Let the conversation go wherever is natural.

BABY CHECKS: WHAT MIGHT COME UP FOR YOU

Patience, Please

While the increasing discomforts of the third trimester and the growing excitement about impending motherhood may mean that you're more than ready to get on with the show, your baby—who is not looking at the calendar boxes being too slowly checked off as you move toward your due date—might deliver a different message. Your baby may or may not share your impatience to meet in person, so to speak.

Thus, when you check in, the message you get from the baby may be different from the message you're getting from your body and soul. "I am doing really well but I still need time," it may tell you. "I know you're anxious for the delivery, but please be patient. I'm not quite ready." This can actually help you to be patient, acting as a reminder to take each day as it comes. When the time is right a moment that scientists still haven't solved the mystery of—the fetus will often let you know that he or she is ready to be born. Until then, enjoy this one-of-a-kind feeling of life wriggling inside you. Your baby will be in your arms soon enough.

Are You Sure You're Ready for Me?

Charlotte's baby was breech at 35 weeks. She was open to trying Dreamagery.

"Why are you not in the right position?" she asked the image of her baby with concern.

The image responded, "I'm not ready to come out yet, and I'm worried and frustrated, too."

"Why?"

"You're not ready for me." Charlotte's voice began to break.

"Ask the image to say more. What does it mean by that?" I prodded gently.

She asked, and then there was a long silence, and a sniffle. "It says I know," Charlotte finally reported. "It says, 'Hey, you left my dad, you don't have any labor support, and we don't even have a place to live right now!' It says it's pretty happy in there and it doesn't want to think about coming out till I get things a little more settled."

Charlotte let the image know that she "got it" and understood. It had every right to feel the way that it did, and I encouraged her to thank it for sharing this with her. After Charlotte returned her focus to the room, I waited for her to speak. "It's all true, you know," she admitted. "Jeff and I broke up a month ago and I moved out. I'm staying at my friend Angie's house till the baby comes, and I have to figure out what we're going to do."

This may sound far-fetched, but it is a true story from one of my patients, and a story I like because it illustrates nicely the point that there may be reasons besides chance that babies do what they do. Whether this baby was breech because of Charlotte's issues or not we will never know. It is possible (though not studied) that the mother's stress can affect the tension of the lower part of the uterus, for example. The hypothesis is that stress prevents the relaxation of the muscles that normally allow for the larger part of the fetus, the head, to settle in, with the result that the smaller parts (feet) present first. Given the mysterious interconnectedness of the fetus and the mother, I also do not rule out a more spiritual or metaphysical possibility—that this baby in particular was not ready to be born and quite literally was headed in the other direction!

Regardless of whether or not Charlotte's life situation was playing a role in her baby's breech presentation, she had issues that needed to be addressed, and the exercise helped her face them instead of expending all her energy ignoring them. She reopened a dialogue with the baby's father and began looking for a place of her own after delivery. She also continued an ongoing dialogue with her baby, which she loved doing. She felt they grew closer every day.

✓ REALITY CHECK: NESTING

How much are you doing to get ready for your baby's arrival? Have you prepared a nursery? How do you feel about the plans for your baby shower? Have you bought or borrowed anything baby-related yourself?

There is no right or wrong way to physically prepare to welcome your baby. In the Jewish culture, for example, it is believed that baby showers or bringing any baby paraphernalia into the home before the child's safe arrival is tempting fate. But whatever your ethnic traditions, a look at the form your nest-feathering takes can be telling by months eight and nine.

Eagerly preparing for your baby's arrival may be a way of doing some of the soul-level work that will help you try on your new role of Mom. Or it may be just a way of "keeping busy" so that you can *avoid* doing the deeper work! Some moms-to-be report a surge of energy and purposefulness about cleaning, stocking up on diapers and food, or some other way of getting ready for their baby. One mom took everything out of her linen closets, refolded it, and organized it by color—for the first time since she'd moved into her home 10 years earlier! This type of nesting behavior often signals that your body and your soul know what is needed and are wired to help prepare you mentally, emotionally, culturally—and practically—for momhood. If you haven't been doing any other prep work, this version of "nesting" can seem to strike like a lightning bolt. Anecdotally, women often (but not always) report experiencing it within a week or so before going into labor. That's really amazing when you think about it, and again affirms the wisdom of our body and soul. Note: If you do experience one of these sudden surges, take care not to overdo things or to do anything unsafe, such as climbing a ladder or using toxic chemicals to clean.

When a woman isn't doing anything to prepare ("I'll deal with it after the baby gets here"), it can be an indication of a certain level of denial. If, as in the Jewish faith, there are cultural beliefs that discourage making ready, you can still gauge the significance of your behavior during this time by doing a little soul-searching: Are you making mental lists or window shopping through a catalog for the kinds of items you'll want and need? Or are you using the cultural prohibition as a welcome escape from emotional as well as practical preparation for the baby?

Be aware of what the idea of nesting brings up for you.

C h a p t e r   1 9

Third Trimester:
The Inside Scoop

∞

What's happening biologically, weeks 29 to 40

WHAT'S HAPPENING WITH YOU:
THIRD-TRIMESTER CHANGES

Awareness and self-care can help you be proactive about physical changes including the following:

HAIR: Normally, individual hairs grow for between two and six years, enter a resting phase for three months, then fall out, to be replaced by new hair. At any given time when you're not pregnant, about 15 to 20 percent of your hair is in the resting phase. But in the third trimester, less than 10 percent of your hair is falling out and being replaced—so you have a thicker and more luxuriant head of hair at this time.

BREASTS: They continue to enlarge. A thick yellow fluid called *colostrum*, which sustains the baby before actual milk comes in, may leak or be squeezed from the nipple. This is normal. Some women find it helpful to start wearing nursing pads at this stage, to absorb leaks. Small cosmetic cotton rounds are also helpful and less cumbersome.

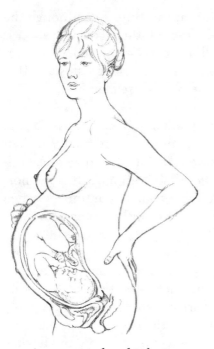

A woman in her third trimester

LUNGS: You may feel that you are breathing harder than usual. The amount of oxygen you need at this point has increased by 15 to 20 percent. To help compensate, the amount of air entering and leaving your lungs in a minute (called the minute ventilation) increases by 30 percent to 40 percent, so that overall you have increased oxygen in the blood of your arteries and veins. There is less carbon dioxide in your blood, which is important because it helps the carbon dioxide from the baby's circulation come across into yours, and you can exhale it. Increased progesterone probably causes these changes. Late in pregnancy, the uterus pushes against the diaphragm and, in turn, the lungs, making it harder to take deep breaths comfortably. At this time it's good not to overstress your lungs; walk slowly and take breaks as needed during exercise.

HEART: Your heart rate has been gradually increasing during your pregnancy and is now 15 to 20 percent faster than the normal pre-pregnancy heart rate. In the third trimester, 17 percent of your blood flows to the uterus, compared with just 2 to 3 percent in the first trimester. Your cardiac output—the volume of blood the heart pumps in a minute—depends on your position. When you lie flat on your back, the enlarged uterus presses against the inferior vena cava (the large vessel that returns blood to the heart), compressing it. This significantly decreases how much blood there is to send back out to the body, including the blood flow to the baby, which is why it's best to sleep on your side. If it's comfortable, make it your left side as this position creates the least compression and allows for the greatest blood flow. A pillow between your legs can make you more comfortable.

BLOOD: It's normal to become anemic at this time. Even though the actual number of red blood cells is increased, their concentration is diluted since the plasma (the noncellular part of the blood) has increased even more. This "dilutional anemia" is usually greatest at 30 to 34 weeks and often improves across the rest of pregnancy.

BLOOD PRESSURE: Blood pressure gradually begins to rise again, returning to nonpregnant numbers by the time you are full term. So if the doctor says that your blood pressure is "rising," this may mean relative to the second trimester; ask so you know for sure. It is *not* normal for blood pressure to rise above pre-pregnancy numbers; when this is the case it can be a sign of preeclampsia or hypertension.

BACK: The lower part of the spine begins to curve, so that your center of gravity stays over your legs, a process called *lordosis*. Imagine if it didn't and you had a very straight back—the bulk of the pregnancy would be way out in front. Unfortunately, lordosis also usually means lower back pain, which increases as the pregnancy progresses. Try some of the recommendations for pelvic pain below to alleviate back stress.

PELVIS: Ligaments in the pelvis loosen to enhance delivery, most likely due to increases in the hormone relaxin. You have a moveable joint at the front of your pelvis, called the pubic symphysis, that widens significantly by 29 to 32 weeks (as much as 3 to 4 mm in width). While this is great for delivery, it can be very uncomfortable. The combination of relaxin acting on the joints, lordosis, and a big, protruding midsection can make you feel "wobbly" in late pregnancy. Pelvic girdle pain—which can feel like a searing ache around the back and stomach—may also develop. A Swedish study of almost 400 mothers-to-be with pelvic girdle pain found acupuncture to be the most effective treatment; stabilizing exercises to improve mobility and strength also helped. Other ways to ease back pain: massage, a cold pack, a warm bath, or pelvic tilts (kneel on all fours, relax your lower back, tilt your pelvis forward and hold a few seconds before pulling your pelvis back until your back is again straight).

STOMACH: The muscle tone of the sphincter between your esophagus and stomach is reduced, so as the baby grows and exerts increased abdominal pressure, you may experience increased acid reflux and heartburn. Gastric acid production rises in the third trimester as well. To lessen heartburn, try eating smaller meals and stay upright for two hours after you eat. Avoid fatty or fried foods, as well as highly spiced dishes. Eat more protein and try chewing sugarless gum after a meal to reduce the acid.

BOWELS: Constipation may worsen as there is increased obstruction from the uterus. Hemorrhoids can also increase as a result of dilation of the vessels. Continue to drink ample fluids and incorporate extra servings of whole grains and cruciferous vegetables which contain natural fiber. Dried fruits like plums, prunes, and raisins also help.

BLADDER: The risk of urinary tract infections increases in the third trimester due in part to the fact that you are now excreting more glucose. As the bladder comes under increasing pressure from the growing uterus, its capacity decreases. Stress incontinence—a small leakage of urine when you cough, laugh, or sometimes just move a certain way—is common. Most pregnant women use sanitary pads at this point, and it's always helpful to know the location of the nearest restroom!

KIDNEYS: Because the ureters are so dilated now, which means more urine is sitting around, kidney infection is more likely. It's not your imagination that you have to urinate frequently. Listen to your body, and lower your risk of urinary tract infection and kidney infection by urinating whenever you feel the need, which will help keep the urine from stagnating in the ureters.

GALLBLADDER: The volume is twice that of its nonpregnant state, and it empties much more slowly. Because of this there is an increased risk of gallstone formation. Interestingly, this seems to rise with each additional pregnancy.

WHAT'S HAPPENING WITH YOUR BABY NOW

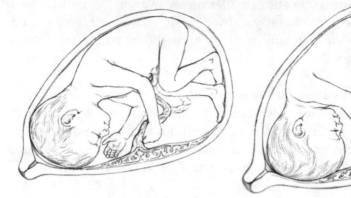

Fetus at 7 months   *Fetus at 8 months*

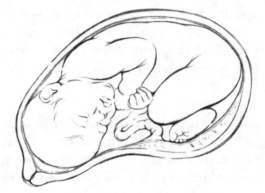

Fetus at 9 months

Month 7 (28 to 31 weeks)

Your baby now weighs between two and three and a half pounds, is more than a foot long, and is essentially fully formed even though some body systems and organs, like the lungs, are still developing. Strong limbs mean strong kicks and stretches, which are easily felt. Your baby's senses are all functioning, too. Eyelids open and close. Hearing is developed, and by birth your baby will show a preference for the sound of your so-familiar voice. While a baby born now is viable, many do not yet have lungs that are developed enough to breathe on their own. A baby born this prematurely would also lack the antibodies and iron his mother continues to provide, putting him at heightened risk of infection, and could experience many other possible complications.

Month 8 (32 to 36 weeks)

Some babies born this early do very well, while others need as many interventions as more premature ones. Every added week in the uterus can make a significant difference in how well the baby does. Your baby really begins to put on weight rapidly now, gaining as many as three or more pounds this month. Typical babies will be about 16 to 19 inches, although individual growth rates vary from midpregnancy on. The downy hair called lanugo begins to disappear and will be mostly gone by full term. Sleep patterns become somewhat more predictable. A baby who has been sleeping may be startled awake by a loud noise—so don't be surprised if you feel a sudden movement or kick to your belly. Most babies assume the head-down position for birth by around 34 weeks.

Month 9 (37 to 40 weeks)

A baby who has reached 37 weeks is considered full term (even though this is a week before the two-week window around your due date). Your baby is fully developed and can function outside of you. The key development that takes place in the last month of pregnancy is the addition of protective fat to keep the baby's body temperature stable, and the transfer of added immunities from mother to baby. The lungs are now filled with surfactant, a substance that helps them stay expanded after each breath, meaning they will be able to function outside of you. Most but not all of the greasy coating called vernix has disappeared. Some remains to lubricate the way down the birth canal.

Normal birth weights range between 5.5 and 10 pounds; normal birth lengths range between 18 and 22 inches.

Fetal Headlines

- At 37 weeks, your baby is considered full term (12.3 percent of babies are born before 37 weeks).
- At 38 weeks, many babies shift lower in the pelvis and settle

with the head firmly in the pelvic bones. This is very typical if it is your first pregnancy and is known as *engagement* or "dropping." This both changes your shape slightly and makes it easier to breathe.

- Remember that you can expect your baby two weeks before or after your due date!
- The average newborn weighs around 7 1/2 pounds and is about 20 inches long. Boys generally weigh slightly more than girls.

Chapter 20

Third Trimester:
Medical Care

❧

An integrative medicine perspective, weeks 29 to 40

BASIC MEDICAL ISSUES NOW

Checkups and Tests: What Happens and Why

Your visits to the doctor or midwife increase in the third trimester. You will typically be seen every other week in the eighth month and then weekly beginning at 36 weeks. (Your care provider may suggest a different schedule for you.) More attention is paid to the medical monitoring of the baby's growth and well-being at pregnancy's end, because complications can develop more quickly and more often now. Be persistent about sharing your own feelings about things that seem bothersome or amiss, and ask questions when you don't understand why something is being done. You have a right to know everything that's happening, including test results—after all, you're the one who's pregnant!

You'll continue to be monitored in the same ways you were previously, with these additional emphases:

- *Fetal position.* Beginning around weeks 34 to 36, your doctor will keep a close eye on how your baby is positioned in your uterus. You might have some idea based on where the kicks are coming from and whether you can feel the large rump, although it's easy to mistake a head for a bottom and arm movements for those of a leg. An experienced obstetrician or midwife will be able to palpate your belly and make a pretty educated guess. Where the heartbeat is heard will provide another clue, although even then because you hear the heartbeat through the umbilical cord as well as the heart itself, it can be misleading. Ultrasound can be used to verify position if necessary.

WHY: To assure that the baby is head down as your due date approaches.

At the start of the third trimester, most fetuses are still flip-flopping around. As time goes on and they keep growing, they begin to have less and less room to make major position changes. By some time in the 34th to 36th week, the shape and tone of the uterus causes most babies to be held in a vertical lie, meaning they lie lengthwise (up and down in the uterus) rather than sideways, and they usually settle into a head-down position (*cephalic*). This is the most common presentation for delivery—more than 95 percent of babies are cephalic by the time they engage in the birth canal, probably because there is more space for the head in this part of the pelvis than at the top (fundus). The move into the head-down position typically occurs in the last few weeks of pregnancy for the first baby, and may happen later in subsequent pregnancies.

About 3 to 4 percent of fetuses, though, may be breech (feet or bottom facing the cervix). Rarely, they can be transverse (horizontal). Position is not a cause for concern until about week 36, at which point, if the baby is still breech, you'll want to discuss your options with your doctor. (See "Breech and Other Presentations.")

Every once in a while, a baby will not settle into any position, but will continue to have significant changes in its position through to the end of pregnancy. This is referred to as an "unstable lie." This is most often seen when the typical conditions that force the baby to settle into one position don't exist. For example, it's sometimes seen if there is an unusually large amount of amniotic fluid, if the baby is unusually small, or if the uterus is unusually relaxed—as occasionally happens with a "grand multips," a woman who has had a large number of babies, and whose uterus lacks the muscle tone that is typically present.

- *Weight check.*

WHY: To be sure you're on track for a healthy weight gain. If you're gain-ing too much in the third trimester, it's an added physical strain—and that much more weight you'll have to lose later. Excessive weight gain in the mother is also linked to high birth weight in the baby, which can create complications in labor and delivery. If you gain several pounds in a short period of time (over a few days or a week, for example), this can be an important flag for preeclampsia, in which case the weight gain is due to retained fluid.

- *Fetal heart tones and fetal movement.* Your doctor will listen to the fetal heartbeat and should ask you the results of your kick counts. If there is any concern about fetal well-being, you'll be monitored further.

WHY: To verify the baby is alive and well.

- *Cervical exam.* In the last month you may have a cervical check to determine whether you are getting ready for labor. Not all practices do this routinely. (I don't.) It's not unusual for cervical dilation to start early and proceed slowly (even weeks before you deliver), especially if you have given birth before. If a checkup reveals you are beginning to dilate, no treatment or change is required unless regular rhythmic contractions are also felt and you are premature.

WHY: To ascertain whether your body is preparing for labor. If there is any reason to suspect a problem, you will definitely have a cervical exam.

- *Group B strep test.* Group B strep (GBS) is a bacterium that's common in the vagina. As many as 40 percent of pregnant women have it and experience no ill effects. A test is the only way to know whether you are a carrier of GBS. This is done using a vaginal swab and takes a few seconds. It's routinely done between 35 and 37 weeks. (Testing ear-lier is not an accurate predictor of GBS at delivery.)

WHY: During delivery, GBS can infect the baby and cause a serious or even fatal infection. You will be given intravenous antibiotics

✓ **REALITY CHECK:** How Big Will Your Baby Be?

Strangers will take one look at your belly and tell you you're carrying a whopper. Your doctor measures your fundal height and palpates your abdomen and says the baby seems "about average." And your ultrasound indicates that the baby will probably only be about six pounds. Who's right? The best answer might be to ask, what do *you* think? One study found that asking a mother how much she thinks her baby will weigh is a more accurate predictor than an ultrasound reading. Another example of the power of your inner wisdom!

You'd think technology had the edge, but ultrasounds as a way to estimate newborn size are far from accurate. They can provide general reassurance that a baby is growing properly, and they can generally assess whether a baby is very large or very small, but they are notoriously poor predictors of actual pounds and ounces. Genetics, your birth weight, and your overall health and nutrition all influence birth weight.

during labor in the following situations: if you're found to have the bacterium; if you've tested positive in a previous pregnancy; if you go into labor before 37 weeks *and* the test has not yet been done; or if your membranes have been ruptured for more than 18 hours.

HOW TO MAKE A CONSCIOUS CHOICE ABOUT . . . POSTPARTUM CONTRACEPTION

Even if you love babies and think you will be ready for another next year, it's a good idea to give your body and soul a break between pregnancies. This allows you to focus on your new baby and your new life and on returning to optimal health. You may find that you are not interested in thinking about another child for a while. This can change dramatically from what you had planned, so be sure to check in with yourself about this one. In any case, you need to think about postpartum contraception. More than one-half of all couples change contraceptive techniques between pregnancies. After your baby is born, what will you choose?

First, reflection. What kind of birth control did you use before you conceived this child? How did you feel about it? Did you conceive this child intentionally or accidentally? How do you feel about the various options for birth control? What do you know about them or what have you heard about them? What are your partner's feelings about different forms of birth control (barrier methods versus hormonal forms versus vasectomy, and so on)?

Do you plan to have more children? If not, you may want to consider a permanent method of birth control (vasectomy for your partner, or tubal ligation for you, aka "having your tubes tied"). If you are contemplating surgical or permanent methods, such as these (which should be considered permanent even though reversal procedures do exist), you should fully explore your feelings in order to make a truly conscious choice. This can help minimize the feelings of grief that some women feel when they decide to give up their chance of having more children. Lost libido may also accompany such a decision, especially if it has not been made with careful forethought. If you know you want more children in the future, or think that you might, you will want to choose a birth control method that won't interfere with your fertility.

Second, information. Learn the pros and cons of the types of contraception that you are considering. Be sure that you understand the full range of options. The IUD, for example, is one you may not have considered previously because of possible discomfort. But women who have been pregnant tend to do very well with IUDs, and it is easily removed when you are ready. If you are interested in birth control pills, there are progestin-only formulations that can be used during breastfeeding. There are also different methods of hormonal contraception, such as the patch, which delivers hormones through the skin, and the ring, which is placed in the vagina.

Ask your doctor for recommendations and/or seek other sources of advice.

Third, action. Make a decision and tell your doctor. If you are considering tubal ligation, you should be aware that if you have a vaginal delivery it will be performed the day after. If you need a C-section, the tubal ligation will be done at the same time that that procedure is performed. So you will want to have made a final decision before you go into labor. For insurance coverage, there are also often papers that you need to sign at least one month prior to your delivery. It's important to know that even if you sign the papers, you can ALWAYS choose not to have the surgery. This has two practical implications: 1) stay conscious about this decision, even after you sign the papers. You may have second thoughts, and you should listen to them and change your decision if appropriate. 2) If you think you *may* want the surgery, given the unpredictability of the timing of your delivery, it is better to sign the papers and continue to process the decision. Once you decide, be certain to tell your physician, and confirm it when you are admitted for delivery.

Then, re-reflection. Unless you opt for a tubal ligation or a vasectomy, your decision can be easily changed. But with surgery, you can't change your mind once the procedure is done, so now is the time for you and your partner to reflect on your decision again.

POSSIBLE MEDICAL ISSUES NOW

Fetal Well-Being

If there is any question about fetal well-being, which most often occurs because you have noticed a slowing or absence of movement, you will be monitored to get further information and hopefully reassurance that all is well.

The standard way to assess fetal well-being is with a *nonstress test* (NST), which can be administered in your doctor's office. This test is noninvasive and simply entails placing two external monitors on your belly while you're lying down. These will electronically monitor both the fetal heart and uterine contractions. This is the same electronic fetal monitor that is typically used in labor. Adults, who have fully mature neurological systems, can move about their daily business without much change in their heart rate. Because a fetus has an immature system, however, every time it moves its heart rate increases. So the doctor is looking for accelerations in heart rate as a sign that the baby is moving and that all is well. This is called a reactive nonstress test. The ability of the fetus to respond in this way depends on how far along it is in its development. Early in the third trimester, even healthy babies will not necessarily have these accelerations. By about 32 weeks, though, every healthy baby should.

If the test does not show a response appropriate to the fetus's age, it is quite possible that the baby is just in a sleep cycle. Your care provider may therefore do something called *vibrational acoustical stimulation*, or VAS. Vibrational acoustical stimulation simply involves using an instrument that produces sound and vibration on your abdomen to prompt a fetal reaction. An acceleration in the fetal heart rate in response to this stimulation is reassuring. When I was in residency we would often accomplish the same goal by simply playing ordinary spoons for a short time on the mother's belly—a low-tech, low-cost way to create sound and vibration!

If your nonstress test is nonreactive—that is, it does not show the heart rate accelerations we would expect, even after prolonged monitoring, or shows other signs that may be worrisome, a *biophysical profile* (BPP) is typically done next. The BPP simply involves, in addition to an NST, watching the baby on ultrasound for thirty minutes. Then the test is scored for five different aspects of fetal well-being: fetal breathing movements, fetal body movements, fetal tone, the amount of amniotic fluid, and the reactive fetal heart rate (as indicated by the NST). Two points are given for each element that is normal, zero for each element that is abnormal, and one point if it's in between. Based on this score and how far along you are in your pregnancy, a plan will be made that may vary from sending you home with instructions to continue with kick counts and return if you notice decreased fetal movement, to having you stay on Labor and Delivery for more monitoring of the baby, to inducing labor or performing a Cesarean section. This plan is individualized, and as such, you should be fully informed of what the tests show, what the doctor's interpretation is, and the reasons for the suggested plan of action.

Preeclampsia (Toxemia, or Pregnancy-Induced Hypertension)

Preeclampsia is a disease that involves hypertension along with other signs and symptoms, and is one of the more common medical complications of pregnancy. It occurs in about 5 percent of all pregnant women. We don't understand what causes preeclampsia, who will get it, or why the progression of the disorder varies so much from woman to woman. It is a growing concern, however, because preeclampsia rates have risen by nearly a third in the last decade. The increased number of pregnant women who are older and who are carrying multiples (often arising from fertility treatments) may account for part of this rise in preeclampsia.

One way of understanding the effects of this disease is to think of it like this: just as it causes your hands or face to retain fluid, swelling can also occur in other parts of your body that you are unable to see. For example, your nervous system (including your brain) may swell, which can cause hyperreflexia (meaning you have overactive "jumpy" reflexes), headaches, visual distortions, or even seizures (at which point your condition becomes a medical emergency called *eclampsia*). The kidneys can swell and start to malfunction, causing a decrease in your ability to make urine, or even a complete shutdown of your kidneys. The liver may swell, causing discomfort or pain and in extreme cases, the liver can rupture. Given these possible changes, you can see why this disease is potentially fatal and merits careful monitoring. The good news is that many of them result in symptoms you notice and in changes in blood and urine readings that your doctor can test for.

PREECLAMPSIA: WHO'S AT RISK

Preeclampsia is more common in:
- Teen moms
- Women over 40
- Women pregnant for the first time
- Women carrying twins, triplets, or higher multiple births
- Women who had hypertension (high blood pressure) prior to pregnancy
- Women who have had preeclampsia in a previous pregnancy
- Women with obesity (pre-pregnancy)
- Women with a history of smoking

Interestingly, women carrying pregnancies conceived in summer months seem to have higher rates of preeclampsia, but we don't know why and this is not considered a medical risk factor.

Women who develop preeclampsia often ask me, "How did this

happen? What could I have done to prevent it?" The short answer is that there's nothing we know that prevents this condition. So let go of any thoughts or feelings that you could have done something to change this. There are numerous clinical reports on different preventive approaches, including calcium, magnesium, zinc, fish oil, evening primrose oil, and vitamins E and C. None, however, have yet demonstrated clear benefit. If you are at risk for preeclampsia, you may want to consume more of these nutrients, although my basic plan for good pregnancy nutrition offers plenty of calcium, omega-3 fatty acids (found in fish oil), and antioxidants such as vitamins E and C.

You've probably noticed that I've made repeated references to the benefits of being aware of the signs of preeclampsia. At the risk of sounding like the proverbial broken record, let me say that it's a perfect illustration of the benefit of staying tuned in to your body. Very often the first signs of this dangerous disorder, which can creep up on you and catch you unawares, is swelling in the face or hands or a jump in weight gain (caused by retaining fluids). These are the very signs that checking in with your body can reveal to you. Early detection can be lifesaving, since the later preeclampsia is caught, the harder it is to manage successfully.

Your doctor will do several things to arrive at a diagnosis if there is a possibility of preeclampsia. These include:

• Taking a detailed history. You will be asked about any hand or facial swelling you may have noticed, headaches, changes in vision, upper abdominal pain, and other possible symptoms.

• Assessing your blood pressure. A diastolic pressure of 90 or above and/or a systolic pressure of 140 or above are considered abnormal and cause for concern.

• Doing a physical exam. Among other things, the doctor will assess edema (swelling), and check the nervous system for irritability. The nervous system is typically more excitable or reactive in pregnancy compared with a nonpregnant state, but with preeclampsia, reactions to stimuli like a knee tap can be much more extreme.

• Looking for protein in the urine. A fresh, clean-catch sample will be used initially. Because vaginal secretions also contain protein, a catheter may be used to obtain the cleanest possible sample. The doctor may also ask you to collect your urine over 24 hours. This allows us to assess this aspect of kidney function over a longer period of time, which is more helpful information than a "spot" check.

- Checking fetal well-being.

If preeclampsia is suspected during your workup, you'll probably be asked to lie down immediately on your left side (called the left lateral decubitus position), the position that keeps your blood pressure at its lowest and allows the best circulation to your organs and to your baby. Your condition will be closely monitored, and your blood pressure will be treated if it gets dangerously high. You may be admitted to the hospital for further observation. Fetal well-being is monitored through a nonstress test. If there are questions about growth, fundal height measurements, or the nonstress test, an ultrasound results.

Since preeclampsia doesn't progress at the same rate in everyone, it's critical that you be evaluated and carefully monitored once a diagnosis is made. If your condition appears mild and stable (not trending toward a more severe state) you may be sent home with instructions to reduce your activity level and relax more; sometimes bed rest is prescribed. Or you may be hospitalized right away, possibly for the duration of pregnancy. If you are full term or close to it, you may be delivered. The goal is to enable the fetus to remain in the uterus as long as possible in order to mature—without threatening the mother's health. And therein lies the challenge.

Once preeclampsia starts, it virtually always worsens, most typically in a slow but steady fashion. The only "cure" is the delivery of the baby. The timing of this delivery will depend on two factors: how sick you are, and how far along the baby is.

If the disease is mild, and the baby is not yet full term or close to term, delivery will most likely be postponed, at least long enough to administer steroids to help with the maturation of the baby's lungs. Some women remain in the hospital for weeks with only mild preeclampsia and go on to deliver a healthy full-term baby.

If you are dangerously ill, or your disease has progressed to eclampsia (see below), the baby will most likely be delivered no matter when your due date is. If the disease is becoming dangerous to you, it is also becoming dangerous to your baby.

While in labor, the mother with preeclampsia is given magnesium sulfate by IV to help prevent seizures. This drug does not reduce pain but sedates the nervous system, making you feel slow and sluggish and possibly slowing labor. On the other hand, the body often knows what is best in these cases and what I often see is that despite the drug, the body works toward a quick labor. If it is possible, a vaginal delivery is preferable to a C-section because preeclampsia can affect the clotting ability of the blood, so major surgery adds risks to an already serious situation.

Deciding on a course of action involves a balancing act between the baby's health and the mother's. What's best for the one is not necessarily ideal for the other. Sometimes I see moms who refuse delivery because they want to give their baby longer to mature. That's well-intentioned but misguided, because they risk losing both their own life and their baby's. Preeclampsia is one situation where management decisions are best made by your doctor. You should of course be fully informed and involved, but ultimately this decision is one based in clinical judgment. This is where you'll be glad you put time and energy into choosing someone whom you trust.

Eclampsia

Eclampsia is not a different condition but rather the most serious form of preeclampsia. If you have a seizure, you have eclampsia. You are much sicker with eclampsia, and the risks can include death of the mother and baby, although with immediate medical attention and delivery of the baby, most survive. If you have preeclampsia you should feel confident that with vigilant, proper care, your condition is very likely to be managed so that it does not progress to this level; only a minuscule fraction of all pregnant women in the United States—0.02 percent to 0.05 percent—will have eclampsia.

> **FEAR:** I'm puffy; I must have preeclampsia.
> **FACT:** All pregnant women retain water to some degree (called *edema*), most commonly in the ankles and feet. But you may also have swelling in your face or hands that is normal and not at all related to preeclampsia. Because the stakes are so high, however, it's always best to report the symptom and let your doctor evaluate you. Pay attention to changes in the swelling—does it stay the same or recede or continue to worsen? If your care provider dismisses the swelling as "nothing" but you can tell that it is worsening or feel real concern, report back again, or seek a second opinion.

SIGNS OF PRETERM LABOR

Staying attuned to what's normal for you now and what feels different can help you identify premature labor (see Chapter 16, pages 232–234). If you experience any of the following symptoms before you're full term, let your doctor know. Don't hope that a worrisome symptom will "go away." Better to get it investigated. If you have preterm labor, there are actions you and your doctor can take to try to forestall labor, and every extra day the baby has to mature can be significant.

Symptoms to report to your doctor include:

- Cramps like menstrual cramps
- Lower back pain, especially if it is rhythmic or comes and goes
- Feeling pressure or achiness in the abdomen, lower in the pelvis, in the thighs
- Mucusy vaginal discharge that's new, especially if bloody or brownish
- Leaking of fluid, which can be a sign of your water breaking and can feel like a small trickle of leaking urine or be a big gush of watery fluid

---

Preterm Premature Rupture of Membranes (PPROM)

The break in the amniotic sac which releases amniotic fluid (the so-called bag of water) is known as the rupture of membranes, or your water breaking. If this happens before the 37th week, it's a serious condition. See Chapter 16, pages 235–240, for a complete discussion.

Premature Rupture of Membranes (PROM)

Most often water breaks during or just before active labor begins and is a normal part of childbirth. This can happen on its own or the doctor may do it, a simple procedure called amniotomy. However, when this happens after the 37th week of pregnancy but before labor begins, it's called premature rupture of membranes, or PROM. When a woman is full term and her water breaks, labor usually begins within 24 to 48 hours. If labor does not begin naturally, she can be induced to prevent the risk of infection, which increases after the membranes rupture and time passes.

Third-Trimester Bleeding

While vaginal bleeding is rare and occurs in about 4 percent of pregnancies, it is alarming if it happens to you. Understandably, patients worry that they are losing the baby or that something is seriously wrong. But as with bleeding earlier in pregnancy, there are many possible causes, some of which are trivial. And because the fetus is now viable, it can often be safely delivered even if the bleeding turns out to be a sign of something serious. Inform your doctor as to how heavy your bleeding is. Is it spotting? Like a period? Heavier than a period? Also report what you were doing when you noticed the bleeding and whether it is accompanied by any other symptoms, such as cramping, abdominal pain, fever, or vaginal irritation. Let her know if you have recently had sex.

Among the possibilities your doctor will consider:

• *A vaginal infection.* An infection that is very inflammatory can cause some spotting or blood-tinged discharge. This is not a cause for alarm, and the infection will be treated by appropriate medication.

• *Cervical irritation.* This is usually caused by intercourse irritating the cervix, which can be delicate and bleed easily at this stage. This kind of bleeding is also usually light, and clears up on its own.

• *The cervix dilating and effacing.* This causes bleeding that is often referred to as "bloody show." It's usually very mucusy and happens when you are in labor.

• *Placenta previa.* The most common reason for late-term bleeding is a problem where the placenta covers all or part of the cervical opening and bleeds as the cervix dilates. It's typically a painless, but serious condition; once bleeding occurs it requires hospitalization, close monitoring, and possibly Cesarean delivery. (See "Placenta Problems" below.)

Placenta Problems

The placenta is an organ that grows only for the purpose of nourishing the baby during pregnancy, and it is delivered after the baby. Most moms never see it, and if they do look at it after delivery, it's inside out. (I recommend asking to see it; it's very cool!) Though most pregnant women never give it a thought unless something goes awry, the placenta is a part of you really worth knowing. (See Chapter 11, pages 136–137.)

On one side, this blood-filled organ is attached to your uterine wall where the fertilized egg first implanted itself (since it, like the baby, was formed out of that fertilized egg), and on the other side it is attached to your body via the umbilical cord. Normally the placenta is implanted fairly high in the uterus. Problems develop when this is not the case. Placenta problems fall into the following categories:

1) *Low-lying placenta*. The least problematic scenario is a placenta that has implanted lower than normal in the uterus but does not cover the cervix. It doesn't necessarily cause any problems. Occasionally a low-lying placenta can cause bleeding when the cervix starts to dilate.

2) *Placenta previa*. In about 1 in 250 pregnancies, the placenta is attached too low in the uterus and covers all or part of the cervix, which poses potential hazards at delivery.

- A *complete previa* means the placenta is covering the entire cervix, blocking the fetus's exit from the uterus and therefore requiring a C-section delivery.
- A *partial previa* is where only a portion of the cervix is blocked; it also requires a C-section because as the cervix dilates, more and more of the placenta becomes detached from the uterus, causing bleeding and decreased oxygen to the baby.
- A *marginal previa* means that the placenta just reaches the cervix. You may still be able to deliver vaginally.

Previa can first be seen on ultrasound in the second trimester, most often during the baseline ultrasound around 18 weeks. It's not usually a cause for concern then, because as the uterus grows, the placenta will usually be pulled upward and away from the cervix. (We often refer to this as the placenta "moving"; see "Reality Check," below.) If a previa is seen in midpregnancy, it will be followed up early in the third trimester to see whether it is still a previa.

All previas must be monitored because there is a risk that as the cervix begins to dilate in the weeks, days, or hours leading up to delivery, the placenta will be stripped away from the place where it is attached to the cervix and cause bleeding and danger for both the mother and baby. In some cases the woman is allowed to remain at home, usually on bed rest, with strict precautions regarding movement (must be limited) and intercourse (absolutely none). If there is any bleeding, however, you will be evaluated at the hospital for a period of time and likely hospitalized until your baby is full term and can be delivered. Depending on when you were diagnosed, this can be a period of weeks or even months. As with preeclampsia, if you are premature and your condition is stable enough to postpone delivery for a short time, steroids may be given to help mature the baby's lungs. You and the baby will be watched very closely, as bleeding can be sudden and life-threatening. Sometimes blood transfusions are necessary, as well as emergency C-section.

✓ REALITY CHECK: A "Moving" Placenta

"I'd like to do some imagery to encourage my placenta to move," a patient with placenta previa told me. While I applaud her wanting to take a proactive role in her situation, Dialoguing and Dreamagery have their limits. Once it is implanted, your placenta can't physically move from one position to another through the power of your suggestion and encouragement. A placenta referred to by doctors as "moving" isn't a free-floating orb. The placenta remains attached to the same place on the uterine wall where it originally implanted, but its position relative to the cervix may change as the uterus itself stretches and grows. Thus a placenta that was too close to the cervix at one point in pregnancy, may very naturally be shifted away as time goes on and the uterus continues to grow. In fact, this is the case in 90 percent of previas.

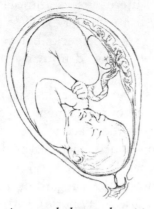

A normal placental position

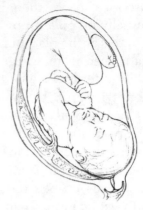

Low-lying placenta

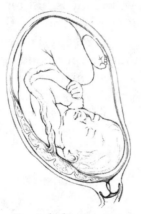

Partial placenta previa

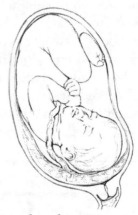

Complete placenta previa

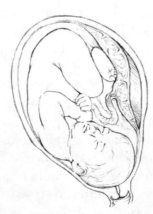

Placental abruption

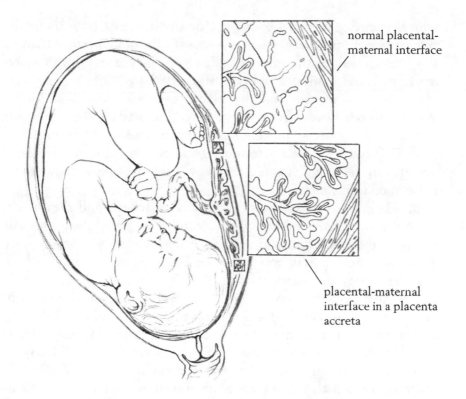

normal placental-maternal interface

placental-maternal interface in a placenta accreta

If the previa is complete, and you therefore know you will require a Cesarean delivery, you may still be hospitalized ahead of delivery so that you can be monitored in case of sudden bleeding. Generations ago, complete previas were a key cause of maternal death. Thanks to ultrasound diagnosis and better monitoring, fewer than 1 percent of cases are now fatal. This is still a large enough number that your doctor will not want to take any chances, which is why you may end up in the hospital for the remainder of your pregnancy. It's rare, though possible, for a complete previa to be discovered only at delivery.

Once you've had a placenta previa the risk of recurrence increases with each subsequent pregnancy.

3) *Placenta accreta.* This rare but difficult complication is turning up more often, 1 per 2,500 deliveries and is a side effect of our rising C-section rates. An accreta occurs when the placenta implants abnormally, most commonly on scar tissue on the uterine wall of a woman

who has previously had a C-section (or any surgery that scars the inside of the uterine wall—such as removal of fibroids) rather than on the smooth wall of the uterus. At delivery, the placenta, which normally detaches easily for delivery after the baby, does not separate from the uterine wall and the placental site continues to bleed. Women who have had two or more C-sections and also have placenta previa have a nearly 40 percent risk of having an accreta, according to ACOG. However, unlike determining the placement of the placenta, accretas are seldom diagnosed ahead of delivery because they cannot be seen on ultrasound.

Bleeding after the birth can usually be managed and the baby is almost always delivered safely, but accretas virtually always require surgical removal of the uterus—in other words, a hysterectomy. Although some cases of accreta can be managed successfully without a hysterectomy, the implantation site of the placenta is usually so extensive that there is no other option. Blood transfusions can also be necessary. If you have had a C-section previously and an ultrasound reveals that your placenta is in a suspicious location (implanted over the old C-section scar low and/or a previa), your doctor will likely acquaint you with the possibility of an accreta and the possibility of a hysterectomy. If this is the case for you, it is an ideal time to do Dialoguing and Dreamagery to help you process this situation. It is possible to have an accreta with no history of a C-section or other surgery, but it is very rare.

4) *Placenta abruptio* (also called abruption). The separation of the placenta from the uterine wall before delivery of the baby is a serious but unusual event. When it happens, it deprives the baby of oxygen and can cause bleeding that may be fatal to both mother and baby. Eighty percent of these occur before the onset of labor. There are three grades of abruption, with grade 1 being the most mild and grade 3 being severe. While the incidence of abruption ranges from 1 in 86 to 1 in 206 births, only 15 percent of these are grade 3. The grades are diagnosed clinically prior to delivery. However, a diagnosis of complete or partial abruption is only made after delivery, based on the inspection of the placenta. Having said this, virtually all complete abruptions present as grade 3, and grades 1 and 2 are typically partial.

A woman having an abruption will typically have vaginal bleeding, contractions, and abdominal pain, and the severity of the symptoms usually correlates with the severity of the abruption. It is possible to have an abruption with no visible bleeding because of what's known as a concealed hemorrhage or concealed abruption, meaning the bleeding is walled off behind the placenta. Abruptions are more common in women with high blood pressure or a history of tobacco or cocaine use. With a partial abruption (partial separation), the most common kind, a vaginal delivery is sometimes still possible. On the rare occasions when an abruption is complete, an emergency C-section must be performed in order to try and save the life of the baby.

FEAR: I've had placenta previa and my doctor recommended "pelvic rest" but I'm not sure how to do it right.

FACT: "Pelvic rest" simply means avoid intercourse or putting anything (such as tampons or fingers) into the vagina. It's crucial for placenta previa (to avoid significant hemmorhage) and PPROM (to avoid infection) and sometimes recommended if you are at risk for preterm labor. Why docs often don't clarify what this actually means, I'll never know.

Coping with a Tough Diagnosis

When you get news of something going awry in the third trimester—such as placenta previa, a breech position, or preeclampsia—you may be extremely upset. Remember that you have a very helpful tool to help you cope: the Feedback Loop. Use it to reflect on what this diagnosis means to you, gather data, and figure out which actions would serve you best. Even if the medical course of action isn't really up to you, the self-care actions you take are.

Breech and Other Presentations

Almost all babies—some 96 percent—present for delivery in the usual head-down position. But what if yours is among the 4 percent who are breech or otherwise in the "wrong" position? Nowadays virtually no physicians will deliver a breech baby vaginally because the risks are too great. Recent studies have documented that outcomes for vaginal breech deliveries are generally poorer than for breech Cesareans. The biggest risk is the head becoming trapped during the process of delivery. This happens because a presenting part other than the head (such as the feet or butt) can deliver through a cervix that is not completely dilated, while the head, which is the biggest part of the baby's body, cannot. A further complicating factor is that when the baby does not come headfirst, the normal flexion of the head, which cleverly allows the smallest diameter of the head to pass through the pelvis, does not occur.

Breeches most often occur when:

- The fetus is small for its gestational age.
- The fetus is premature and hasn't had time to get into the "right" position.
- The fetus has an abnormally large head.
- The uterus has an irregular shape.
- There are fibroids that may interfere with the fetus's ability to be head first.
- The placenta is implanted low (leaving less room for the fetus).
- There is too much amniotic fluid (polyhydramnios).
- The muscle tone of the uterus is weak (which sometimes happens in women who have had multiple pregnancies or pregnancies very close together).
- There are twins. If the first twin is cephalic, however, its delivery will cause the cervix to dilate completely, which may make vaginal delivery of the second twin—the breech twin—possible. The risks of delivering a second twin that is breech is not the same as with a singleton and does not carry the same risk.

So what can you do if your baby is not in the proper position for delivery? You have choices.

HOW TO MAKE A CONSCIOUS CHOICE ABOUT . . . TURNING A BREECH BABY

Learning that you have a breech baby presents you with a number of options to explore.

First, reflection. So you've just received the news that your baby is breech. How does this make you feel? Is it no big deal? Are you anxious? Sometimes the discovery of a breech presentation churns up other preexisting fears about labor. A woman who was nervous about everything proceeding normally may take it as "confirmation" that she was right to be fearful.

What are your preconceived notions about having a baby that is breech? Do you know anyone who has had one? Have you ever heard any stories about them? Does this knowledge reassure you? Make you nervous?

Being aware of your feelings gives you a starting point for thinking about how to proceed. As you review your options, keep these feelings at the fore.

Second, information. There is no right or wrong way to handle this situation. If you are early in the third trimester, say 32 weeks, there's no hurry to do anything and conventionally you will be told that there is "nothing you can do." About 37 percent of women identified as having a breech in the third trimester will ultimately require a C-section. Why not all of them? In part, because many babies who are breech at this gestational age (about 15 percent between 29 and 32 weeks) will turn on their own before it is time to deliver.

The great thing is that there are also actions you can take that may facilitate the turning of the baby. By 34 to 36 weeks (or earlier if you prefer), consider the following possible courses of action. In order of invasiveness from the least to the most invasive, you can:

• Wait and watch. Do nothing, and hope the baby turns. If it does not, you will most likely need a C-section, since this is the current standard of care for breech presentations.

• Try mind-body approaches. Hypnosis and guided imagery may be helpful. In hypnosis, you are given the suggestion at a very deep level of relaxation for the baby to turn. A good hypnotherapist should make a recording of the session so that you can replay it at home, and I would recommend that you do that once or twice daily. In a study of 100 women between 37 and 40 weeks who used hypnosis for versions of breeches, significantly more (81 percent) of their babies flipped compared with those of a control group who did not use hypnosis (48 percent).

Interactive guided imagery is similar to Dreamagery, but done in concert with a trained professional. It provides the opportunity to have a conversation with the fetus about what's going on. You ask the fetus why it is not in a vertex position, what it needs, whether it would be willing to move, and so on. You also express your thoughts, feelings, and desires to the baby. (You can also try this yourself at home using Dreamagery.)

• Explore physical exercise, such as the pelvic tilt. There is no downside to trying this and it makes physiologic good sense. The concept is that it may allow the baby to lift out of the pelvis and make it easier to turn. Exercise also improves body awareness and posture, which may also help.

• Try moxibustion, an Oriental-medicine therapy that uses heat from the burning of an herb to stimulate acupuncture points associated with turning breeches. (It's similar to having fat incense sticks held near your pressure points.) A promising study of moxibustion reported in the *Journal of the American Medical Association* showed that when done at 34 weeks, it was associated with a 75 percent rate of breech babies turning vertex. (Some of these babies would probably have flipped on their own, but in the control group, only 48 percent flipped.) It's an inexpensive, noninvasive, painless therapy, with a quite impressive success rate in early studies. Moxibustion is often combined with acupuncture, which appears to be safe when in the hands of someone skilled in treating pregnant women. Individualized treatment with an Oriental-medicine practitioner will most likely have even better results than just using this one isolated approach.

• Consider external cephalic version (ECV). This procedure, which is usually performed by ob-gyns, is typically done between 36 to 38 weeks. That's far enough along to be fairly certain the baby won't turn on its own, or turn back to breech if it is successfully "verted" or flipped, yet hopefully still early enough so there is room in the uterus to move the baby. About two-thirds of versions are successful (reports range from 35 percent to 85 percent). Almost all successful versions stay in the correct position (93 percent). If this is your first pregnancy, the chances of ECV working are far less than if you have delivered previously. The presentation of the baby also affects the success rate; for example, if it is not engaged in the pelvis and if there is a good amount of fluid around the baby, it's easier for it to flip.

To do a version, the mother's belly is oiled and the practitioner, working with a partner, manipulates the fetus through the abdominal wall in an effort to rotate it into the cephalic position. If that sounds difficult, it is. It can also be very uncomfortable for the mother-to-be. Usually, if a version is going to work, it does so fairly quickly. The fetus is monitored closely before the procedure and then after for signs of distress. Version should be done in a hospital in the rare event of a complication requiring immediate C section. For this reason, some doctors will place an IV prior to the procedure. Some also administer a drug to help the uterus relax, believing that this will facilitate the procedure. (Whether or not this actually makes a difference has not been studied.)

On the one hand, the huge benefit of external cephalic version is that it's a *relatively* noninvasive way to avoid major surgery. On the other hand, it is not entirely noninvasive. Possible problems include separating the placenta from the uterus, uterine rupture, hemorrhage, and fetal distress. And it may not work! Even if it does, remember that in 7 percent of successful versions, the baby still reverts back to breech prior to delivery. Although it is standard practice to attempt a version, I believe that it's not a decision a mom-to-be should make lightly, especially when there are less invasive options worth exploring first. Overall success rates are about 65 percent at term.

Third, action. No choice within these scenarios precludes trying the others, so attempt one or more—in your mind or in actuality. Imagine for a day that you are going to do an ECV. The next day, imagine doing nothing. See how you feel about these opposing scenarios or any of the others in between.

Then, re-reflection. How did the courses of action you tried in your imagination feel? Or, if you used a low-tech alternative approach and it didn't work, what would you like to explore doing now? If one of the choices works and the baby is now head down, you then face another choice: If you are full term, will you wait to go into labor naturally and hope the baby won't turn to breech again before you do, or will you have labor induced now so that the baby has no chance of flipping back? In making this decision with your doctor, spend some time reflecting on what your body, soul, and baby are all telling you. Dialogue with the baby: What do you think? Are you good where you are or are you ready to be born? See what comes up for you and for your baby.

Stillbirth (Intrauterine Fetal Demise, or IUFD)

Fetal death is a very rare event, and always extremely traumatic. When it does happen, it's almost always in mid- to late pregnancy. The reasons may be related to uncontrolled diabetes or hypertension, a problem with the umbilical cord, or genetic abnormalities. Often we never know what the reason is. IUFD is almost always diagnosed before labor. (If the fetus experiences distress during labor, we can usually detect this and act to deliver the baby quickly and safely. A catastrophic event resulting in an unexpected stillbirth in the delivery room, such as might be caused by a complete placental abruption or uterine rupture, is so unusual that I have only seen it happen twice in my entire career.)

One of the things I don't understand in modern obstetrics is the standard approach to the tragedy of IUFD, namely induction of labor. The woman, still reeling from the shock of hearing that her baby has died and just beginning to deal with her grief, is typically told she must deliver her baby vaginally. Even with Pitocin, this can sometimes take more than a day, because her body has usually not yet begun the birth process (a softening cervix, practice contractions, and so on). Then she must endure the same contractions and pain that all laboring women do, all the while knowing that, unlike them, she will not be delivering a live baby. There will be no joy at the end of this process. Even when everyone around you is treating you with great compassion, it can be grueling.

This approach makes no sense to me. Here we live in an age when women can elect to have tummy tucks and breast enlargements under general anesthesia, or even choose to schedule a C-section for reasons of convenience, and yet a woman whose baby has died is not typically offered the option of a C-section. The professional rationale is that she should not be subjected to the risks of surgery for a baby who is no longer alive. That way of thinking places all of the emphasis on the body and none on the rest of her.

Everyone who experiences this kind of tragedy should be offered,

✓ REALITY CHECK: Overdue Baby

Nowadays, it's rare for a baby to be truly overdue. Remember, your due date is plus or minus two weeks. So you are not offi-cially "overdue" (referred to medically as being "postdates") on the day after your due date, but when you hit *two weeks after your due date*. Because this is also the time at which the risk of fetal death increases significantly, most physicians will discuss inducing you prior to this time. We don't fully understand the physiology behind the dangers of an overdue baby, but one fac-tor is that the placenta may no longer function optimally. To be on the cautious side, if you haven't delivered by 41 weeks (one week past your due date), most obstetricians will want to verify fetal well-being, most likely with an NST (nonstress test) and/or an ultrasound. Depending on your personal situation, your ob-stetric history, and often the ripeness of your cervix, your doctor may discuss induction with you at this time.

There are no right or wrong answers about how to proceed. This is an ideal opportunity to check in with your body, soul, and baby, and use this information to help clarify a course of ac-tion. Once you hit your due date, kick counts and tuning in to your body are extremely important. Work with mind-body ap-proaches, such as relaxation and Dialoguing. Virtually no physi-cians (and very few midwives, who will most likely already be in partnership with a physician) will allow a pregnancy to go past 42 weeks. Use this time to prepare for and become comfortable with whatever is going to happen next. Try to treasure these last days of pregnancy. See movies! Sleep! Before you know it, life will be very different and you may wonder why you were in such a hurry.

I know it can be hard not to fixate on your due date; you've had it in your head for nine months. Yet it's so helpful if you can reframe delivery as a fluid space in time instead of a deadline. I think babies are probably laughing at us adults setting "due" dates in the first place, as if they were term papers needing to be turned in. Only your baby, your body, and your soul will decide when the time is right—and it won't be because someone cir-cled a date on a calendar.

and use, counseling. I also give such women a choice of delivery options. For some women it can be helpful and provide closure to go through labor. A woman may also prefer not to have a C-section because of the increased likelihood that her next pregnancy would be delivered by C-section, or to avoid increased risks that accompany any surgery. These are legitimate and very personal choices. But for many women, automatically being told she must go through labor to deliver a baby that has died in utero creates further trauma.

Plato wrote, "This is the great error of our day in the treatment of the human being, that physicians separate the soul from the body." I couldn't agree more.

Chapter 21

Third Trimester:
Self-Care

∞

Centers of Wellness modifications for weeks 29 to 40

For some women, nurturing your five centers has become second nature by late pregnancy. Others may discover that paying attention to
each becomes more challenging, either because of fatigue and the
sheer physical demands of being so "great with child," or because an
unexpected complication has made the whole pregnancy more stressful and/or frightening. Those scenarios can actually be eased by paying closer attention to self-care now. In addition to looking for ways to
meet the goals set out in Chapter 4, consider the following for the
third trimester:

MIND

Relaxation is paramount now—to give your body a break, to soothe
your anxious soul, and to start preparing yourself for the work ahead
in childbirth.

• *Pay attention to your stressors and whether they are changing.* People may respond to you differently as you grow more visibly pregnant.

What do you enjoy most about this? Least? How would you rate your level of stress now compared to first and second trimester? Do you have a sense of why this has shifted?

• *Activate the relaxation response twice a day or more.* If once a day still works for you, great. But give twice a day a try. You may find that the added escape is helpful as stresses mount.

• *Take more mental vacations.* Use this visualization tactic, described in the Basic Self-Care Plan for Pregnancy, whenever you find yourself growing weary or impatient for pregnancy to be over. As the mother of a baby, I can attest that this is a wonderful stress-reliever after you deliver, too.

• *Indulge in baby-related plans, if they relax you.* Some women find focusing on baby plans to be soothing—especially simple, mindless tasks such as addressing birth announcements, writing shower thank-you notes, reading baby catalogs, trolling the Web for possible baby names, or washing and folding baby clothes and blankets. If such activities stress you out, on the other hand, let them slide.

• *Get plenty of sleep.* Here are some tips on how: If you have trouble finding a comfortable position, experiment. Most women find it comfortable to lie on their sides with their knees bent. Pad your body with lots of pillows—between your knees, along your back, and under your belly when lying on your side. Make sure the room is not too warm and that you aren't using too many blankets. Your increased body heat may necessitate fewer blankets than usual. And don't forget that you should never lie flat on your back at this point in the pregnancy. If getting good sleep is still an issue, try hypnosis. Keep the tape by your bed and use it before sleep and if you wake.

• *Catnap.* The simplest activities—walking to your car in the parking lot, grocery shopping, a normal day at work—can be taxing by late pregnancy. Listen to your body and allow it to sleep and rest as much as it wants.

• *Begin to mentally prepare for labor and delivery.* You can use many mind-body techniques to do this, including imagery to actively imagine the kind of experience you're hoping for, hypnosis to help align your unconscious mind with your conscious desire for this experience, and Dialoguing to prepare and get all parts of you in sync. Make time to read the chapters on labor and delivery well in advance of your due date. Take a childbirth education class (see pages 244–246) by the middle of this trimester.

NUTRITION

Many women are surprised to discover changes in this domain. Both your changing body and your changing soul can prompt you to eat differently now, so don't stop eating consciously, no matter how tired you may be getting of being pregnant.

• *Pay attention to how this domain is changing for you.* As the baby grows a great deal, you are liable to notice differences from week to week, especially since your digestive system has a front-row seat to the changes.

• *Eat smaller meals.* If gastric reflux or heartburn is a problem, you'll be less likely to have difficulty if you eat smaller meals. Keep snacks on hand that you like and that are also nutritious—fruits, nuts, whole-grain crackers or muffins, hard-boiled eggs, yogurt, vegetable sticks—so that you're not tempted to reach for junk foods. Think of the snacks you eat as mini-meals.

• *Don't eat a lot close to bedtime.* Your slowed gastrointestinal system may mean you'll be kept awake when you'd rather be sleeping.

• *Focus on omega-3s.* Continue to include oily fish (such as salmon and sardines) in your diet. If you dislike fish, look for omega eggs or try flaxseed. Your reserves of omega-3 fatty acids get expended a lot faster in the last trimester, because they are used in the development of the central nervous system. There is evidence that babies born to mothers who have a diet rich in omega-3s have better visual acuity as toddlers. It is also being investigated whether a lack of omega-3s after delivery predisposes a woman to postpartum depression. (See the omega-3 chart on pages 51–52.)

• *If UTIs are a problem, drink cranberry juice.* It's been shown to be good for the bladder and decrease the incidence of UTIs.

MOVEMENT

Caution is the watchword at this point in pregnancy. Listen to your body's messages. Even if your exercise routines have not been much changed by pregnancy so far, you can expect to make certain accommodations before you deliver.

• *Listen to your body and don't try to override it.* Some women have a tendency to push a little harder late in pregnancy, despite feelings of wanting to slow down. You're feeling that way for a reason! If your body wants to take things more slowly, let it.

• *Beware the shift in your center of gravity.* Falls are more common in pregnancy than at any other time in life. Wear good supporting shoes to counteract the effects of a shifted center of gravity and loosened pubic bones. Consider taking a Tai Chi class, which can increase body awareness and help you improve your sense of balance.

• *Avoid deep bending.* Because the loosening of ligaments creates the greatest instability in your joints now, you need to be careful not to put too much stress on them. Take extra care when lifting objects. Be sure you have both feet firmly planted on the ground shoulder-width apart, and bend from the knees, not the waist.

• *Continue Kegel exercises to strengthen the pelvic floor.* The physical changes of both carrying the pregnancy and the labor and delivery process are hard on the muscles of the pelvic floor. Doing Kegel exercises will strengthen these muscles and help protect them. The stronger they are, the less likely you will have problems down the road like pelvic prolapse (where the organs that sit in the pelvis—bladder, bowel, and rectum—can drop down into the vagina) or urinary leakage (incontinence). You should continue these exercises through postpartum and beyond.

• *Try perineal massage.* Although there is no evidence to prove this, perineal massage is thought to improve the elasticity and tone of these tissues so that they will stretch more easily when you deliver the baby, helping you to avoid an episiotomy. To do this, gently rub and stretch the skin at the opening of your vagina. Some women find it comfortable to do this in a warm bathtub. You can also use a natural oil (like olive oil) to lubricate the tissues. This can be done daily, by either you or your partner. Be sure hands are clean and nails are trimmed.

FEAR: If I raise my arms over my head, the umbilical cord could strangle the baby.

FACT: There's no connection between your arm muscles and what's taking place in your uterus. Legitimate reasons not to reach too much, however, are the danger of losing your balance and the risk of twisting your back muscles.

SPIRIT

Having a child brings all kinds of new connections into your life. Welcome them and explore them. You may ultimately decide that not all of them work for you, but you won't know until you try.

• *Spend some mom-time.* As you begin to mentally step into the role of mother, your thoughts are probably turning to the way that you were mothered. Many women find it rewarding and instructive to spend special one-on-one time with their mothers now. If your mother is no longer living, seek out people who knew her while she was mothering you, or spend time with her using imagery. You might also spend time with women you are close to, or women whose relationship with their children seems like a good model to you.

• *Line up postpartum help.* What is the plan after your baby is born? Ideally a new mom should not be left all alone with a new baby; although this is becoming a modern norm thanks to scattered families and tough work schedules. This is not the way of new motherhood for most other cultures or even for most of history in our own culture. Think about who you want to be there to help you. Will your partner take off from work and if so, for how long? Do you want your mother? Your mother-in-law? A sister? A friend? Someone with experience with newborns can be especially useful. Give some consideration to how you interact with this person and whether they will be a helper or a stressor, and what boundaries you think would work best for you and your family.

• *Talk about the baby with people who want to hear your thoughts and feelings.* Thoughts of the baby and impending motherhood may consume you, and dominate your preferred conversation. Seek out those who want to share such conversations. Women who don't have children and aren't pregnant, for example, might not relate and only leave you frustrated. Pay attention to how you feel around people and then honor those feelings. Journaling about this topic can also be great.

• *Enjoy your baby shower.* Moms-to-be have many different reactions to this rite of passage. Some look forward to it; others dread it or find it corny. While it's worth reflecting on why you have the reaction you do (especially if it's a strong one), think hard before opting out completely. Baby showers serve lots of purposes. Ostensibly, they're a way to furnish your household with the baby items you'll need. But they also serve as a bridge to parenthood. They allow friends and family members to participate in your pregnancy. They're an opportunity to learn from others about labor, delivery, and new motherhood. And they're another way for you to try on the idea of becoming a mom.

HOW TO MAKE A CONSCIOUS CHOICE ABOUT . . . LABOR WITNESSES

One of the more surprising trends I've seen in my obstetric career is the growth of labor as a spectator sport. A couple of decades ago fathers were exiled from the delivery room; now the pendulum has definitely swung in the opposite direction. Not only do we have Dad right next to Mom's bed, but at times we also have the doula, the expectant grandparents, the older kids, the stepkids, the best friend, and a host of other labor supporters and observers. I've walked into delivery suites that look like parties, with ten or more people milling about.

Sometimes, no one's even paying attention to the laboring woman. For every exaggerated birth scene portrayed for laughs on movies and TV, I've probably seen a real-life counterpart. I've seen card games in progress, the TV on, picnics, and even heated arguments. I've also attended births where all the guests are completely focused on the impending birth, though they can be just as unconscious about what they're doing. They crowd around the bed, touching the mom and shouting like a cheerleading squad, "Push! Push!" This can not only override any personal experience the laboring mom may want to have, it almost certainly precludes her ability to focus on her baby and her body. It also presents a safety issue when the doctor cannot clearly communicate with the patient or the other care providers in the room. Labor is definitely a time when everyone truly involved needs to be communicating well and on the same page. I've had to get right in front of my patient's face and say, "You need to look me in the eye, no matter what else is going on. You listen only to me, and I listen only to you." Doctor and patient are a team, especially in childbirth. There needs to be clarity and connection, without distraction.

This trend is the result of a number of factors, one being the widespread use of epidurals. This means that the majority of moms-to-be are more distanced from labor pains, and often also from the labor experience itself. It is therefore easier for them to be more sociable, and their labors are easier for others to watch. In the 1990s, the popularity of TV shows depicting labors (e.g., *A Baby Story*) showed many situations of laboring before a group, reinforcing the idea that this was the norm.

The question of whether or not to have loved ones around you during this sacred time is a highly individual choice. *As an integrative medicine obstetrician, I want you to not just have the event, but I want you to have the experience.* I want you to feel supported, relaxed, and conscious. I want to feel that you and I are connected and working as a team with your body, your soul, and your baby. So before you invite friends and family to watch your delivery, get conscious about your motivations and your true feelings about this choice:

First, reflection. What do you want this experience to be? Who do *you* want to be present at this momentous time?

Consider the "why" behind each person you're considering having present. Why do you want them? Because they asked to participate? Because they connect with you deeply and help you relax?

Because you feel like you're supposed to have friends and family around you? Because you don't want to let anyone down?

Consider the individuals. Can they appreciate the difference between being a spectator and being a supporter? Can you count on them to respect that difference in the heat of the moment? If you change your mind during labor about desiring their presence, will they be upset or argue, or gracefully wait somewhere else? Do they share and value your view of this life experience?

Reflect on the labor experience you envision. Does having others support or hinder that vision? How? Consider how you feel about having these individuals see you at your most naked (physically and psychologically). Use visualization to give you an idea of what it will be like. Imagine your delivery with the person in question present. Then check in. How do you feel on the levels of body, soul, and baby? Does your body feel relaxed knowing they are there, or tense? Does your soul feel content with this connection, or unsettled? Does your baby love the thought of this person being part of the birth experience, or recoil from it?

Reflect on what you want the moment of birth to be like. Do you want to share the baby with everyone right away? Do you want to make a space for you and your partner to be alone with the baby?

Second, information. Find out about hospital policies regarding birth witnesses. Some institutions may specify a limit, others may have age restrictions. There may also be rules about where witnesses may go and how they can interact with hospital staff. Having too many people in the way poses a safety risk; birth attendants need to have access to equipment and to the patient.

Consider getting a variety of perspectives, such as from your care provider or others who have labored with and without a variety of labor supporters.

Discuss the possibility with the people you are thinking about inviting. Sometimes women assume that, say, Grandpa-to-be wants to be in the room when he'd really rather meet the baby once it's cleaned up and not watch you deliver. Be sure that the person understands that you won't know how you are actually going to feel once you're in labor, and that you may change your mind.

If you are considering having a child present, consider the child's age and maturity. While all children are different, typically those under age eight can't understand the pain of labor or appreciate the magic of the event. They can be a distraction. Bear in mind that unless you're having a scheduled C-section, you won't know what time of day you'll be laboring or for how long. If a child of any age is present, an adult who is not the primary birth supporter should be present to care for the child. Children of all ages benefit from being counseled about birth beforehand. (Actually, I believe adults do as well.) If bonding is a concern, a wonderful option is to arrange to bring the child to the hospital soon after the baby is born, giving the mom some time to recover but still allowing the child to feel like a part of the experience. Many hospitals do not allow children on labor and delivery (L&D) floors as an infectious-disease precaution.

Also be aware that at any point the doctor may ask people to step out or leave, depending on what's going on and what's in your best interest. Your health and your baby's, after all, are the priority. You should be informed, however, why such a request is being made.

Then, action. Make a decision. You will feel better about whatever choice you make if you have done so consciously.

Finally, re-reflection. This step is essential. After you've made your choice, it's never too late to change your mind. Things change. First re-reflect after you decide and before you share this decision. If it feels right, let those involved know. But again remember that even once you're in the delivery room, the option is yours to disinvite those whom you no longer want present, or to invite someone else in. This is not a party, after all; it's a sacred life experience—your life, your experience.

SENSATION

Pamper, pamper, pamper. This center takes on higher value than ever in the third trimester. Okay, maybe you're not feeling too sexual (although many women still do). On the other hand, you are apt to feel especially female, lush, and sensuous—at least when you're not achy, crabby, and tired. The third trimester is a perfect example of when mind over matter can make all the difference in how you perceive each day.

• *Make sure your maternity clothes fit well.* Yes, it's possible to out-grow them. If your waistband or bra is digging into your skin, this can exacerbate physical problems and discomforts (such as heartburn). Even though you may tire of wearing the same limited wardrobe over and over, you'll feel better about your clothes if they fit. If money is an issue, look into secondhand shops or barter with another pregnant mom (or one who recently delivered) to refresh your look inexpensively. If you're debating whether to make a purchase, remember that you'll probably continue to get use out of it for the first month or two (or longer) after you deliver.

• *Wear a maternity bra at night.* For extra support, if it feels comfortable.

• *Keep exploring ways to indulge all five senses.* You may get into certain routines involving a particular scent of candle that you like, or the nubby feel of a particular sweater. Keep experimenting with new pleasures. The seasons have changed since your pregnancy began, and so have you; different things may appeal to you now.

• *Prepare some labor tunes.* Having music you enjoy hearing during labor can be very soothing. Spend time now trying out different tunes and consider making a special tape, CD, or MP3 playlist.

• *Don't worry about the baby during sexual activity.* It bears repeating, because I am asked about it so often: Your fetus is extremely well-cushioned in your body. Your abdominal wall is thick, then there is the even thicker wall of the uterus, and finally your baby is floating—even at the very end of pregnancy—in the sac of amniotic fluid. Intercourse won't affect him or her in the least.

DECISIONS TO MAKE AS YOU START YOUR THIRD TRIMESTER

• *Start shopping for a pediatrician.* It's better to do this task while you have time. Ask friends and your doctor for recommendations. As you did when finding a pregnancy-birth partner, look for a professional who is philosophically aligned with you. Other pluses: an office located near your home, admitting privileges at a local children's hospital, convenient hours (ask about what happens if you need care after hours and on weekends), and coverage by your health plan.

• *Make a conscious decision about circumcision.* Circumcision is often done the day after delivery in the hospital. I am always surprised at how many people shrug as if they are considering this important choice regarding their son's care for the very first time. Use the Feedback Loop tool to help you and your partner think through and feel comfortable with your decision. Everybody has a starting "story" or preconceptions about circumcision, even though most people have never really spent any time thinking about it before. For some people, the choice to circumcise is deeply rooted in religious or cultural traditions. For others it's just considered the default thing to do (or not do). Many people argue that removing the foreskin decreases sexual pleasure and that it is a cruel practice. On the other hand, there is data that not being circumcised can increase the spread of certain STDs. Medically it's a wash; the American Academy of Pediatrics says the decision should be a personal one. Considering that circumcision is a medical intervention and potentially traumatic, and that any intervention involves a modicum of risk, I think it's best to really understand your "whys" and feel good about them. This is a good topic to discuss with not only your obstetrician, but also your future pediatrician. It is a good way to get to know one you would like to use for your child, and begin to get a sense of his or her style.

• *Consider whether you would like to do cord-blood banking.* After delivery, your baby's umbilical cord blood (the blood left in the cord) can be collected, frozen, and stored in a blood bank for possible use later in the treatment of certain diseases such as leukemia and sickle-cell anemia. This has become a popular step in recent years since umbilical cord blood was found to supply the same kinds of blood-forming (hematopoietic) stem cells as found in bone marrow. In the event that your child needed radiation that destroyed bone marrow, for example, cord blood could be used in place of a bone marrow transplant. Cord blood is a rich source of stem cells that are "pluripotential," which means that they have the potential to develop into any number of cells, from heart and blood cells to liver cells, nerve cells, and so forth. Unlike most conventional medicines, treatments based on stem cells replace or correct damaged and diseased cells in our bodies. As of today, stem cells are used to treat over 40 life-threatening diseases. In the future, it is possible that cells from a single unit of cord blood could be multiplied, allowing the stem cells to be available for multiple uses. Children with cancer, certain genetic diseases, and some blood disorders can use the cord blood of their full siblings. Cord blood can also be donated so that it can be used for individuals in need of a transplant who cannot find a match elsewhere.

Cord-blood storage does remain somewhat controversial. The American Academy of Pediatrics does not recommend that parents store their children's cord blood for future use as "biological insurance," citing a low likelihood that most children will ever need a bone marrow transplant. If the child developed cancer or a genetic disease at this time, his or her own cord blood would not be used for transplantation. Private storage can be expensive, as much as $1,500 to $2,000 for collection and the first year of storage (banking) plus an annual banking fee that can run $100 plus per year. There are some concerns about private banks' processing procedures, as they do not have to follow FDA standards.

I recommend considering cord-blood banking to all of my patients who are eligible. (People with family histories of cancer in a first-degree relative cannot donate to public banks because they are at slightly higher risk of the baby developing a malignancy.) You can also donate your child's cord blood to a nonprofit public cord-blood bank for use by others, if you deliver in a hospital that has been set up as an established collection site linked to a public bank. If you choose this option you can't retrieve your baby's own blood for personal use later.

The research in this area is continually advancing, and the life of your child will hopefully be a long one. This year at Duke, cord-blood transfusions were used on an experimental basis for two babies who had anoxic brain injury (brain damage due to lack of oxygen). Whether this will prove to be of benefit in these kinds of situations remains to be seen, but it does illustrate the kind of advances that are being explored.

• *Make sure you (and your partner) know the drill.* Work out plans regarding communication and transportation for when labor begins. These can change from day to day depending on schedules. Have backup plans, too—for example, identify a neighbor who is willing to drive you to the hospital, or the number of a reliable taxi service. (Don't plan on driving yourself to the place you'll deliver!) Be reassured, though. Labor rarely happens as suddenly and dramatically as portrayed on TV. Most moms have plenty of time to get ready and get to the hospital calmly.

GET-READY GUIDE

Well before the third trimester ends, you'll want to take care of the following:

• *Pack your hospital bag.* You'll want basic toiletries; warm socks (labor rooms can get cold); slippers (for walking in your room or the corridors); pajamas and robe; something comfortable to labor in if you don't want to use a hospital gown (caution: it will probably get bloody); a hairband for long hair; a change of clothing for leaving the hospital (maternity clothes from mid-pregnancy; you will not be your pre-pregnancy weight or size); clothing for the baby to go home in; and any labor aids you want to bring. (Read Chapter 25, "Labor and Delivery: Self-Care" for ideas.) You may also want your cell phone or telephone calling card, a list of key numbers to call with the news, a camera, nonperishable snacks (for Dad or after you deliver), and cash (for Dad to get food). If you wear contacts, you'll also need your glasses. Keep a running list of items you're using now and can't pack (glasses, journal, iPod, certain toiletries) so that you won't forget them if you have to leave quickly or so that someone else can gather them for you. If you write a birth vision statement, have it ready to go too (see pages 370–374).

• *Preregister at the hospital.* You'll save frustration and time at admittance if your paperwork has been handled in advance.

- *Buy an infant car seat.* It's the law in every state that a baby must travel in one. Purchasing yours ahead of time makes one less thing your partner needs to do before picking you up at the hospital to go home (and gives you some say in which model is selected). You may want to start with the lightweight models made especially for babies under 20 pounds; models designed for older babies or toddlers are big and cumbersome. If you get one that is easily removed from the car, you can use it to transport a sleeping baby. The middle of the backseat is considered the safest place to secure a car seat. And definitely figure out how to put it in ahead of time—the last thing you want to slow down your homecoming is struggling with the car seat in the hospital parking lot! Most fire stations will teach you or check them as a community service.

Part Six

Labor and Delivery

The Miracle of Birth

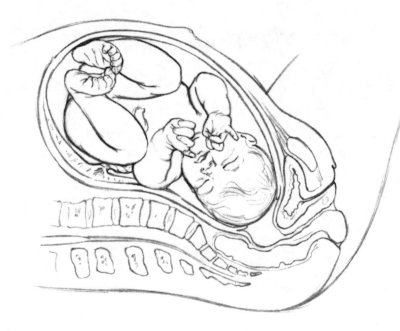

Chapter 22

Labor and Delivery:
Reflection and Observation

∞

Checking in with body, soul, and baby about childbirth

Having a "conscious labor and delivery" means bringing the same level of body-soul-and-baby awareness and involvement to the culmination of pregnancy that you practiced in all the months leading up to it.

What kind of labor do you want? What do you envision? How events transpire is not entirely your call, but you still have a powerful degree of influence over the experience. Now, more than ever, being aware can make all the difference.

There are two big reasons why a conscious labor is such a worthy goal: First, although many decisions during childbirth must be made by medical professionals, ideally they should be made in partnership with you. Labor does not unfold in an automatic sequence that's identical for everyone, and it's not "managed" in a single, universal way. Even more so than with prenatal care, labor and delivery is as much art as science, with many options for handling most circumstances. When you're aware and involved, you can help make the choices that are best for you—yes, even in the excitement of labor.

Second, and equally important, consciousness during labor gives you the power to own and define the experience. Regardless of whether you have a drug-free natural delivery or a C-section under general anesthesia, whether you labor for a full day or for a few hours, your birth *experience* will be more than just the sum of its mechanical details. Owning your birth story means that no matter what kind of labor you end up having, you will be at peace with it. You'll be content that you did your best in the circumstances—and instead of simply being "glad that it's over," you will most likely emerge from labor transformed by this miraculous event.

Planning for your labor is a little like planning a wedding. In neither scenario will you be able to control every detail. No matter how much time you spend color-coordinating the gowns and flowers and arranging place cards on the tables, you can't control the weather, obnoxious Uncle Albert, or a clumsy caterer dropping the wedding cake. But you do have a choice about how to respond to what comes up. The best approach is to prepare for labor as best you can and then embrace what unfolds, surprises and all. It's your birth story, unique to you.

Compare the diverse experiences of two women:

Jenna's Story: Unconscious and Disappointed

Jenna hoped for a vaginal delivery because the idea of a C-section frightened her. She was so fixated on a natural delivery that she refused to pay attention to the discussion of Cesareans in her childbirth class. "I don't want to jinx myself," she told her partner, Bob. She read everything she could about natural childbirth and felt psyched and ready.

Her water broke one week before her due date. After Jenna had been laboring for 20 hours, she was 5 cm dilated. She was given Pitocin to increase her contractions, along with an epidural, because she was finding it harder to get through each contraction.

Several hours later, her dilation seemed stalled at 8 cm. This can happen for several reasons; in Jenna's case, it was determined that the baby was in a difficult position for an easy vaginal delivery. Even after good contractions for two hours, she did not dilate further, and her doctors proceeded with a C-section. Jenna was in tears about this decision, and was given some sedation to help calm her. A healthy 7 pound, 14 ounce son arrived minutes later.

Jenna was relieved to see him, but couldn't stop thinking about how her delivery plans had "gone wrong." *How could this have happened? There must have been something I could have done differently, or the doctors could have done,* she ruminated. She was so caught up in these internal conversations that she wasn't able to be fully present for her son's birth, and didn't feel elation or joy in that moment. Part of her was still back in the labor room, second-guessing herself and her doctors. Everything felt dimmed by a pervasive sense that she had failed her carefully prepared birth plan. "If only I hadn't been so tired," she kept saying. "If only I had kept on a little longer."

Taylor's Story: Connected and Content

Taylor, too, wanted a natural delivery. She had chosen her doctor and birthing center in part because they had low rates of Cesarean delivery. She and her husband, Paul, took childbirth-preparation classes and tried to do everything they could to prepare themselves emotionally and practically. For Taylor, that included following a conscious pregnancy plan for the entire nine months.

As she Journaled and reflected on her thoughts about labor itself, she became aware of just how strong her aversion to the idea of a C-section was. Rather than compartmentalizing this concern and avoiding thinking about it, Taylor met it head-on. She Dialogued with the fear, asking, "What are you afraid of? Tell me your worst-case scenario." Through this dialogue, she realized that, as a woman who prided herself on fitness, she dreaded the possibility of being "incapacitated," and that the thought of having to recover from what is after all major surgery seemed overwhelming. Once she had articulated this worry, Taylor did some reading about what the postpartum phase was like after a C-section, and she began to feel better. Yes, there is a longer recovery time with a C-section, but the recovery would be complete, and she'd soon be back to her former level of activity. She realized that while she still hoped very much for a vaginal delivery, everything would be fine if for some reason she ended up with a Cesarean.

During her labor, Taylor continued to check in with herself on body, soul, and baby levels. Everything went beautifully for the first eight hours. Then, when Taylor was 7 cm dilated, she fell off her labor curve. Two hours, then four, passed without progress. Taylor wanted to keep trying, but after the last labor check, the baby's heart-rate tracing was beginning to show signs of distress. The doctor advised a C-section and Taylor, who had been aware and informed at every stage of labor, agreed. She felt a momentary stab of disappointment, but she also knew she had done everything she could. She checked in with her body, soul, and baby, and at each level she realized that she was at peace with this decision. Her focus across all three dimensions quickly shifted to the imminent delivery of her baby.

It was wonderful to see her in the OR, fully present, connected to Paul and the medical team. When their son was handed to Paul and he brought him to her side, they both brimmed with joy. *I did it*, Taylor thought. *I'm a mom! And he is sooo amazing!*

REFLECTION AND OBSERVATION:
BEFORE LABOR BEGINS

When thinking about labor, we tend to focus on the physical aspects of labor, and understandably so—after all, it's called "labor" for a reason! We talk a lot about the "miracle of birth" in reference to the physical act. But the spiritual dimension of childbirth is almost never discussed, and certainly not by most obstetricians. But as much as childbirth is a major event for the body, it's also a transformative event for the soul just as significant as your own birth and your own death. You've had this life within you for all these months, nurturing it and growing it. You are the conduit for bringing a new soul into the world. That's huge!

The processes of separation (of the baby from your body) and new beginning (of your shared journey as mother and child) can inspire complicated feelings. Reflect on this dimension of the birth process in your third trimester, as your due date draws near.

SUGGESTED TOOLS:

Journaling Your Journey (tool #6)

What are your preconceptions about giving birth? Whether you're aware of it or not, your ideas about childbirth have been fed by a lifetime of stories—stories based in fact, fiction, and everything in between. We've all seen countless "births" on TV and in the movies, for example. Chances are good that throughout your pregnancy, friends and perfect strangers alike have come forward to share their own birth experiences. Unfortunately, most of the stories moms to-be often hear are the horrible ones, not the beautiful ones. Gaining a realistic understanding of the birth process is one thing; hearing lots of scary stories is something else entirely. Don't get "hexed" into a negative perception of birth by listening only to such dramas. Tell these storytellers (whether they are well-intentioned or not), that it's "doctor's orders" that you not listen to negative birth stories. As an obstetrician who has attended thousands of deliveries, I can assure you that there are many more wonderful births than nightmarish ones.

Whatever you've picked up about labor and delivery from your reading, your care provider, your childbirth class, and your partner (who has his own lifetime of collected birth stories) affects your expectations and desires. These are the images that will fuel your own experience of labor—or drain it. First become aware of them, then shift them or rearrange them to align with the hope and intention you have in your heart. The power of intention is huge. Aligning your body, your soul, and your baby, along with your partner and/or labor supporter and your physician to the same vision is an important step.

1. Before you write, make these stories conscious. Think about your images of labor and delivery, wherever they may have originated. What parts have stuck with you (whether positive or negative)? What are you expecting? What are you hoping for? What are you fearing? Feel free to write as you explore.

2. Now Journal about the labor story you would most like to have. Envision what you want to unfold. Make it more powerful by including as many details as possible. Don't, for example, simply say you want to be "confident and eager." Step in to it further. How do you *feel*

as you are entering into labor and delivery? Close your eyes and feel the eagerness, the confidence. Feel it in your body, in your soul, and in your baby. Have the experience you are hoping for. Who's there? What's the room like? What's happening with your body? How does it feel to finally deliver this baby and look in those eyes? The more you flesh this out, the better.

Dreamagery (tool #9)

You can also use visualization to connect with your feelings. Invite an image that represents your labor and delivery experience. Notice everything about it. What does it have to say to you? What does it need? What do you have to say or ask it? What do you need? Let it know what you are hoping for, and ask what you can do to help realize this scenario.

PRE-LABOR CHECK-INS: WHAT MIGHT COME UP FOR YOU

I'm Terrified.

I met Momoka when one of the other ob-gyns was on vacation. "So, how are you feeling about labor and delivery?" I asked, routinely.

"I don't know. I'd rather not think about it." She then added that she'd had an uncomfortable feeling about labor almost from the time she discovered she was pregnant. She changed the subject anytime anyone began sharing their own birth story and avoided asking her care provider any questions about it. She didn't want to read or hear any labor tips, nor did she sign up for childbirth preparation classes.

"Why do you think this is?" I asked her.

"It just scares me. So I don't dwell on it. It's not like there's anything I can do about it anyway."

"Here's the good news. There *is* something you can do," I suggested. "While it may sound counterintuitive, if you explore these feelings rather than run from them, in the end it won't be so scary." I introduced Dreamagery, so Momoka could have a conversation with her body to see what it had to say about labor.

First we did some breathing exercises to get into a relaxed state. Then I asked her to imagine a place where she felt comfortable, at peace, and safe. She chose a favorite beach. She spent some time just noticing everything about this place—and really enjoyed being there. Once she was comfortable and ready to proceed, I asked her to invite an image that represented her labor. "The first thing that came into my head was a basketball," she said. "That's too weird. I don't even like basketball. I'm not even an athletic person." I encouraged her to stick with this first image and see where it took her. "Spend some time just noticing everything about this image—what it looks like, how it feels, how it smells," I guided her.

Then I asked her to engage the image in a conversation. What does it want to tell you?

The image's answer: "I know what *I'm* doing. You don't have to do it. Your job is to support me, not be afraid of me."

Momoka continued to feel alienated from the image that had appeared. "It feels strange and unfamiliar," she said. I asked her to share her thoughts and feelings directly with the image. She did, and the basketball explained that it was okay that the concept of labor felt foreign to her, just like the ball itself did. It's okay that she felt like she didn't know how to "play," and that she was fearful that she wouldn't do it "right." They continued to have dialogue back and forth, with Momoka expressing her fears and doubts, and the image responding. The basketball reassured her again that what might not seem natural or instinctive to Momoka, was completely natural and instinctive to it, that it loved to play basketball, that that was the very thing it was made to do! And all it needed of Momoka was trust. It wasn't her job to be something she wasn't, it was simply her job to support her body in what it was designed and meant to do.

Momoka was surprised by her body's bluntness, but the answer made sense to her. "I am not a jock," she admitted. "I was the kid who always got picked last for teams, and I nearly didn't graduate from high school because I couldn't pass the swimming test. I have just been dreading having to do something this physical. But I think I get what the image is saying to me. This is altogether different from me learning to swim. What a great thought that there is a part of me I don't even know that not only knows how to do this but wants to do it!"

I encouraged Momoka to honor all of these feelings, and to listen to her body's vote of confidence. The physicality of childbirth, an act that your body is biologically wired to do, is different from the physicality of a sport that you have to learn. The relationship between one's comfort level with one's body and readiness for labor is a complicated one. Some women who are not generally physically confident nevertheless feel very psyched for labor, while very athletic women sometimes have fears. I suggested that Momoka actually get a basketball and that she spend a little time every day holding it, smelling it, getting familiar with it. It would be a great physical reminder, a symbol of her body's message to her. And of course I asked her to continue her conversations with it. She continued to release her fears and grew excited about the prospect of supporting her body in doing something it wanted and knew how to do. It was the first time in her life that she felt like she was working in partnership with her body and with confidence in its abilities. It was interesting to watch this evolve and deepen over the weeks of her Dreamagery.

When the time came, Momoka wound up pushing for three hours, and delivered a perfect daughter. "I don't know where my strength came from," she said later. "But I feel great. It was the hardest thing I have ever done, and I did it!" I do know the origins of that strength: By trusting her body, believing in it and supporting it, she ended up feeling more connected to it and to its power than ever before in her life. That's still evident today, three years after she had her baby, in the way she holds herself, the way she moves, and in her general sense of confidence. The labor she had feared so greatly was a huge blessing.

Excited but Nervous

Feeling a combination of eagerness and anxiety prior to labor is completely normal. Even though the body is quite ready to bring forth the baby growing within you, the soul can be a little apprehensive. The body can be apprehensive, too—perfectly natural, since, if this is your first pregnancy, your body hasn't actually done this before.

If mixed feelings are the case for you, simply be aware that this is your starting point and then ask yourself what you need to feel more comfortable. For some women, reading about labor or going to visit the labor and delivery unit where they will deliver only increases their anxiety. They don't want more knowledge or more facts; however, they may be more open to exploring their feelings. Other women feel that the more information they can get, the better. They may even think that watching an actual delivery would be helpful. For them, the real-life deliveries that can be viewed on TV shows such as *A Baby Story*, on The Learning Channel are a wonderful resource. Ask yourself where you fall on this spectrum, and then appreciate your own wisdom in knowing what works for you.

✔ **REALITY CHECK:** Common Fears About Labor

Fear of the unknown is very human, and especially for the first-time mom, labor is a big unknown. Whatever your specific fear, the process is the same: Make it conscious. Use the tools such as Journaling, Dialoguing, and Dreamagery to "greet it at the front door," if you will, so it doesn't keep trying to come in the back way. Thank the fear for showing up and then get to know it. Your goal should be to understand the fear as deeply as possible, rather than to vanquish it or make it go away. By honoring the uneasy feeling rather than repressing it, you're much more likely to make it constructive rather than destructive or distracting. Tip: Ask your body and your soul directly to help you understand the fear and what it needs to help let go of it.

Common labor fears include:

• *Fear of losing control.* You may run life by your BlackBerry and have color-coordinated closets, but labor is not about controlling events. It's about going with the flow. Sometimes women are worried about losing personal control, afraid they'll swear or scream during delivery (both perfectly normal responses to the experience). Others have difficulty with the idea that they cannot plan how everything will turn out. A woman counting on a VBAC (vaginal birth after [a previous] Cesarean) dreads another C-section. A woman who wants a natural delivery can't bear the idea that she might need drugs. Since loss of control can be an especially threatening situation for women who have been victims of molestation or rape, it can be particularly important to explore this if you have been in those situations.

• *Fear of failure.* A woman who has struggled with trying to have a "perfect" pregnancy—gaining the right amount of weight, eating all the right foods, exercising, wearing the most fashionable maternity clothes—may worry that in the clutch she'll somehow fall apart and not be able to "do" childbirth "properly." This kind of fear is closely related to fear of losing control and thus of failing to live up to some imaginary ideal or standard. It may come from her partner, her parents, her childbirth class, her social circle, or deep within herself.

• *Fear of pain.* Anticipating the pain of childbirth is difficult because no one can tell you ahead of time exactly what it will feel like. Human beings all seem to register pain differently and have different thresholds for it. What's more, the position of the baby, the use of Pitocin, and other factors mean that the amount of pain can vary from labor to labor.

• *Fear of hospitals.* Some women I see simply don't like the medical environment. They may pride themselves on never taking aspirin and understandably associate the gleaming white halls and antiseptic odor with sickness, rather than health. For someone who has been through serious medical situations themselves or with a family member, this can be a strong association. Others are apprehensive about the loss of modesty, privacy, and autonomy that accompany hospitalization.

• *Fear of an emergency.* Sometimes when women process their fear, the bottom line is a deep concern that something might go wrong. The concern may center on something going awry with the baby, even if everything has been fine up to this point, or of something happening to the mother herself. The latter is a fear that a woman's partner often also feels as the woman gets closer and closer to the great unknown of delivery. Of course childbirth *was* once a life-or-death experience, before we knew about handwashing and antibiotics and how to handle common complications. Maternal death today is exceedingly rare and almost always occurs in pregnancies that were known to be at very high risk for specific problems.

A Prisoner of Preconceptions

Sometimes it's not exactly fear that influences how we approach labor, but a set of expectations imposed on us from outside. Doctors can have a particularly powerful impact, which is why it's so important to choose a doctor whose childbirth philosophy is in line with your own. When Caroline was seven months pregnant with her first baby, she needed an ultrasound to check the location of the placenta. Everything was fine, and her doctor told her that it looked like she would have a big baby. At first, she didn't think anything of it. She and her husband, Tyler, are both tall, and if anything, she was glad to know their son would probably be tall, too. His size seemed to signal his good health.

At her next checkup, the ob repeated the ultrasound and said again that the baby was measuring big. This time he added that she would probably need a C-section. This message was reinforced to her at each visit thereafter. Naturally, that was the story that Caroline then held in her head: My baby is big, and I need a C-section. She began to accept it as fact.

When I was introduced to her at a social function, she was already 39 weeks along, and she mentioned that she was scheduled for a C-section in three days. No, she wouldn't have a trial of labor, she told me matter-of-factly. Her doctor said the baby was "too big."

In actual fact, however, the only reason to go straight to a C-section for a first-time baby who looks large is if the mother is a diabetic and the baby measures *very* big. These macrosomic babies of diabetic moms (those with a very high birth weight) are at higher risk of shoulder dystocia (getting their shoulders stuck during delivery) than large babies of nondiabetic moms. But if the mother is not diabetic, the optimal standard of care is to go through a trial of labor first; if labor stalls, then you can go to C-section. I've done vaginal deliveries of countless healthy nine- and ten-pounders. What's more, late ultrasounds are notoriously unreliable in estimating fetal weight. I've attended many deliveries where the estimated fetal weight was very high, but the actual birth weight was only average.

Because Caroline wasn't my patient and she was so close to delivery, I didn't think it appropriate to second-guess her doctor. But it felt unfortunate to me that she had been cheated out of the opportunity to make choices, to engage fully in this big decision about how she would give birth. This was because her physician drew the "too big" conclusion early on, stated it as fact to her repeatedly, and did not share information about the options available to her.

As it turned out, Caroline's son was big: 9 pounds, 7 ounces. But was he too big to have been delivered vaginally? I doubt it. But we'll never know. And even if she'd had a trial of labor and wound up with a C-section, does this mean that her doctor's decision to go straight to a C-section was the "right" one? I feel that it was not, because there's nothing really "right" about an unconscious choice made by a physician and "delivered" to a patient.

Veteran Moms: "Here We Go Again!"

Body and soul check-ins can be especially vivid for women who have gone through labor before. That's because in a first pregnancy, the stories you've heard about childbirth originate outside yourself. In subsequent pregnancies, you have a history. And your body holds memories of those deliveries, as does your soul, and they will draw strongly on that prior experience.

If you had a good experience, your body may feel quietly confident: "Been there, done that, let's go." If this is the case for you, acknowledge that, but also try to dig a little deeper. Explore whether there is anything you would like to do differently this

---

✓ **REALITY CHECK:** Expectations

There's a delicate balance between being clear about your intentions and hopes, and becoming overly attached to them. When a woman locks in to a position, digging in to make her expected plan come true no matter what, this is every bit as unconscious as having no plan at all. She may have arrived at her choices via a very conscious process but if she is unable to adjust them when necessary, they've become just a stance. They don't honor the dynamic and mysterious nature of the birth process.

Common examples of being hostage to one's expectations:

- demanding an epidural as soon as you get to the hospital or as soon as it's offered
- vowing not to have any medication at all
- being determined not to have a Cesarean, no matter what
- insisting on a VBAC no matter what

If you have faith and trust in your medical partners and know they understand your wishes, if you check in with yourself often, and if you remain an active participant in the process, what ultimately *needs to happen*, will. It may not be the same as what you expected, or hoped for, but it will be a situation you can appreciate and feel good about.

---

time (such as different positions for labor or delivery, different people present, or new relaxation techniques to try). Often, second and subsequent births are wonderful opportunities to open up to the whole experience, because veteran moms have already been through the Great Unknown, and they tend to be much less distracted by fear.

If you had a difficult first delivery, however, that will be your body's and your soul's reference point, even if circumstances are entirely different this time. Bethany, for example, had a very long labor during her first pregnancy. The delivery was then complicated by severe postpartum hemorrhaging due to uterine atony (i.e., lack of tone, a condition where the uterus does not contract after delivery of the baby). She needed multiple transfusions and came close to dying. It had been an extremely traumatic experience for her and her family. By an unfortunate coincidence, when she arrived at the labor and delivery suite for her second delivery, it turned out to be the exact same suite she had been in the first time. Immediately she tensed and felt anxious—and it's little wonder, since she had nearly died in that room. And although there was nothing to indicate that history would repeat itself here, she felt transported, within both her body and her soul, back to that first delivery. So did her husband. The fear in the room was palpable.

Even if you think you've fully processed and grieved over a traumatic event, returning to the scene of a bad experience often triggers memories and emotions. It's therefore especially important to spend time reflecting on your past experience. Be conscious of the strong feelings you hold concerning it. Use the tools to put closure on the last experience and to rewire your body and soul for this new and different one. You don't want to wait until you're being wheeled into the delivery room to realize that you have unresolved feelings from your last delivery. Also explore what different choices you can make, and what role you can play to make it a different experience.

Bethany had done everything she could think of to prepare herself for her second delivery. She hired a doula to offer her extra support during labor. She worked with a hypnotherapist to help "rewire" the feelings and beliefs around labor and delivery that were imprinted from her first delivery. She and her husband visited the labor and delivery floor several times in advance of her labor, so that she could "desensitize" herself and feel comfortable and safe there. And once she was in labor and found herself in a room that held such bad memories, she politely but firmly asked to be moved to another room. Because she had consciously confronted the feelings from her first delivery, she was clear about what she needed and strong enough to make sure she got it. The second delivery went smoothly and she delivered a healthy daughter completely uneventfully. Interestingly, months later Bethany told me that she realized that many of her psychological wounds from her first experience had been healed through the preparations she made the second time.

REFLECTION AND OBSERVATION:
DURING LABOR

Reflecting on labor and delivery well before your first contraction is key to making the most of this amazing experience—but don't stop there. It's even more important to stay connected to your body, soul, and baby while you're actually *having* the experience. Quick Pics are an ideal way to keep you focused and engaged.

Women often ask me, "How on earth will I be able to check in with myself when I am busy laboring?" Or, "Don't women lose focus in labor? How will I be able to concentrate on anything?" But consider who's doing the laboring—you. You can very naturally check in with yourself because you are already focused on yourself. You're not really doing anything "extra." During the final intense phase of labor, you may find it easiest to run quick check-ins with yourself between the contractions.

SUGGESTED TOOLS
(THROUGHOUT LABOR):

Body Quick Pic (tool #1)

Check in frequently once labor has begun. Notice all you can about the contractions themselves. In early labor, is the pain easier to work with when you are standing or sitting? Can you keep breathing or are you inclined to hold your breath? Does it help or hinder to be touched? Is there anything that you need to make things work more smoothly? Anything your body needs?

Though your focus tends to zero in on contractions during labor, don't ignore the rest of your body. Are other places holding tension or pain? Are you cold or hot? Be aware of what is most helpful and comforting. And be aware that this can change dramatically throughout labor, which is why Quick Pics should be ongoing.

Soul Quick Pic (tool #5)

Are you feeling comfortable and connected to the process? Is your soul engaged and present? Is there anything that it needs or would like? Most women feel the energy of the soul during labor to be focused and centering.

Baby Quick Pic (tool #8)

It's said that the most significant life event for any human being is birth. Childbirth is a long and complicated transition for a baby. The soft plates of the baby's head compress and overlap, and bang against the pelvic bones. The baby's folded-up body needs to assume a series of positions as carefully choreographed as any ballet in order to exit its mother's body. Much happens in a relatively brief space of time as the baby makes the transition from a snug uterus to a contracting one, from the uterus to the birth canal, and finally, from living within your body to life outside of it, and taking that very first breath. Your baby, understandably, has its own viewpoint about labor and delivery.

Almost always (unless there is sudden fetal distress), the feedback you'll get from your baby is readiness and eagerness. We now think that the baby plays a critical role in determining the timing of labor, issuing hormonal signals that ready the mother's body for delivery. This can be reassuring and inspiring as you do your own work to help your baby be born.

LABOR CHECK-INS: WHAT MIGHT COME UP FOR YOU

This Is Going to Be Great!

Anita was putting her feet up late one evening 10 days before her due date when she felt a "pop" followed by the slow dampening of her sweatpants. Her water had broken. Although she had not yet experienced a strong contraction, she wasn't entirely surprised by this development. Over the past several days, she'd noticed an increasing number of Braxton-Hicks "practice" contractions and her discharge had recently been thick and mucusy. She recalls, "I said to Mom [who was her labor coach], 'This means we'll have a baby soon!'"

After calling her doctor to inform her of what had happened, Anita was told to come to the hospital. She ran through her Quick Pics and discovered that she felt rarin' to go—especially physically. "I was exhausted when I sat down to watch some TV, but suddenly I felt adrenaline shooting through me." Checking in with her body, soul, and baby, she got "three thumbs up." Says Anita, "It's as if my whole self was saying, 'I am so up for this—it's going to be great!' "

Induce or Wait?

Vi noticed a persistent trickle of wetness that didn't seem like urine. She came in to have it checked, and sure enough her membranes had ruptured. Like most doctors, I prefer to deliver babies within 24 to 48 hours of the water breaking, in order to avoid infection. Vi, who had been hoping for a natural delivery, was already 3 cm dilated; chances were good that she would soon begin active labor. On the other hand, she'd had a rough several weeks. It was the hottest summer in years, and Vi felt unusually sluggish. Vi and her partner, Alix, had twin toddlers who were very demanding, one of whom had broken her arm two weeks earlier.

"I don't like the idea of inducing," she said. "I want to do everything all natural this time."

I encouraged her to check in with body, soul, and baby to verify how they felt right now. Her body was ready to get on with delivery, she noted, but her soul still felt inclined to give it more time, and the baby was content to wait, too.

So Vi went to an antepartum room, with reminders to check in every couple of hours or so with herself, knowing she could change her mind at any time.

Eight hours later, she called the nurse to say she was ready to be induced. "My contractions have slowed down but my body in every other way is feeling like, 'Let's get on with it,' " she said. "Since I might wind up being induced anyway, it doesn't feel right anymore to wait and see. It feels right to get started." There's no way to know whether she would have gone into labor on her own before the risk of infection from her ruptured membranes grew significant. What's important in this case is that she felt aligned with the course of action that she took, although it was not what she had expected to do. She felt happy and relieved with the decision.

Ready for My Epidural?

When Ann arrived at the hospital, she was 4 cm dilated and having regular, steady contractions. She had used the consciousness processes all through pregnancy and it was beautiful to watch how relaxed and attuned to her body she seemed to be. Ann had spent time during her pregnancy thinking about medical pain relief and felt positively inclined toward it, especially epidurals. All her friends had had them and raved about them. The idea of blocking out the worst of labor pain sounded good to Ann.

Her husband, Matt, seemed a little anxious as she worked with each contraction. It can be hard to watch the woman you love experiencing pain of any kind, even the "good" pain of labor. "What about the epidural?" he asked the labor nurse. "She wants one."

The nurse looked at Ann. "Okay, you're dilated enough. Ready?"

Ann shook her head. After her contraction ended, she paused to do some quick check-ins. Her body felt pretty good; the pain was intense but not as bad as she'd feared. Her soul felt psyched and still energetic, and the baby felt good. "I don't know if I need anything yet," she said. Matt looked surprised but didn't say anything.

"Okay," the nurse said. "If you change your mind, let me know. We'll check your cervix again in two hours."

Ann's labor progressed steadily. Two hours later, she was 6 cm dilated. She used a combination of breathing exercises that she had picked up in childbirth class plus the 4/7/8 breathing she had used all through her pregnancy to relax. Every so often she checked in with herself, and found that things were more manageable than she'd expected. Again, she didn't feel ready yet for the epidural, which she had decided to think of as a crutch to lean on when the pain felt too challenging.

By her next labor check, Ann was deeply involved with her

labor. The room was darkened and quiet. It was as if she were somewhere deep within herself and far away from the rest of us. Matt stayed by her side, wiping her forehead and sometimes gently rubbing her back. He watched the monitor and told her when each contraction began to subside after its peak. No one asked Ann whether she wanted her epidural anymore, as she had made clear that she'd request it when she was ready. Now the contractions were coming faster.

After a particularly long one, Ann whispered, "I think I need that epidural now."

"Well, guess what?" the nurse said to her. "You are 9 cm and almost ready to start pushing. At this point, it's better for you and the baby not to have an epidural."

Ann seemed startled, then another contraction began. Although her body was tired from the hard work, Ann felt exhilarated and energized by the news that she was almost fully dilated. She decided to focus on reaching 10 cm and not think about the epidural anymore. Sure enough, she was ready to push a half hour later, and 45 minutes after that, her daughter, Stella, was born.

"I'm shocked that I didn't have an epidural and none of my friends can believe it," Ann said later. "I thought I wanted one. And I would have just agreed to it if I hadn't kept checking in with my body. But I was so into the whole thing that my body was doing that I just kept thinking I'd have it later. And then it was time to push! I felt like I was doing what I was meant to do. It was very cool!"

Push a Little Longer?

Jenny had one of those extremely long labors that makes me feel such empathy. She'd come to the hospital twice during the week of her due date, hoping she was in active labor when she wasn't. When it finally looked like the real thing, two days after her due date, everything seemed to happen in slow motion. When she arrived at the hospital, she was 4 cm dilated. And there she stayed for the next four hours. She was given Pitocin to stimulate contractions, and then began to slowly but steadily dilate to 10 cm.

By the time she began pushing, Jenny had been monitoring

her contractions for 24 hours—but it felt like a week when she factored in the false alarms. She stayed in touch with herself and the doctor throughout her labor, and although tired, she felt good about how things were going. She'd planned to deliver in a squatting position, only to find that she was too exhausted even to be supported in this way. Her pushing was not very effective. "I just couldn't get the hang of it," she said later. "My body kept saying, 'Come on, work with me, we can do it,' but my soul was like, 'Man, you've been working really hard and you're flattened.' " When the crown of the baby's head was within view, and Jenny was so close but obviously exhausted, we offered to use forceps. Jenny reflected on this. "My body said, 'Okay, help me out here!' and I knew it would be fine." With the assistance of the forceps, little Adrian was delivered in a flash and Jenny's work was done. She looked into his eyes and everything else melted away.

Chapter 23

Labor and Delivery:
The Inside Scoop

∽

What's happening biologically during childbirth

One of life's great mysteries is the exact mechanism by which birth is triggered. Does the mother's body say, "Okay, time's up?" Does the fetus decide, "Now!" Or do they work in symbiotic concert to orchestrate the moment? We don't completely understand it. In some species, including rabbits, rodents, dogs, and cats, the mother has the predominant role in the initiation of the birth process. In others (cows, horses, goats, sheep) the fetus does.

In the primate family, mother and child both seem to influence the onset of labor. The latest thinking is that labor is set in motion when, deep in the fetal brain, the hypothalamus sends a message to the pituitary gland, which in turn unleashes a cascade of hormonal reactions that cross the placenta and prepare the mother for labor. Whatever their origin, these hormonal messages have effects throughout the mother's body: Collagen in the cervix starts to break down, making the cervix easier to stretch; painless Braxton-Hicks contractions begin to efface (thin) the cervix, preparing it to dilate; oxytocin is released in pulses, locking on to the oxytocin receptors in the uterus, which are now 80 to 100 times more plentiful than they were in early pregnancy; and finally the uterus is cued to contract, which dilates (opens) the cervix, then propels the baby through the birth canal.

SIGNS OF LABOR

The following changes indicate that labor is nearing (though not necessarily immediately):

Engagement (Lightening, or Dropping)

The baby's head engages, or settles deeper, into the pelvis in preparation for birth. This allows the mother's lungs to expand more fully be-

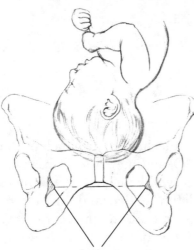

ischial spines

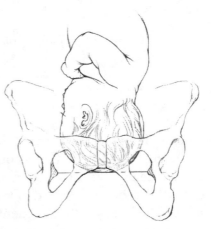

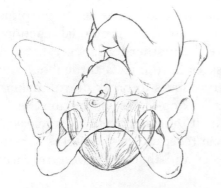

Stations of the Baby *Where the top of the baby's head is in relation to the ischial spines is referred to as the station. Station is measured in numbers, from -5 (the baby's head is still high in the pelvis, above left illustration) to 0 (the baby's head has dropped into the pelvis and is at the level of the ischial spines, above right illustration) to +5 (the baby's head is at the opening of the vagina, also called crowning, left illustration).*

cause they have less pressure against them—there is literally more "breathing room," and the shortness of breath that is sometimes felt late in pregnancy eases. You may, however, feel the need to urinate even more often, because now the bladder is more compressed. In addition, your profile may look slightly changed.

For a first baby, engagement usually happens by 36 weeks. For subsequent births, it may not occur until you are actually in labor.

Passing of the Mucus Plug

During pregnancy, a thick gathering of mucus collects at the cervix to help block bacteria from entering the uterus. In some women, as the cervix starts to thin (efface), this plug—which looks like thick discharge, not like an actual cork or plug—becomes dislodged. The discharge, called "show," may be clear or blood-tinged and it's thick, not watery. Ask your doctor if you have questions about any unusual discharge you notice in order to be sure it is the mucus plug and not your water breaking. The latter requires medical attention, while passing your mucus plug does not (see below). The passing of the plug can occur hours, days, or even weeks before labor begins. Some women never notice the passing of the plug at all.

Rupture of Membranes ("Water Breaking" or "Bag of Water Breaking")

The amniotic sac usually breaks at some point during labor or is broken by your doctor to facilitate labor. When the sac breaks or leaks before labor gets under way in a woman who is full term, this event is known as premature rupture of membranes (PROM). (If your water breaks before you are full term, this is premature preterm rupture of membranes, or PPROM.) Chances are good that you will go into labor spontaneously within 12 hours or so of your water breaking. If labor does not begin within a certain window of time specified by your doctor—usually 24 hours—you will likely be induced, because you and your fetus are now at increased risk of infection.

It can be hard to identify ROM yourself. The liquid may be a small trickle or a more substantial gush. Because amniotic fluid constantly replenishes, the leakage can be a continuous drip. Leaking urine, vaginal discharge, or the mucus plug can all be mistaken for water breaking. You will not necessarily notice contractions immediately.

If you experience any leakage of fluid in any amount before you feel any contractions, see your doctor to have it checked. The only way to verify that it's amniotic fluid is for a health professional to examine you and the fluid. A vaginal exam will look for pooling of fluid in the vagina. Then the pH of the fluid is checked. (Amniotic fluid has a different pH from vaginal secretions.) Finally the fluid is examined under a microscope; when dried, amniotic fluid shows a telltale "ferning" pattern (it actually looks like ferns) caused by crystallization of the salt in the fluid.

Although many pregnant women worry about the potential embarrassment of having their water break while they're in a public place, in reality only 1 in 10 women experience rupture of membranes as a first sign of labor. Even if it did happen to you, the leakage wouldn't necessarily be noticeable by others.

Contractions

For most women, contractions are the most noticeable sign that labor has begun. A contraction is the involuntary tightening and release of the long muscles that wrap around the uterus. As these muscles contract and shorten, they pull on the muscles at the very bottom of the uterus around the cervix, causing it to widen. Imagine your uterus as an inverted wine bottle, whose neck is the cervix. In order for your baby to be born, the neck must widen, changing the jar's shape to that of a wide-mouthed mayonnaise jar. When the mouth of the jar (your cervix) expands to 10 centimeters, the point at which no cervical tissue can be felt at all, you are fully dilated and ready to begin pushing.

Contractions are intermittent, because it is the relaxation phase that allows oxygen to be delivered to the fetus. The force of the contractions must increase over time so that the soft tissues of the cervix and birth canal can continue to stretch. Labor contractions come at fairly regular intervals that get ever more frequent over time.

Women often ask me, "How will I know when contractions start? What do they feel like?" You'll know it when it happens, though exactly how you experience it depends on your body and your stage of labor. During the third trimester, many women experience painless "practice," or Braxton-Hicks, contractions. These help prepare your body for labor without actually dilating the cervix. Braxton-Hicks contractions may cause the muscles over your abdomen to tighten, but they don't actually hurt or take your breath away. Nor do Braxton-Hicks contractions follow a regular pattern; they often stop when you change position. Because they can appear weeks ahead of delivery, they are not an indicator that labor is about to begin, the way that regular contractions are.

(See "True or False Labor?" on page 369 in Chapter 24.)

The All-Important Cervix

The cervix is a neck-shaped structure at the opening of the uterus to the vagina, which dilates (opens) during pregnancy to allow the passage of the fetus. For all the emphasis that is placed on uterine contractions, the real key to labor is the changes that are happening to your cervix. If you're having contractions but your cervix hasn't started to "ripen," or become softer, you're not really in labor, because the cervix will not begin to dilate. Once the softening has begun and you are having contractions, your labor progress will be measured periodically by checking the cervix.

To check your cervix, a doctor, midwife, or nurse inserts two fingers into the vagina in order to feel it. She will try to do this in between contractions so that the exam is more comfortable for you. Three changes to the cervix are monitored as signs of progress:

1. *How effaced (thin) it is.* Effacement is the thinning out of the cervix. In a first pregnancy, the cervix typically effaces (thins) before it dilates (opens). Imagine a cuff-like membrane stretching over a baby's head; the more the membrane stretches to accommodate the head, the thinner it becomes in the process. The cervix is said to be "50 percent effaced" when it is half its original thickness; it is "100 percent effaced" when it's paper-thin. This does not mean you're ready to deliver, although inexperienced residents sometimes make the mistake of thinking that a woman who is having her first baby and who is fully effaced is ready, because the cervix is so thin they can feel the baby's head right through the thin membrane of cervix that remains. The woman of course gets excited that her delivery is so near, only to have those hopes dashed when a subsequent exam finds her only a centimeter or two dilated!

In women who are giving birth for the second time or more, the cervix never gets paper-thin. When it is as effaced as it is going to get, it can still be 1/2 to 1 cm thick.

2. *How dilated it is.* This is a measure of how open the cervix is. The spectrum ranges from fully closed, to fully open and ready to accommodate the baby's head for delivery. Dilation is measured in centimeters, from 0 (not dilated) to 10 cm (fully dilated). Usually your measurement is simply referred to by numeral. For example, you may hear that you are "at 6" (6 cm dilated) or "up to 9" (9 cm dilated). When you are 10 cm dilated—often referred to as "complete," as in completely dilated—you are ready to begin pushing.

In a first labor the cervix does not usually begin to dilate until labor has begun, although it can happen. But the cervix of a woman giving birth for the second time or more may begin to dilate before labor. In fact, it's not unusual for such a woman to walk around 2 or 3 cm dilated for two or three weeks before she delivers.

3. *The position of the cervix.* As you labor, the cervix moves from the posterior, or far back of the vagina, to the anterior, or front, of it. (This is why cervical exams when you are not very far along in labor can be much more uncomfortable than later in labor.) Eventually, the cervix moves far enough forward that it aligns with the vaginal opening.

FEAR: Cervical exams will hurt.

FACT: By performing the exam between contractions, the care provider will minimize discomfort. You can play a role in alleviating any potential discomfort, too. If you're tense, your pelvic muscles will be tight, which can cause pain at any point in labor. Right before a cervical check, do a quick relaxation technique such as deep breathing. Talk to your body, and let your knees fall all the way to the side. This position helps the muscles of the pelvic floor relax. The further along you are in labor, the more comfortable the exam will be.

YOUR BODY IN LABOR: THE STAGES

Labor isn't one big event that suddenly happens, but a series of phases during which many processes occur. These are known as the "stages of labor."

Knowing what to expect in these phases enables you to work with them effectively. Also, viewing labor as a series of steps rather than one long ordeal, can make it less overwhelming. You can relax as much as possible into the rhythms of each phase and take encouragement from your sense of progress over time.

Don't worry too much about exactly when you move from one stage to another. The following textbook-based descriptions of the stages of labor are somewhat artificial divisions of a fluid and naturally unfolding process.

First Stage of Labor: Dilating the Cervix

The first stage of labor begins with effacement (thinning of the cervix) and ends with complete dilation (the cervix opening to its full diameter of 10 cm). This stage—by far the longest—is what's usually referred to when we talk about "labor," though it's not the whole story. (See box entitled "How Long Does Labor Last?" on page 357.)

The first stage of labor is subdivided into early and active phases:

Early (Latent) Labor

The beginning of labor is marked by the start of cervical change in the presence of regular contractions. This is when you realize that you're in labor, though it is rarely physically challenging. It usually lasts until you are 2 to 4 cm dilated.

What you may experience: Though these contractions are obvious, they're not necessarily painful. They tend to be spaced at intervals of 10 minutes or more, with the length between contractions growing shorter. Most women can talk and move about during early labor, even during contractions. You may feel excited or apprehensive, full of energy or, depending how long this stage lasts, increasingly fatigued. Other common reactions include loss of appetite, slight cramps, backache, or diarrhea. You may notice increased mucus or your water breaking during this stage.

What to do:
- Try to continue with your normal activities for as long as you can. Although you don't want to exhaust yourself, walking around, doing the dishes, and other routine activities can help you relax. If it's the middle of the night, you can rest in bed as long as is comfortable to conserve energy, although racing adrenaline may get you up anyway.
- Eat a light snack for energy.

- Tell your labor partner and anyone else who needs to know that you are in labor.
- Check your suitcase early to see that you have everything you need.

Active Labor

This is the "working" part of labor. There is an increasing pace of cervical dilation, usually beginning around 2 to 4 cm. An oft-quoted measure is that active labor begins when you reach 4 cm dilation. But in fact, you can't actually pinpoint when your active labor began until well after you're in it. Then your doctor can look back at the chart of your labor (see "Your Labor Curve" on page 358) and see where dilation began to progress at a much faster rate. By definition, *that's* when you entered the active phase of labor, whether or not the dilation of your cervix measured 4 cm.

Active labor is itself further subdivided into three progressive phases:

1. *An acceleration phase.* Contractions come closer together and become longer and stronger as you enter the active stage of labor. This phase of your body shifting gears, if you will, from the latent to the active stage is referred to as the acceleration phase.

What you may experience: It's difficult to do anything else, even carry on a conversation, while you're having a contraction during this phase. Each contraction typically builds in intensity to a peak and then subsides. Back pain is possible, depending on the position of the baby and how your body is responding to labor.

What to do:
- Follow the Centers of Wellness Self-Care strategies in Chapter 25.
- Try to remain on your feet or sitting upright as long as possible.
- Vary your positions to see what's most comfortable. Note that this may change as labor progresses.
- Focus only on yourself and your needs and tune everything else out.
- Rely on your labor partner for anything you need, from physical support to ice chips to a foot rub.
- Empty your bladder periodically as you feel the urge.

- Allow yourself to rest fully between contractions. Take a deep breath and release it slowly to signal to yourself the end of each contraction.
- Continue to do your Quick Pics.

2. *The phase of maximum slope.* This is the longest phase of active labor, and is the time during which your cervix dilates the most, typically from about 4 cm to about 9 cm.

What you may experience: Your contractions will continue to be strong and regular. (You're not likely to notice any distinction between the acceleration phase and this phase in terms of how contractions feel.) It is as if your body is now warmed up and the contractions are able to have their greatest effect.

What to do: Follow the same advice as for the acceleration phase above.

3. *The deceleration phase, also known as transition.* Sometimes the most challenging part of labor, this is when the cervix dilates the final 1 to 2 cm. This phase is characterized by longer, more intense contractions that are only two to three minutes apart and that can last several minutes, peaking several times during each contraction. This final centimeter or two takes longer than the dilation in the previous phase.

What you may experience: You may be nauseated, may alternate between feeling hot and cold, and may be getting increasingly tired. Back pain may intensify now or be felt for the first time. Psychologically, this can be a challenging time as each contraction is longer and stronger, and your cervical dilation slows. You may feel distressed, disoriented, or unable to continue much longer, although you will also discover reserves of energy you didn't know you had as your body rises to the challenge. Often women seem to be in a completely different place when they are wholly connected to the mental and physical demands of transition—a beautiful thing to witness.

What to do:
- Try crouching, moving onto your hands and knees, or another position that rounds the back to ease pressure.
- See the tips for back labor (box).

- Remind yourself that transition is a short phase which means you have the longest work of labor behind you and the birth of your child almost right ahead of you.
- Use imagery during each long contraction to imagine your body opening up, like a flower, to reveal your baby (or any imagery that comes to mind).
- Surrender to the process as fully as you can. Your body knows what it's doing; allow it to come into the fullest expression of its powers and support it.

BACK LABOR

Sometimes labor pain feels concentrated in the lower back. The pain can persist even between contractions. It's widely believed that back labor is most often due to the position of the baby and most common when the baby is "sunny side up" (faceup instead of the usual facedown position), but the evidence for this is mostly anecdotal. Back pain can be most intense during transition. To alleviate the discomfort of back labor:

- Experiment with different positions to see if one better reduces the pressure.
- Try positions where the back is rounded, such as on all fours resting on your knees and elbows or lying on your side.
- Have your partner massage the area where the pain is worst.
- Have your partner apply counterpressure to the area (by pressing the back with the heel of the hand, for example).
- Put ice packs or a heating pad on the affected area. (Some women respond better to heat, some to cold.)
- Use Dialoguing, if you feel you can, to "communicate" with your back and ease the sensation that you are locked in a battle with it.
- Ask for an over-the-counter pain reliever if the pain is prolonged and intense. Your baby will not be negatively affected.
- If hypnosis and/or acupuncture are available, take full advantage!

Second Stage of Labor: Delivery of the Baby (Pushing)

This stage begins at 10 cm dilation and ends with the birth of the baby. It's known as the pushing stage, because that's what you have to do in order to help move the baby down the vagina to be born.

What you may experience: Your body feels a strong urge to bear down, almost as if in a bowel movement. You may also feel a corresponding rectal pressure. Contractions last a minute or longer and can be anywhere from two to five minutes apart.

By pushing during the contractions, your whole body works with the uterine muscles to aid the descent of the baby. Many women report that the contractions are easier to handle now, especially following transition, because they feel more in control, more like they are "doing" something productive. It's also common to feel excitement and a renewed sense of progress. However, if pushing lasts a long time or you are tired from a long, active labor, you may become frustrated or discouraged.

As the baby's head approaches the opening of the vagina, "crowning," there can be a brief but strong sense of pressure and burning that lasts until the baby's head emerges. The speedy, slithery delivery of the body follows in short order.

What to do:
- Recognize that if you are feeling exhausted this is perfectly normal.
- Because you are nearing the last real stage of delivery—the pinnacle of the process—take a few moments to refocus your energy and intention. Some women like to pause to notice the sensation of their baby inside their bodies for the last time. Check in with your body. Do you feel like you are in a comfortable and productive position to start pushing?
- Rely on your labor partner or nurses to help support your body as needed.
- Follow your doctor's or midwife's guidance. Good communication with your labor attendant is essential. I ask the laboring woman to give me her full attention and to tune out the other voices in the room. A slow and controlled delivery is the goal—one in which the baby is literally eased out.

Your attendant may therefore ask you to stop pushing or to give only gentle, smaller pushes immediately before birth.

- Use the techniques you've learned in your childbirth classes. Take care not to hold your breath during each push.
- Use visualization to help you focus and stay engaged. (See "Baby's First Dance" for a description and illustration of the birthing process.)

Third Stage of Labor: Delivery of the Placenta

Most new moms think of delivery as ending when the baby is born—but there's one cool part left. The third stage of labor is the delivery of the placenta (also called the afterbirth). Contractions usually stop immediately after the baby is born and then resume minutes later, with less intensity, in order to deliver the placenta. These contractions help the placenta to peel away from the uterine wall where the embryo attached nine months ago, and then to be expelled, usually in one easy push. The third stage usually lasts less than 10 minutes, but can take as long as 30 minutes.

Once the placenta is delivered, and the obstetrician is assured that your uterus is contracting and your bleeding is slowing, she will examine the placenta, the membranes, and the umbilical cord. This is to assure that it appears "intact"; i.e., that no pieces of placenta or membranes were left inside, to assess the general appearance and health of the placenta, and to see that the umbilical cord had all three of its vessels—two arteries, which are small and thick-walled, and one vein, which is bigger and thinner-walled. A cross section of a normal cord looks like a smiley face, with the umbilical arteries the eyes and the vein the mouth! I like to show patients what the placenta looked like when it was inside the body protecting and nourishing the baby by flipping it to reveal the meaty, fleshy part that was attached to the wall of the uterus. It's an impressive organ—it kept your baby alive for nine months—and worth a quick look.

Following the delivery of the placenta, the uterus will continue to contract. These contractions, which are mild compared to those that delivered your baby, cause the uterus to involute, or shrink, back toward its pre-pregnancy size. Blood vessels are being closed off as the uterus shrinks, reducing the odds of excessive bleeding. These contractions can cause slight discomfort (but rarely actual pain) and are

HOW LONG DOES LABOR LAST?

The length of labor can vary widely and still be normal.

Research has shown that women who do not receive an epidural and who are in labor for the first time have labors that look like this:

Latent phase of first stage: average 6.4 hours; 95 percent of laboring women will have completed this phase within 20.6 hours

Active phase of first stage: average 4.6 hours; 95 percent will complete this in 11.7 hours

Rate of cervical dilation during active phase: average 3 cm/hour; 95 percent will progress at a rate of at least 1.2 cm/hour

If a woman falls within the ranges for the 95 percent population, typically their obstetrician will not intervene. Once you are beyond that, taking action should be considered, because there is most likely a reason progress is not happening more rapidly.

Second stage (pushing): average 33 minutes, 95 percent in 1.9 hours (If you have an epidural, you are typically given another hour to push before it is considered out of the norm [i.e., roughly 3 hours instead of 2])

Third stage: average 5 minutes, 95 percent in 30 minutes

Women who are giving birth for the second (or more) time have shorter labors, as follows:

Latent phase of first stage: average 4.8 hours, 95 percent will complete in 13.6 hours

Active phase of first stage: average 2.4 hours, 95 percent will complete in 5.2 hours

Rate of cervical dilation during active phase: average 5.7 cm/hour, 95 percent 1.5 cm/hour

Second stage (pushing): average 8.5 minutes, 95 percent in 46.5 minutes (If you have an epidural, you are typically given another hour to push before it is considered out of the norm [i.e., roughly 2 hours instead of 1 hour])

Third stage: average 5 minutes, 95 percent in 30 minutes

known as afterbirth pains or "afterpains." You may continue to feel them occasionally for several days.

What you may experience: For the most part, in the excitement of having delivered, this stage is barely even noticed except for the moment of the placenta actually delivering. You'll feel a lot of pressure, but no real pain. Your care provider may massage your abdomen to check the uterine progress both before and after the placenta is delivered. The afterpains can be strong, although they are more like intense menstrual cramps than the contractions of active labor.

What to do:
- Continue your breathing exercises; this helps you relax during the delivery of the placenta and during abdominal massage or when you feel afterpains.

Your Labor Curve

The progress of your labor is often plotted on a graph known as a labor curve (or Friedman's curve, after the man who extensively researched the normal course of labor). It's basically a chart with time running on one axis and centimeters of dilation on the other. (See diagram, page 359.) I like using these graphs because they make it so clear when to take action and when to leave things alone. The labor curve plots your individual progress against what we would expect, or like to see. It is indeed a graphical representation of every aspect of your labor—your cervical progress and the baby's descent and position, all plotted against time.

No two women have the same labor curve—which is pretty remarkable when you think about it! If your doctor uses a labor curve graph, you may very well want a copy to include among your birth mementos. It is the medical story of your labor and delivery.

YOUR BABY IN LABOR:
THE SEVEN CARDINAL MOVEMENTS

During active labor and pushing, the baby descends into position in the birth canal (as the vagina is referred to in childbirth). About 95 percent of fetuses are in the optimal position for delivery when labor begins:

head first. People often think that the baby shoots straight out like a circus performer out of a cannon. In reality, for the fetus, maneuvering the birth canal is like following the steps of a choreographed dance—with Mother Nature as choreographer. It's the shape of the maternal pelvis that largely dictates these motions. (See illustrations on the next page.)

Sample Labor Curve Chart

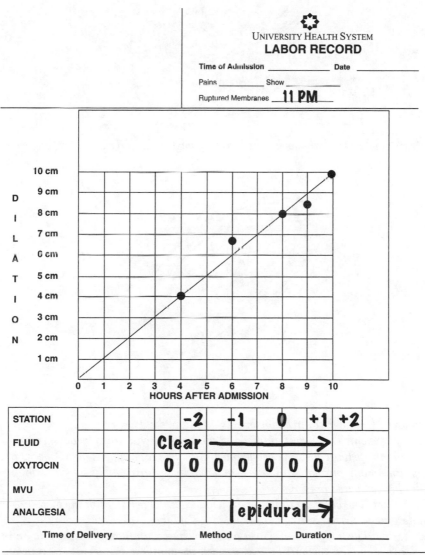

UNIVERSITY HEALTH SYSTEM
LABOR RECORD

Time of Admission _____ Date _____

Pains _____ Show _____

Ruptured Membranes __**11 PM**__

STATION				**-2**	**-1**	**0**	**+1**	**+2**	
FLUID			**Clear**				→		
OXYTOCIN			**0**	**0**	**0**	**0**	**0**	**0**	
MVU									
ANALGESIA						**epidural** →			

Time of Delivery _____ Method _____ Duration _____

Labor Record
BCHD# 162 NS REV. 12/99

Original – Mother's Medical Record
Yellow – OB Department

Chart Order #
OB-361

Baby's First Dance: The Cardinal Movements of Birth

There are seven "cardinal movements" a fetus must perform to be born—a tricky dance worthy of great applause! They happen very fluidly, but here you can get a sense of them:

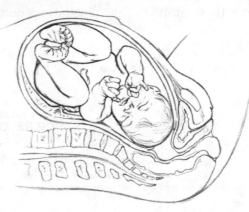

This is what the baby looks like before labor begins and the head is engaged.

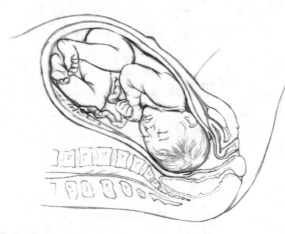

Now you see the first three movements taking place. They are:
1. Engagement: The widest diameter of the baby's head drops below a certain place in the pelvis called the pelvic inlet. This usually happens by 36 weeks in a first-time mom, but not until later—or sometimes during labor—for a woman who has delivered previously.
2. Descent: The baby continues to drop lower in the pelvis, with the fastest rates of descent occurring during the second stage of labor.
3. Flexion: The baby's head moves onto the chest with the chin tucked down in order to allow the portion of the head with the smallest diameter to pass through the dilated cervix.

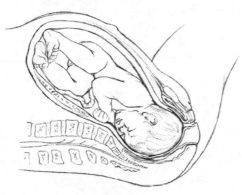

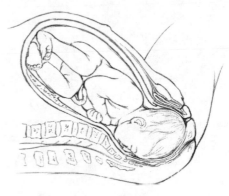

4. Internal Rotation: The head rotates from its original position so that the shoulders, the widest part of the baby's body, can enter the pelvis at its widest part. The baby's descent continuos.

5a. Extension: This head extends upward as the birth canal curves.

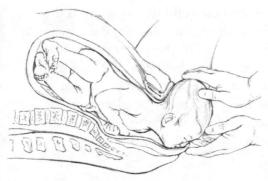

5b. In this stage of extension the head begins to deliver.

6. External Rotation: Also called restitution, this refers to the return of the baby's head to its original position relative to the torso. This happens as the head is delivered.

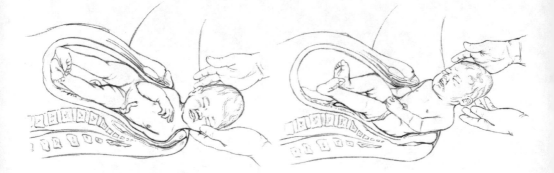

7a. Expulsion: The rest of the body rotates, starting with the anterior shoulder (the one under the pubic bone)
which is delivered.

7b. In this stage of expulsion, the
other shoulder (the posterior) is delivered, after which the rest of the baby
quickly follows.

Once the baby's head is out, the doctor or midwife will immediately run her fingers up inside the birth canal to check whether the
umbilical cord is wrapped around the baby's neck, a situation called a
nuchal cord. If this is the case, the cord will be "reduced," which simply means brought down around the baby's head. After the cord is
checked but before the body is delivered, the baby's nose and mouth
are suctioned so that when she or he takes her or his first breath the
nasal passages are clear.

Now the baby is greeted by the obstetrician and welcomed into the
world (my favorite part!). After the delivery, the doctor or midwife
takes care to hold the baby at about the level of the perineum so that
neither too much nor too little blood moves between placenta and
baby. Then the umbilical cord is cut, and if the baby is crying (a sign of
health) and looking good, he or she will most likely be placed on the
mother's belly. That's where the nurse will dry the baby, while continuing to observe his or her transition to the outside world.

CUTTING THE CORD

In a normal vaginal delivery, the brand-new dad or labor partner is given the opportunity to cut the umbilical cord. This can be a wonderful moment, but understandably not all husbands and partners care to do it. There is no judgment of anyone who prefers not to cut the cord. If the answer is "No thanks," the labor attendant will do the job.

I'm often asked: Should cord cutting be delayed until the umbilical cord stops pulsing? There are no formal guidelines about how soon after delivery the cord should be cut. In a full-term healthy baby we don't know if it makes a difference whether the cord is cut immediately or not, and it is safe either way. There is certainly no need to rush. In the case of a distressed baby (i.e., one that is not breathing well, has a low pulse rate, etc.), the obstetrician is likely to want to cut the cord immediately so the baby can be turned over to the pediatrician for needed care. But in premature babies a slight delay (30 seconds to two minutes) in clamping has been shown to reduce anemia and improve blood pressure. Birth partners who want to cut the cords themselves may prefer such a delay, too, to fully absorb the event they just witnessed rather than focusing on a task.

AFTER DELIVERY:
WHAT HAPPENS TO YOUR BABY

Keeping Warm

It takes a while for a newborn to regulate temperature properly, so keeping the baby warm and dry is a priority. The ideal situation in a normal vaginal delivery is for the baby to be placed immediately on your belly. Not only does this allow you to meet and hold your child from the first seconds of life, but your body heat will warm him. A knit cap will also help warm the baby, preventing the loss of heat through the head. If immediate medical attention is needed, the newborn will be placed in a warmed bassinet. A bassinet is also used immediately after birth if you have had a C-section; this is where the baby is checked, cleaned off, dried, wrapped in a blanket—and then brought to the mother.

Apgar Assessments

A standard scoring system known as an Apgar test is used to evaluate a newborn's condition at one minute after birth and again at five minutes. Apgar is the name of the pediatrician who developed the test, Dr. Virginia Apgar, and has also been used as an acronym for the elements that are evaluated—Appearance, Pulse, Grimace, Activity, Respiration. Apgar scoring can be done while you are holding your baby. In the thrill of those first minutes together, you probably will not even be aware it's being done.

The following items are scored on a scale of 0–2:

Appearance (skin color), which shows how well the lungs are
    working to supply oxygen to the blood
Pulse, which measures the rate and regularity of the heartbeat
Grimace, which assesses reflexes in response to stimulation
Activity (movement), which evaluates muscle tone
Respiration (breathing), with crying earning the top score

An Apgar score of 7 to 10 indicates that the baby needs only routine post-birth care. (Few babies ever score a 10 within one minute of birth because even in a perfectly healthy baby, the hands and feet rarely achieve the fully "pinked up" blush color that is later characteristic of all healthy babies, including those of color. A score under 7 means the baby needs observation and perhaps help, usually oxygen or more suctioning. A score below 5 indicates a baby in distress who needs additional intervention. The five-minute score typically stays the same or improves; its purpose is used to assess how well the baby is adjusting or is responding to intervention. A baby whose second Apgar is below 7 may be assessed every five minutes until the team is certain she is responding well to their intervention and has successfully transitioned to life outside of you.

Weighing and Measuring

Birth weight, length, and usually head circumference are all recorded by a nurse or pediatrician. This baseline will be essential in monitoring how well your newborn grows in the days, weeks, and months to come.

Taking a Footprint

Your baby is identified for posterity within moments of birth. If you deliver in a hospital, an ID bracelet will be attached to his ankle or wrist, usually one that matches your own to eliminate any possibility of mix-ups. Your baby's footprint is also recorded in ink. If you like, ask to have a second footprint impression made right into your baby book. This can be a lovely keepsake. Often a copy is automatically made for your use.

Antibiotic Eyedrops

To prevent eye infections from bacteria your baby might have been exposed to during birth, these drops will be given to the baby within an hour of birth—as required by law.

Later Treatment

Before discharge your baby may experience the following as well:

- A PKU blood test. Taken through a prick of the heel, this blood screen is required to test for phenylketonuria (PKU) and other disorders. It's done when your baby is 48 hours old.
- Genetic screenings. These vary by state law, although every state requires testing for some number of genetic disorders and other health problems. To find out what your state requires, you can check http://genes-r-us.uthscsa.edu/resources/consumer/statemap.htm.
- A hepatitis B immunization. The first shot in the series is usually given before discharge, and is definitely given within 12 hours of birth if you are a hepatitis B carrier or are not sure. This is one of the prenatal labs that you had done at your first prenatal visit.
- Hearing assessments. Some but not all states require them.
- Circumcision. This is performed on a son a day or two after birth if you request it. (See "Make a conscious decision about circumcision," page 319.)

AFTER DELIVERY: WHAT HAPPENS TO YOU

Immediately after your baby's birth, the physician monitors your blood loss, facilitates the delivery of the placenta, evaluates the size of the uterus (which should be contracting), and assesses your perineum. If you had any tears or if an episiotomy was done, these will be repaired at this time. Most women are barely aware of most of what is going on, as their attention is on their newborn child, and local anesthetic is used for any necessary stitching. The sutures that are used are absorbable and therefore do not have to be removed later.

Once the placenta is delivered, you will be given Pitocin through your IV (if you have one) or via an injection to the thigh muscle. Sometimes patients who did not wish to use Pitocin to induce or augment childbirth are alarmed to hear about this postpartum use of Pitocin. But it is the standard care in obstetrics to give a one-time dose of Pitocin (whether or not you had Pitocin during labor) to help the uterus contract after the delivery of the placenta. This is done because the contraction of the uterus is the primary mechanism for controlling blood loss after delivery. Uterine atony—failure of the uterus to contract appropriately following delivery—can lead to postpartum hemorrhage (excessive bleeding). This is a very serious condition, and it can occur very quickly. If medical management fails, a hysterectomy may be needed to save the woman's life. Prior to the use of medications for the treatment of uterine atony, this was the most common cause of hysterectomy. Pitocin used after delivery of the placenta helps prevent that unhappy outcome.

The nurses will continue to monitor your vital signs to check for fever and other signs of potential complications. You're also examined frequently for two other important reasons: 1) to ensure vaginal bleeding is not excessive and 2) to verify that the uterus is contracting properly. The nurse palpates your abdomen to check that your uterus is remaining contracted and has descended to about the level of your belly button. If it does not feel firm, she will massage it to help it to contract. While this may not be comfortable, it is a very important part of your immediate postpartum care. You should feel free to massage it as well. It should be easy to feel.

After several hours, you'll be checked less frequently. If you did not deliver in a LDR room (labor, delivery, and recovery all in one place), you may be transferred to a postpartum unit for recovery.

In the absence of any complications, discharge follows one to two days after giving birth vaginally, and a day or two longer after a C-section.

Chapter 24

Labor and Delivery:
Medical Care

∞

An integrative medicine perspective on childbirth

BASIC MEDICAL ISSUES NOW

When to Go to the Hospital

The first question most moms-to-be ask me regarding labor is "How do I know when to go to the hospital?"

Your care provider will give you guidelines about "when it's time." These can vary by provider and by the individual case. In general, you will be directed to go to the hospital or birthing center if:

• *there is any question as to whether your water has broken*. Are you leaking some kind of fluid but not sure what it is? You need to have it checked. If your membranes have indeed ruptured, you and the baby are at increased risk for infection because the barrier between your sterile uterus and your not-sterile vagina has been broached.

• *you are starting to experience regular, painful contractions.* "Painful" means that they are strong enough that you have to stop what you're doing in order to breathe through them. I tell first-time moms who are full term (37 weeks or more) to come in when they have three to five strong contractions within a 10-minute window, and veteran moms to come in when they notice any strong and regular pattern (even if there are only two or three contractions per 10 minutes). Second labors tend to progress more quickly, and once you detect a pattern to contractions you are likely in active labor. Call and ask your provider if you're unsure. If you are not full term but are experiencing regular contractions you will be asked to come in for an evaluation. (See "Signs of Preterm Labor," page 294.)

Of course you should also call your doctor if you have any indication that something is wrong, such as decreased fetal movement, fever, chills, nausea, or vomiting.

Stay at Home as Long as You Can

Because first labors tend to be long, your goal should be to spend the early stages at home. As eager as you may be to get to the hospital—the "staging area" for the big event—and as concerned as you may be about making it there in time, there are some good reasons not to rush in. Labor is going to unfold in its own way. At home, you'll be better able to relax. You can walk around, dance, or rock in a rocker. You can check in with yourself. You can make sure everything's ready with your overnight bag, make phone calls, eat a light meal, and relax, relax, relax. And this is key: the longer you hang out at home, the longer you're out of the hospital.

Don't get me wrong. Hospitals are great places. I've logged more than half my life in them! But they're no place for a woman who is not in active labor (or who does not have some other condition requiring monitoring). Let me explain why.

Once you get to the hospital, you will be evaluated to determine whether you are actually in active labor or not. If you are, or if your water has broken, you'll be admitted. If you are not, you'll be sent home. If you're not in active labor but seem far enough dilated that you might be soon, you may be told to walk around for two hours and come back for a recheck. It's the amount of time, rather than how you spend it, that's the key behind this prescription. If you really are in active labor, in two hours your cervix will be further dilated, whether

TRUE OR FALSE LABOR?

Often first-time moms eagerly present themselves at the hospital only to be sent home, not to return again for days or even weeks. How can you tell if what you're feeling is real labor or false labor? Here are some general guidelines:

- *How regular are contractions?* In labor, the intervals between contractions usually grow consistently shorter; for example, every 10 minutes apart, every 8 minutes, every 5 minutes, every 2 minutes. False labor pains are sporadic and follow no pattern.
- *How long does each one last?* In labor, contractions last 15 to 30 seconds in early labor and get longer as labor progresses. In false labor, they're more irregular.
- *Where do you feel the contractions?* True labor pains are usually felt high up in the abdomen, radiating throughout your stomach and lower back. (This reflects how the uterine muscles tighten.) False labor pains often present in the abdomen or groin.
- *Do the contractions change when you switch position?* In active labor, contractions keep coming regularly whether you are sitting or standing, walking or still. If they stop or slow down when you change what you're doing, it's not the real thing yet.
- *Can you talk?* A real, active labor contraction will usually require all your concentration. An early labor or a pre-labor Braxton-Hicks contraction might catch your attention, but its gentler squeeze will leave you able to chat right through it.

you've been walking or sitting. If your dilation hasn't progressed, you're still in early labor, and you'll be sent home.

I always feel for the patients who come in so eagerly, only to be turned away. It can be a real mental letdown—not the greatest frame of mind for building the momentum you would like. So why not just admit you? Because, in addition to taking up a hospital bed unnecessarily, you increase the risk that somebody will do something to you that you don't want or don't necessarily need, such as hooking you up to an IV, starting you on Pitocin, or rupturing your membranes. Believe it or not, these things are often done because we medical folk often feel the need to do *something* just because you're there. Often these actions come with the justification of "We'll just get your labor going" (which understandably sounds pretty good!) regardless of whether or not your labor would move along just fine without such measures.

So if your philosophy is that pregnancy is a natural process that you'd rather have supported than controlled or overridden, do yourself a favor by staying home during early labor.

Write a Birth Vision Statement—Not a Birth Plan

Patients often ask me whether they should do a birth plan—written documentation of their preferences for labor and delivery—and what should be in it. I don't believe in birth plans. Though they've grown very popular among informed moms-to-be, I find they too often distract from genuine consciousness around childbirth. It's as if the focus turns to the many individual trees, and the forest is missed. You *can't* plan a birth; there are simply too many factors that are in the hands of nature. However, you *can* create a vision and an intention for your birth experience.

What this means is that instead of drawing up a long and detailed document describing your preferences for each step of labor and delivery, you write your birth vision statement, which is shorter, more general, and more philosophical in nature than many of the birth plans women are often advised to set down on paper. It should grow out of conversations you have had with your doctor or your midwife, during which you have come to a basic understanding and agreement on your preferences. The birth vision statement allows you to further clarify what is important to you, and to express this both to your care provider and to any other health professionals you may encounter.

Why do I discourage the "birth plan" approach? Because too often I've seen women enter L&D with incredibly detailed plans that they regard as their gold standard; any deviation from the birth plan means "failure" in their eyes, and potential conflict with the staff. While such a patient has made a lot of choices about her desired labor and delivery, it's as if she never went any deeper in her envisioning of the birth process than creating a checklist of specific preferences for each step in the process. When events don't match her hopes or preferences for each stage, she feels disappointed or frustrated. She risks getting caught up in this negative energy rather than the energy of bringing a new life into the world. Even if everything *does* go according to her specified plan, she may miss out on the full experience, she may fail to realize that what is happening is not a series of technical choices to be crossed off a list, but the birthing of a new life. Miracles can't be scripted in advance, but have to unfold in their own way. Honoring and respecting this process is at the core of a conscious birth.

A birth vision statement should be short—no more than one concise page that can be placed in your chart. Being brief also forces you to focus on what really matters most to you. Rather than making a list of dos and don'ts, make your birth plan an expression of the essence of what your intention is for this experience. Ironically, the more detailed it is, the less likely it is that it will be used as a guide for your care providers, in part because it's difficult to remember so many details in the heat of the moment. Experienced providers also know that doing everything according to a foreordained plan is impossible in childbirth, leading them to tune out an instruction list. More crucially, a woman who has created a document spelling out every eventuality will often bypass direct communication with her nurses and other care providers because she feels as if she has already said it. Establishing open and ongoing verbal communication with your labor team is absolutely essential.

A birth vision statement has three parts:

1. Your intention. Start by writing in one sentence your intention for this transformational experience in your life.

Example:
I intend to be fully involved in and aware of every aspect of my baby's birth.

2. Your philosophy. Then list any guiding principles that are important to you.

Examples:
* *to be as active and engaged as possible in all aspects of the process*

- *to have everyone in the room honor the sacredness of this event*
- *to have my medical team be as minimally invasive as possible within the realm of providing the best medical care*

3. Specific preferences. Be specific only about the things that are really important to you. You may want to include your initial preferences about the following (while keeping in mind that any or all of them may change when you are actually in labor):

- Who will attend you (and who won't, if there are specific people you don't want in the room)
- Your thoughts on pain management
- Your environment: music, lights, scent, and other aspects of your surroundings
- Mobility (Do you plan to remain upright as long as possible? Use a tub? Sit?)
- Labor positions, especially for pushing and delivery
- What happens immediately at birth (Do you want to hold the baby immediately? Begin to breastfeed right after delivery? Does your partner want to cut the cord? Do you want to see the placenta?)
- Cord-blood banking (see pages 319–320).

Example:
Once I enter the second stage of labor, I want to be as quiet and focused as possible, with only my husband and people who are essential for the delivery in the room with me. I want to avoid pain medication for as long as possible and plan to use breathing exercises instead. After the birth, I want to hold the baby as soon as possible and stay with her for as long as possible.

Give a copy to your doctor at one of your visits and see if she is comfortable with it or has any questions. Also put copies in your hospital-bound suitcase so that you can give them to your labor nurse for your medical chart at the hospital, and to any other medical personnel you may encounter.

As you think through these topics, remember that birth vision statements, as well as birth plans, are not binding contracts or order forms. Hospital personnel are probably not going to post your birth preferences on the wall and tick off each item as it happens—nor should you want them to!

Many women choose not to write any preferences down. What matters most is that you have reflected on your feelings and intentions, and shared them with your provider and your labor partner, regardless of whether you have committed them to paper.

✓ **REALITY CHECK:** The Myth of "Standard" Labor Care

Every woman tends to believe that the way she is cared for in labor is The Way. Later she compares notes with friends, and they discover just how variable the medical management of childbirth can be. Many patients are surprised when I tell them that there is not, in fact, one gold-standard way to manage labor and delivery. Even from one academic medical center (where doctors are trained) to another, labors are managed very differently. In fact, there are many options about how to monitor a woman and her fetus, when to intervene, and how.

Each physician falls somewhere along a spectrum of approaches to labor care. At one end are those who view childbirth as a natural process and do nothing unless absolutely necessary, and at the other extreme are those who see childbirth as a medical condition that should be aggressively managed (some might say overridden). The former is a healing-based approach; the latter, like much of modern medicine, is a disease-based one. The difference boils down to how the physician views his or her role: to support a natural process, or to take over and control the process.

My strong preference is toward the healing end of that spectrum. I don't believe that one-size-fits-all health protocols are appropriate. Individuals are different in too many ways—especially in the dynamic and variable situation of childbirth. Doing nothing for too long can be very dangerous; it's in part why complications and death were once much more commonplace in childbirth. Likewise, intervening when it is not essential (such as certain inductions or elective C-sections) may be standard protocol in a given institution, but can introduce unnecessary complications. In the healing-based approach that I use, I medically intervene when there is a reason, such as when the patient has "fallen off the labor curve" (see pages 358–359), she has developed an infection, or her baby is showing signs of fetal distress. Otherwise I don't—why override a natural process, just because you can? I do not, however, consider pain management a medical intervention, and I support whatever methods a woman feels work best for her.

By choosing a care provider who has views of childbirth that align with your own, you can minimize the possibility of unpleasant surprises in your medical care during labor.

Stay Involved: Working with Your Medical Team

Your doctor's or midwife's role in labor is to make medical decisions regarding your delivery. Ideally you'll make most of them together, although it's always possible that an emergency situation will arise in which you need to defer to his or her expertise. It's not, however, the care provider's job to make decisions about what your *experience* of childbirth will be. Will you feel like the central player in the miracle of your child's birth? Will you feel fully engaged, alive, and present? That's up to you.

Some advice on working with your medical team in labor:

• *Don't hand over all authority the moment you enter the hospital or birthing center.* You do have a voice, an important one, especially now. Feel free to speak up—to your care provider, labor nurses, and other hospital staff. They may work there all the time, but this birth is a once-in-a-lifetime experience for you. Hopefully you have already established this kind of collaborative relationship with your care provider, and that working relationship can be carried into the labor suite as well.

• *Always be sure you understand the rationale for any course of action taken.* If your care provider declines to give you an answer and just expects you to do it because he or she is the one in charge, chances are that he or she is acting unconsciously—following a rote way of doing things without bringing an understanding of "why" to the decision. Asking why (and why not) actually helps everyone bring greater consciousness to the choice, and assures that you are a part of the process.

• *Ask about all of your options, as well as why a particular one is being recommended or chosen.* Be sure you understand the risks and benefits of each option. There is rarely only one course of action. An emergency C-section is the only case I can think of where there is little time for discussion and you need to trust your doctor's judgment.

• *Do give your care provider credit.* Hopefully you have chosen this person, and this birthing place, because you trust their knowledge and expertise. Although you shouldn't count yourself out of the decision-making process, you do need to recognize that there are points at which the expert knows more than you. A good doctor or midwife wants to work in partnership with you because you each bring unique expertise to the occasion. The health care provider knows obstetrics, but you know *you.*

• *Make sure that your partner, and any support people you may have involved in the process (such as a doula), understand your preferences.* You should discuss this well before you go into labor. Share your birth vision statement with them (see pages 370–373).

• *Make your preferences clear to medical staff as well.* Ideally, you and your doctor or midwife have already discussed your feelings about key issues like C-sections, pain relief, inductions, and other interventions, and your preferences and philosophies are written in your chart. Give a copy of your birth vision statement to the staff when you arrive at the hospital, especially your labor nurse. She will be a key person in your experience, and may be someone you have not previously met. (You may meet more than one labor nurse if you have a long labor, as shifts change. Repeat the conversation—or have your partner do this—with each new face attending your delivery.) So many medical professionals take C-sections for granted these days that when there is a borderline question about whether to do one— and there are many gray areas—how quickly they move toward surgery may be very influenced by the preferences you made known to them.

• *Be realistic.* You can't control everything that happens in labor—nobody can. Medical emergencies can develop no matter what kind of preparations you've made. You'll feel better about your birthing experience if you don't fixate on a certain kind of delivery but focus on being open-minded and connected to the process.

• *Don't get so wedded to the labor you desire that you miss the experience of the one that's actually happening.* (See "Write a Birth Vision Statement.)

• *Don't forget to check in with yourself—body, soul, and baby—throughout labor.* It only takes a moment to turn your attention to how each dimension is doing at that moment. Between contractions is a great time to realign your focus.

Remember this advice is not coming from some outsider renegade; I'm a hospital-based obstetrician. As much as I respect medical professionals, I also deeply respect the laboring woman. The power of this incredible experience—this experience that is taking place within your body and your soul, and is happening to your baby, too—is yours to claim and to own.

> **FEAR:** I'll be prepped for labor in ways I don't want.
> **FACT:** The days of all labor patients having perineal hair shaved, receiving an enema, and showering are long gone as these measures have been found unnecessary and intrusive. The standard prep for a vaginal birth today happens right before delivery; the vaginal area is quickly "washed" with Betadine or some other type of soap. And that's about it.

AT THE HOSPITAL: MONITORING LABOR

At the hospital or birthing center, fetal health, your health, and your labor progress will be checked periodically. Here's how:

Fetal Monitoring

There is some debate over how beneficial it is to be monitored (that is, to have the fetus's heart rate monitored) in labor. The value, of course, is that doing so confirms fetal well-being. The problem is that monitoring is not perfect. Because it alerts us to *possible* problems, rather than definite ones, it introduces the risk of unnecessary interventions. Some medical professionals argue that the less monitoring done, the better. Others prefer to err on the side of caution and monitor throughout active labor. In fact, continuous fetal monitoring once a woman is in active labor is typical in almost all hospital settings and most birthing centers. This is also how I practice. "Continuous" doesn't have to mean nonstop, though. I encourage my patients to walk during labor if they feel like it, on the condition that they lie down periodically in order to let us monitor fetal heart rate.

A normal fetal heart rate is 120 to 160 beats per minute. A faster or slower rate can be an indication of a problem, though it doesn't necessarily mean there *is* a problem. When there is a deviation from the normal range, your care provider may do one of several things to correct the situation, including asking you to change positions, giving IV fluids, or adjusting medication. If there is concern that the baby may be in danger, an emergency C-section can have the baby out literally in a matter of minutes.

There are several ways fetal monitoring can be done:

• *External monitors.* These monitors are strapped against your abdomen with two big belts. The most common kind of monitoring, they can be used continuously or periodically. They track two things: the fetal heart rate and the length and frequency of contractions. They are the same as those used for nonstress tests.

• *Internal monitors.* Internal monitors are used if it is not possible to adequately monitor you externally, for example with obese patients. They are also used if more exact information is needed, such as if labor is not progressing well and the strength of the contractions needs to be quantified. If there are twins, and it is difficult to track both on external monitors, one may be monitored internally and the other externally.

The amniotic sac must be ruptured to use an internal monitor.

There are two monitors, a thin wire with a small electrode attached to the fetus's scalp to monitor its heart rate, and another called an intrauterine pressure catheter (IUPC), which is a thin tube with a pressure-sensing device on its tip, to measure contractions. The IUPC lies in the uterus next to the baby, but is not attached to anything internally. Once an internal monitor is in place, the mother is usually restricted to bed.

• *Doppler ultrasound and fetoscope.* Although they are not a part of standard ob care, some physicians and midwives sometimes rely on two other devices to listen to the fetal heartbeat in labor. A Doppler is a small, handheld ultrasound device that uses sound waves to "hear" the heart, the same device typically used at your prenatal visits. A fetoscope is a stethoscope used to listen to the baby through the belly and was regularly used before the Doppler became available.

It's easy to get caught up in the flashing numbers and readouts on the monitoring equipment, but interpreting the data is best left to your doctor or midwife. A decrease in the accelerations of the fetal heart rate, for example, doesn't necessarily mean that the fetus is in distress. Often this simply happens because the fetus is sleeping. (Yes, even while you're working hard and pumping with excitement!) In this case, the labor attendant may stimulate the baby to see if the heart rate accelerates. Basically, the doctor wakes the baby up. This can be done in one of several ways: 1) by use of a buzzer on the abdomen called vibrational acoustic stimulation (VAS), 2) by the "poor man's version of VAS," clapping spoons together against the belly to make a similarly loud sound, or 3) by the doctor manually scratching the baby's head gently while doing a cervical exam.

The bottom line is that the assessment of fetal well-being is your labor attendant's job. Your job is to focus on staying connected to your body, soul, and baby.

Maternal Monitoring

Your vital signs (heart rate, respiratory rate, temperature) are routinely taken and assessed. Other maternal assessment depends on the specifics of your condition. Your heart rate is typically tracked on the fetal monitor, along with your baby's, but other vital signs will be specifically noted on a regular basis.

Monitoring Labor Progress: Cervical Exams

A cervical exam involves inserting two fingers into the vagina to assess the thinning, dilation, and position of the cervix, as well as the position of the baby, in order to help gauge how far along your labor is. The exam only takes a few seconds. (For more details on how the cervix is evaluated, see Chapter 23.) While cervical exams are a handy way to monitor labor progress, they're not without risk and therefore should be done sparingly. Anytime anything (including fingers) is put into the vagina, there's a risk of introducing infection, especially after the membranes have ruptured.

Try to avoid the situation where the labor nurse checks you, then the medical resident comes in a few minutes later and checks you again, and then the attending physician does the same, unless there is something unusual going on for which they are trying to get multiple opinions. Be proactive and when you are about to be checked, ask why, especially after your membranes are ruptured.

In active labor, cervical checks are not normally necessary more than once every two hours. If your cervix has dilated adequately in those two hours, meaning by at least 1 cm per hour, labor is proceeding normally and can be checked again in two more hours. Once you are in active labor, if your cervix has not dilated at this rate after two hours, this is often referred to as "falling off the labor curve"—meaning labor is not proceeding as expected and the doctor needs to investigate why. Other reasons for cervical exams would include fetal distress or if you have the urge to push.

FEAR: Labor will be terribly painful.

FACT: Most women experience some degree of pain, it's true. But what that pain feels like is quite variable. There is a paradox in that pain is a natural by-product of the progression of labor, but pain can also inhibit labor. How can this be? Credit something called the fear/tension/pain cycle. When you are afraid, the normal response is to tense up; when you are tense, you feel pain more acutely, which increases your fear. Therefore it's to your advantage to be as relaxed as possible, either by helping your mind and body work with, minimize, or block out the contractions and/or by taking medications.

✔ **REALITY CHECK:** What Is Labor Pain?

Labor hurts. However, unlike the pain caused by an external injury, which is a threat to your health and well-being, this is pain from internal forces working exactly as they were meant to. What you're feeling is the contracting (squeezing) of the uterine muscles as they work to ease your baby out. I've never heard of anyone passing out from her own labor pain. In fact, your body actually prepares itself to deal with the pain by secreting adrenaline and feel-good endorphins, the same kinds of hormones also responsible for "runner's high."

It may help to remember my favorite insights about labor pain:

• Labor pain is not a signal that something is wrong. Pain actually serves a function in labor, acting as a kind of guidance system; generally, the positions and activities (such as breathing exercises to relax) that most ease pain are those that will help your body work most efficiently.

• Labor pain occurs within a joyous context. That's another way pain caused by contractions is unlike pain caused by injury. In labor, you're fully engaged in a creative process of the highest order, surrounded by loving support, and looking forward to an exciting, imminent end goal—meeting your child.

• While the force of a contraction can make you feel practically turned inside out, all sensations of pain disappear between contractions. You're not going to experience four or eight or twenty nonstop hours of pain.

POSSIBLE MEDICAL ISSUES NOW

Pain Management

The decision is yours, not anybody else's (including your doctor's), when it comes to choosing how you will manage the pain of labor.

Eight in ten women choose some form of pain medication. This is an entirely legitimate choice to be honored, especially when made consciously. I've seen many women derive confidence and relaxation from pain relief. However, as pain relief has become a standard part of ob culture, I've seen many women say "yes" when it's offered without giving the question much deliberation. They're using it automatically, and often before they need it.

A natural (nonmedicated) delivery, if it works for you, is perhaps the peak physical experience a woman can have. While comparatively unusual these days in the US, there is no reason why any woman with a normal pregnancy who wants this experience should not have the opportunity to try it. Like pregnancy itself, a natural vaginal delivery provides the opportunity to feel and do something that your body is expressly designed for. The experience may leave you with a sense of inner strength, confidence, and accomplishment you have never felt before, revealing capabilities you never imagined you had. Any woman can have these feelings about any childbirth experience, but I most often hear such descriptions from those who have had natural deliveries. So if this idea appeals to you, I encourage you to discuss it early with your doctor and to take labor-preparation steps that support this goal, such as childbirth classes that focus on this goal, or working with a hypnotherapist. As with choosing pain relief, choosing an unmedicated delivery should be made with full awareness, not because somebody is telling you that that's what you ought to do.

There's a lot we don't understand about pain, and why some people seem to have very different pain thresholds than others. Some things we do know: A large baby who is pressing against your spinal cord, for example, will cause a different kind and amount of pain from a small baby in perfect position for delivery. But in the end, every woman brings her individual history into the labor room. That history, along with how her labor presents itself, will influence how she experiences and responds to pain and whether she opts for pain relief. Of course, in the event of an emergency, there may be little choice; if a C-section is needed, you'll need some form of anesthesia!

Because you can't know in advance what's in store for you, it's a good idea to understand the possibilities and be open-minded—be conscious—about what may turn out to be right for you.

(Nonmedical pain relief options you can practice on your own are covered in the next chapter, "Labor and Delivery: Self-Care.")

Medical (analgesic) pain relief falls into three main categories:

- *Systemic medication* (sedation delivered intravenously)
- *Regional approaches* (such as epidurals, spinal blocks, and combined spinal-epidurals)
- *Integrative medical approaches* (including acupuncture and clinical hypnosis; there are also mind-body techniques that can relieve tension and pain but don't require medical assistance, which are discussed in the next chapter)

Many physicians don't have a preference one way or another about what kind of pain management you choose. But they will likely have an opinion about *when* in the labor process you are offered each type. As the saying goes, "Not too early and not too late." There are many factors to be considered. For example, regional medication given during the latent phase of labor risks slowing it down, and given too late can make pushing less effective. It's standard not to give regional medication before a dilation of 4 cm or after the point when it appears that the woman will deliver within the next hour. Obviously that still leaves a pretty large window of time in which you can consider whether or not you want it. Alternative approaches can be adapted to any stage of labor—one of their many advantages.

Systemic Medication (via IV)
IV medications are useful in early labor because they can take the edge off pain without tending to stall labor, as an epidural can if given too early. Commonly used examples include Stadol and Demerol. If you're feeling especially anxious about delivery, perhaps because of fear of the pain, these drugs can help ease anxiety and minimize pain, making you better able to relax and helping your body do what it's supposed to do. Sometimes, this can even allow you to sleep through some of your latent labor, which can be a welcome opportunity, especially if you've been at it a long time.

Relief is generally felt relatively quickly and lasts about two hours. Often, each succeeding dose feels less effective than the one before it.

On the downside, because IV medications are systemic, they deliver medication to your entire system at once. Rather than targeting the area where you feel pain, they sedate all of you. This makes you relaxed, but it also makes you feel sleepy and generally dulled. If you've ever had a strong pain reliever of any kind, you may have experienced this feeling. What's more, "all of you" includes your fetus, as these drugs cross the placenta. Systemic drugs are not given close to delivery in order to avoid sedating the baby, which can impact the baby's ability to breathe effectively on its own.

Regional Pain Relief: Epidurals

Epidurals are the most widely used kind of regional anesthesia. Medication inserted through a thin plastic catheter in the back dulls or numbs the sensations in the lower part of the body, while you remain awake and alert. Epidurals are managed by an anesthesiologist or, less often, a specially trained obstetrician. (One reason why epidurals are more routine at large hospitals than at those that deliver fewer than 500 babies a year is that smaller hospitals may lack trained staff to provide them, or lack the 24-hour coverage needed to monitor and manage the epidurals once they are placed.)

It can take 20 minutes to place the epidural catheter and about 30 minutes for you to begin feeling the effects. Most doctors don't like to use epidurals until the mom-to-be is clearly in active labor, so as not to slow labor's progress. If your history indicates a possible need for a C-section (which will require complete numbing), a catheter for an epidural may be placed earlier, even if you intend to labor naturally for as long as possible.

More than half (59 percent) of all laboring moms in the US get an epidural today. In large hospitals, their use tripled between 1981 (22 percent) and 1997 (66 percent). In smaller hospitals, their use doubled in the same time frame. This varies regionally, however. By some estimates, 90 percent of New York City moms get them, compared with 20 percent in Boulder, Colorado. In Canada fewer than half of women receive epidurals (45 percent), and in England the rate is only 12 percent.

Part of the popularity can be accounted for by newer, less heavy formulations that, unlike the epidurals of the past, do not leave a woman completely without sensation during her labor and delivery or for long afterward. In medical parlance, we talk about how "dense" (how potent) an epidural is. Originally they were so dense that they cut off all sensation. While this may sound wonderful to someone worried about pain, it makes pushing very difficult or even impossible, often leading to otherwise unnecessary forceps deliveries or C-sections. It also makes it nearly impossible to have a conscious experience—to deliver a baby vaginally with no sensation at all is the

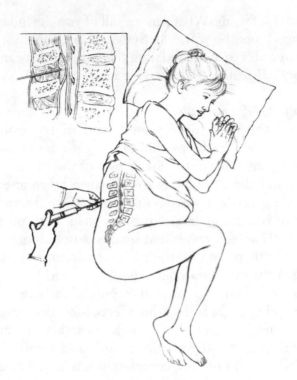

Inserting an epidural

To have an epidural catheter placed, you typically lie on your side curled into a ball. In this position, there's more space between your vertebrae, making it easier to insert a needle into the epidural space, which is an area within your spinal column. After the area is cleaned and numbed with a local anesthetic, the needle is inserted (see diagram) and then the catheter is threaded through the needle. After the needle is removed, the catheter stays in place, allowing medication to be supplied continuously throughout labor via a pump operated by the anesthesiologist.

ultimate disconnect! Ideally, an epidural should take the edge off the pain but still allow you to know when you are having contractions and to feel pressure so that you know when it is time to push. A so-called walking epidural is so light that a patient can actually walk around after it's been placed and dosed. Because this kind of formulation must be managed by a specially trained anesthesiologist with expertise in obstetric care, it is less widely available in community hospitals. They are an option in almost all academic and major medical centers. With most kinds of epidurals, however, the mother stays in bed.

There's some controversy over whether epidurals slow labor down or speed it up. You'd think this would be obvious one way or the other, but there are data to support both sides. The most recent *ACOG Practice Bulletin* states that use of epidurals increases the average length of second stage (pushing) by 20 to 30 minutes. But this varies tremendously from woman to woman. My guess is that in situations where intense pain or high anxiety or fear is creating significant tension, an epidural speeds labor by minimizing the pain and fear that can accompany it, thus allowing labor to progress. In labors where the woman does not experience excessive pain or anxiety, an epidural may very well slow labor by decreasing the effectiveness of her contractions, slowing them or reducing their intensity. The only thing we really know for sure is that responses are highly individualized.

Although the majority of women wind up thanking their epidural more than complaining about it, the procedure is not without risks. In about one in ten cases, a drop in the woman's blood pressure occurs soon after the epidural is placed, which can cause fetal distress. Another common side effect (1 to 3 percent of cases) is a spinal headache, which is essentially a severe headache after delivery that can follow an otherwise uncomplicated epidural. This happens because the epidural needle accidentally punctures the spinal membranes, causing a leakage of spinal fluid, which changes the pressure around the brain. Rarely, the epidural can be placed incorrectly, so that the medication gets into a blood vessel rather than the epidural space, putting the patient at risk for cardiac arrest. It's also possible, though extremely rare, to have a complication referred to as a "high spinal" because the paralysis goes past the uterus up to the chest, leading to respiratory arrest. This occurs only in less than 0.03 percent of epidurals. Some of the epidural's drugs pass through the placenta to the baby, although to what extent and whether this is in any way harmful has not been conclusively evaluated. (See "Fear/Fact" below.)

Epidurals have also been linked to a greater use of forceps or vacuum extraction and C-section, felt to be due to inefficient pushing. Other problems include inadequate or irregular pain relief (you can have "spots" where you still feel pain), nausea, fever, muscle weakness, and—rarely—allergic reaction to the medication.

HOW TO MAKE A CONSCIOUS CHOICE ABOUT . . . HAVING AN EPIDURAL

As with all pain relief, make your choice about whether to have an epidural a conscious one. Because epidurals are de rigueur these days, I'd like to make a few points about choosing one in addition to the information provided in "How to Make a Conscious Choice About . . . Pain Relief," on pages 390–391. Some doctors routinely give epidurals simply because a patient is in active labor or once she reaches an arbitrary point of dilation (often 4 to 5 cm). This is a pretty unconscious way to practice medicine! Don't let someone practicing medicine on autopilot interfere with your own approach.

Long before labor begins, be sure you understand the pros and cons of epidurals. On the pro side: If you are in pain that you cannot tolerate, an epidural can often provide very effective and relatively fast pain relief. And once the severity of your pain is moderated, you may find that you are able to have a more conscious birth, and to be more focused and present. Risks and side effects of the procedure include: incomplete or spotty pain relief; so much pain relief that you feel disconnected from your body, are less able to push effectively, and feel like the experience is not really happening to you; and the physical risks listed in the epidural explanation above.

If medication is offered before you have requested it, check in with your body and your soul to help you decide what *you* really want to do. Is the pain bearable? Not too bad? Getting to be more than you can handle? If you're not sure, you can always wait and evaluate yourself again later. The only time that you may be told it's "too late" for an epidural is when you are nearly completely dilated. Another way to prepare yourself is to run this decision through the Feedback Loop now, before your labor begins.

Regional Pain Relief: Spinal Block
This form of pain relief is similar to an epidural. It's administered with a needle directly into the fluid of the spinal space, which renders pain relief much faster. It's a one-time injection, and is very quick to take effect. Spinals are most often used for C-sections.

FEAR: The baby will be affected by the pain relief drugs.
FACT: This is a possibility, although mainly a consideration with

systemic medication which is unknowingly given close to the time of delivery. Problems are rare because doctors try to minimize the amount of medication and avoid giving it near the time of delivery. If there are problems, they can include the baby being sedated and not breathing well at birth. Even if there is a miscalculation and you do unexpectedly deliver soon after receiving medication, which sometimes happens, the baby will be watched for signs of sedation and can be given a drug to reverse the effects, if necessary.

Integrative Medical Pain Relief: Acupuncture
While not mainstream medical practice in the US, acupuncture for pain relief in labor is routinely used with near-universal success rates in many Asian countries. To give you a sense of how effective this is, it's often used in China as the *only* anesthesia during C-sections, without any assist at all from pain relief medications. In a six-year study of acupuncture for anesthesia in C-sections in more than 16,000 cases in China, it was found to be 99 percent successful, with excellent stability of both the mother's and the baby's heart rate and respiration. Although it's doubtful that anesthesia consisting of acupuncture alone will ever become the norm in the US, I see this method gaining greater acceptance as an adjunct to anesthesia.

Acupuncture is based on the theory that there are energy channels called meridians that run through the body and that the free flow of energy, or qi ("chi"), along these channels is what creates health. Acupuncture involves stimulating specific points in the body (acupressure points) located along these meridians by puncturing the skin with a very fine needle, which is typically kept in place for a short period of time (under 30 minutes). The traditional explanation for its effectiveness is that the insertion of needles restores normal flow of qi through the body, which stimulates its natural healing ability. One theory (as yet unproven) that conventional medicine has put forth to explain acupuncture's effectiveness is that the needles stimulate the nervous system to release chemicals that alter pain perception and influence the body's internal regulating system. This theory makes me smile—it's always so much easier to use our own paradigm to explain "foreign" phenomena than to entertain the possibility of a new paradigm. My hope is that as we learn more, each system will inform the other.

There are many distinct styles of acupuncture, including the kind used in Chinese medicine, as well as Japanese Manaka style, Korean Hand Acupuncture, and the Worsley Five-Element method. Body points can also be stimulated without needles simply by using pressure (acupressure) or heat (moxibustion). Electroacupuncture delivers low-level electrical stimulation through the needles.

Western studies have shown that acupuncture significantly reduces labor pain with minimal side effects, making it a good choice if you want to avoid or reduce the use of medical pain relief. One study also found that acupuncture shortened the length of labor, though this may be related to the reduced use of epidurals in these patients, which would be an indirect effect of the acupuncture rather than a direct effect. A 1997 summary statement by the NIH regarding acupuncture in general stated that the data supporting its use are as strong as those for many accepted Western medical therapies, and the incidence of adverse effects is substantially lower than that of many accepted medical procedures used for the same conditions. The primary potential side effect is infection, which is now avoided by the use of sterile, disposable needles.

In my experience, patients have the best results in labor when they have worked with an acupuncturist previously in the pregnancy; for example, many of my patients consult with a Chinese medicine practitioner for fertility help before they conceive, or see one as part of an overall integrative plan. These patients seem to have the easiest time in labor and noticeably less pain. But wouldn't it be great if one day any woman in labor could enter the hospital and be asked whether she prefers to have IV drugs, an epidural, or acupuncture?

If you are interested in incorporating acupuncture into your labor plan, you will need to check the policies of the hospital where you intend to deliver. In most states, a practitioner must provide proof that he or she has attended and graduated from an accredited school or a school in the process of being accredited by the Accreditation Commission for Acupuncture and Oriental Medicine, and also have privileges to work in your chosen birth setting.

Another option is to work with an acupuncturist during your pregnancy but not have that person in the labor suite with you. In this case, the acupuncturist can place "tacks," tiny tack-shaped needles that stimulate the acupuncture point, or affix small balls over the acupuncture points with adhesive. Throughout labor you or someone else can gently press the tacks or balls into your skin, stimulating the acupressure points.

Integrative Medical Pain Relief: Clinical Hypnosis
I highly recommend using hypnosis for pain relief during labor, as well as for facilitating both delivery and recovery. Hypnosis is a state of deep relaxation and focused attention that allows you to bring the full energy of consciousness toward your goal. The hypnotic state resembles sleep, but you're alert and completely in control. While this form of pain management during labor is not in wide use in our culture, there are no real impediments to a woman who is motivated to use it.

Hypnosis has been shown to speed labor and reduce pain. It can be so effective that it's even been used by women undergoing C-sections as their only form of pain relief, an impressive testimonial to the power of the mind and to the ability of hypnosis to channel that power. If a woman can undergo abdominal surgery using hypnosis with no anesthesia at all, you can imagine how effective it could be at basic labor-pain management in a vaginal delivery. One large study associated hypnosis with a shorter first stage of labor in first-time moms—6.4 hours on average   compared with 9.3 hours in the control group, which did not use hypnosis; the pushing stage was also slightly shorter. While this study had certain weaknesses and better, larger studies are needed, I consider their findings very interesting. Coupled with the individual cases I've seen of patients using hypnosis in labor, the case for trying it is quite compelling. I'd love to see hypnosis tapes handed to every mom-to-be as she was admitted!

Most women, of course, have had no experience with hypnosis. Many patients, on first hearing the idea, think hypnosis means that someone else will control their mind or their experience. In reality this is a technique for harnessing the power of one's *own* mind to help achieve a desired outcome. Although the American Medical Association approved hypnotherapy as a valid medical treatment back in 1958, we still don't completely understand how it works. One theory is that hypnosis causes the brain to release enkephalins and endorphins, natural hormones that are one of the body's mechanisms for dulling the sensation of pain. There may also be other explanations if we look outside of the biomedical model.

If you wish to use hypnosis for pain relief during labor, start working with a hypnotherapist early in your pregnancy—the earlier the better—and discuss your plan with your obstetrician. As with any therapy, the work you do with a hypnotherapist becomes more individualized as you get to know each other, and hypnosis can be invaluable for a myriad of issues that may arise during your pregnancy. The ideal scenario, admittedly not available to everyone, is to work with a hypnotherapist during pregnancy and to also have that person present with you in the delivery room. Having the person at your side can be particularly reassuring and give you much greater confidence. Having said that, this is far from necessary. Many individuals have undergone surgery with only hypnosis done presurgically and using a tape during the procedure. It's a wonderful idea to do this if you are having a scheduled C-section, as the therapist can tailor your hypnosis to your specific situation (your own preconceptions, previous experiences, or degree of your fear, for example). Presurgical hypnosis has also been shown to speed healing. Although it's possible to undergo a C-section using hypnosis only (some hospitals permit it, when planned in advance), most women use it as an adjunct to their surgical pain management, not as their only pain management.

Whether you have a Cesarean or vaginal delivery, you can rely on what you learned in earlier sessions with your hypnotherapist and/or bring tapes made in previous sessions especially for labor. The sessions will be individualized to you and your desired outcomes. To locate a hypnotherapist, check with your physician or health care facility, or use the American Society for Clinical Hypnosis (ASCH).

HOW TO MAKE A CONSCIOUS CHOICE ABOUT . . . PAIN RELIEF

Will you use some kind of medical analgesia, and if so, what kind? This is something to think about—but not make a final decision about—before you hit the delivery room. To come to the hospital declaring either "I won't use any drugs, period" or, "I need my epidural ASAP!" is the unconscious route, because you're not making the decision on the basis of how you actually feel during labor. You're merely sticking to a stance, which is different from making a mindful assessment of your needs in the moment.

It's a big decision, and not one you want to make a snap judgment about—either before the first contraction or 10 hours into them. Here's what to do before labor starts:

First, reflection. Consider your preconceptions about pain relief in labor. What stories have you heard? What's your initial response to the thought of medical pain relief: Welcoming? Cautious? Curious? Not interested? Are there specific fears or concerns that you have about the various options?

Second, information. Be sure that you understand your pain-relief options, both medical (including both conventional drugs and integrative methods such as acupuncture and hypnosis) and nonmedical (see next chapter), and how they work. Ask your doctor or midwife about anything you don't understand. Factors that can affect the progress or intensity of labor, and in turn your perception of pain, include a large baby, twins, labor that is induced, or a baby in an abnormal position.

Collect firsthand stories. If it's of interest to you, seek out women who have gone through labor without any medication or who have tried an alternative approach. Although we don't often hear about them given the focus on medical management of labor, there are many who feel that natural childbirth allowed them to experience the miracle of birth and the power of their bodies in a fuller, more life-affirming way. Likewise, because acupuncture and hypnosis are not commonly used for pain relief in labor, we don't hear much about women who have used them, either.

Third, action. You shouldn't make the actual choice until you are in labor. Remember that there is no right or wrong answer. All that matters is that you are comfortable with your decision. If you start with the least-invasive approaches, you can always change your mind and request medical pain relief, right up until you are almost 10 cm dilated.

Then, re-reflection. This is an absolutely essential step, especially in labor. Use the body-soul-baby check-ins described in Chapter 22. If you feel like you might want something for the pain, ask: Is this something that my body wants and needs right now? Is it okay to continue without any pain medication for a while longer? Some women use the Dialoguing tool to "talk" to their body for input.

POSSIBLE LABOR SCENARIOS

Sometimes labor doesn't go as expected and you will need an assist of one kind or another beyond pain management. The following scenarios are common reasons that interventions are used in labor.

When Labor Doesn't Start

When you are not in labor on your own but it is time for you to be delivered, either because you are past your due date or because there is some kind of problem such as severe preeclampsia, a decision will need to be made about the best route of delivery. Your medical history, the reason that you need to be delivered at that time, and your personal preferences will all be taken into account to make this decision. If together you and your doctor decide that you will attempt a vaginal delivery, your labor will be induced. If you decide on a surgical delivery, a C-section will be performed.

When Labor Stalls in Stage One: Arrest of Dilation

What happens when labor starts fine but does not follow a normal labor curve? That is, the cervical dilation fails to progress at the usual pace or progresses normally for a while and then stops? The doctor will then investigate why. We consider the three main suspects, or "the 3 Ps of labor": power, passenger, pelvis. Here's what we look at and what we can do, depending on what is found:

- Is there a problem with the *power* of the uterine contractions?

If the force of the contractions is not powerful enough, it makes sense that the cervix may not dilate. The only way to confirm that this is a problem is to place an internal monitor (IUPC) to measure the pressure of each contraction. If contractions are determined to be inadequate, Pitocin can be given to stimulate them. If this is the only issue, the added help of this drug usually puts labor back on track. Ideally, only enough should be given to put contractions back within the "adequate" range. Giving Pitocin to encourage more or stronger contractions increases the risk of uterine rupture, which is very rare but possible. (See "Augmentation of Labor," page 400.)

If contractions are measured and found to be adequately strong, no

Pitocin is given, because labor must be failing to progress for a different reason. (An illustration of the adage that more is not necessarily better!)

- Is there a problem with the *passenger* (the baby)?

The position or size of the baby can impede delivery progress. There is virtually no baby too large to be delivered vaginally—not even 10- or 11-pounders. Often the real culprit is the position of the baby's head, making it too big relative to his mother's pelvis. Two babies of the same size in mothers whose pelvises are identical can have different birth outcomes depending on the angle of the baby's head. If the head is not angled so that the presenting part is the narrowest part of the head, as normally happens, this can make vaginal delivery much more difficult, regardless of the overall size of the baby. (See diagrams below.) That's just one illustration of how the baby's position can interfere with labor. Other examples include the way the baby is facing (faceup or facedown), where the arms are, or whether the body is simply not "lined up straight" for an efficient exit. The result can be that labor stalls. When arrest of dilation occurs and it is due to the "passenger," the physician will need to do a C-section.

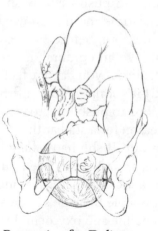 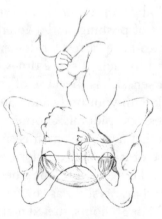

Presenting for Delivery: Good Position

Notice how the baby's head is positioned: When the head is flexed and chin tucked, the smallest possible diameter of the head is lined up to fit through the pelvis.

Presenting for Delivery: Another Angle

Compare the position of this baby's head. When the chin is not tucked down, a much wider part of the head approaches the pelvis first. Often what's thought of as a baby "too big" for the mother is simply one not optimally positioned for an easy vaginal delivery.

- Is there a problem with the *pelvis*?

If labor is not proceeding, another possibility is a structural issue. Women often worry that they are "too small" to deliver. That's actually quite rare. Females are built to bear babies. The shape of the pelvic bones, however, can influence how an individual baby comes through at delivery. There are four different pelvic shapes. Your doctor assesses your pelvis early in pregnancy to scout for abnormalities and to understand your baseline. It's extremely rare that a woman would be told at the outset of pregnancy that she needed to have a C-section because of a pelvic problem. The more important aspect is the relationship of the baby to the pelvis. In other words, if the baby, due to position or size or both, is such that a delivery through the size and shape of your pelvis is unlikely, this is referred to as CPD, or cephalopelvic disproportion.

When Your Labor Stalls in Stage Two: Arrest of Descent

It's possible to labor normally, dilate completely, and then run into trouble pushing the baby out. You push, and push—and push. Still, the baby won't come out. Typically a first-time mom is allowed two hours of pushing, and a veteran mom one hour, before she's considered to have "arrest of descent." If you have an epidural, an hour is added to each of those times, simply because if you cannot feel all of your sensations (because of the epidural) it's simply more difficult to work with your body and your contractions to push effectively.

Besides epidurals, another common reason for a stall at the pushing stage is that the woman is simply worn out. If she had a long latent phase of labor and/or a long active phase, and then has been pushing for an hour or more, she's been through a lot physically. If things got started just as she was going to bed, it's possible that she's been awake for 24 or 36 hours, fueled mainly by adrenaline and oxytocin! Doctors will also assess the possibility of cephalopelvic disproportion.

Depending on the diagnosis, different actions will be taken. Some examples: If the mother is exhausted or unable to push effectively and the baby is low in the pelvis, forceps or vacuum extraction will be considered. If the problem seems to be the relative size of the baby to the pelvis, a Cesarean delivery will be recommended. If the baby is showing no signs of distress, and the mother is exhausted, simple rest (taking a break from pushing) may be the course of action.

When the Baby Is Stressed

When fetal monitors indicate possible signs of distress in the baby, such as decelerations in fetal heart rate or other signs that the baby could be stressed, such as the presence of meconium in the amniotic fluid (see the bottom of page 396), the doctors will investigate. Most likely, the baby is not getting enough oxygen, for one of many different reasons. Among the causes of fetal distress:

• A problem with compression of the umbilical cord. This can be due to:

the baby lying on the cord.
the umbilical cord being wrapped around the baby's neck.
the cord having a knot (probably created weeks ago when the baby still had space to move around).
the prolapse of the umbilical cord. In this rare event, the umbilical cord descends out of the birth canal before the baby and gets compressed between the baby's head and the birth canal. A prolapsed cord can happen when the amniotic sac ruptures and the cord is pushed outward by the rushing fluid, or it can happen—rarely—at other times. An immediate C-section is required.

• A chronic (ongoing) placental problem. Some women have problems with the placenta across the pregnancy, most commonly associated with hypertension. When such a problem is diagnosed ahead of time it is called chronic placental insufficiency. Often in such cases the placenta functions well enough for nonstressful times, but during labor, a high-stress period, it cannot function adequately and results in fetal distress. (See "Placenta Problems," pages 295–301.)

• An acute (sudden) placenta problem. Rarely, the placenta pulls away from the uterine wall (an abruption), interfering with its ability to get oxygenated blood to the fetus.

• A uterine problem. When the uterus is contracting, blood does not flow freely into the placenta and to the baby. With normal contractions, the baby recovers between contractions. When the uterus is not resting enough between contractions—because they are too frequent or too strong—the baby can receive too little oxygen and experience distress. Though this can happen in an unmedicated delivery, much more often it happens because a woman has received too much Pitocin. Uterine rupture is another example of a uterine problem, albeit one that's both extreme and rare.

• A maternal problem. The most typical situation in this category is that the woman's blood pressure drops, which is not uncommon after the initial dosing of an epidural. When this happens, the amount of oxygenated blood getting to the placenta and the baby drops, too. Another example might be if the mother had an underlying medical condition that impaired her ability to oxygenate blood (heart disease or lung disease, for example), which would also affect the oxygenation of the baby.

• A problem with the baby. Rarely, the fetus is sick or has some underlying problem that interferes with its ability to tolerate the stress of labor.

Please realize that hearing the words "fetal distress" in your labor room does not necessarily mean you will be rushed off for an emergency C-section. As a matter of fact, we are moving away from that term. You are more likely to hear "nonreassuring fetal testing," which is far more accurate. We cannot know if the baby is distressed; we only know that the testing is not reassuring and there is cause for concern. Many causes are transient and/or correctable. For example, changing position can move the baby off a compressed umbilical cord. A drop in the mother's blood pressure can be corrected by giving some additional IV fluids. Overly intense contractions can be lessened either by turning the Pitocin down or off, or by giving a drug that temporarily relaxes the uterus.

Meconium is actually what is excreted from the bowels of the baby, that is, baby poop! This does not typically happen before delivery unless the baby is stressed. Meconium is present in about 5 percent of all deliveries. It changes the amniotic fluid and reduces its antibacterial activity thereby increasing the risk of infection for the baby. If it is inhaled by the baby, it can cause serious damage to the infant's lungs. If meconium is noted while you are laboring, the attendant will assess how concentrated it appears and will look for other signs of stress in the baby. She may try to dilute the meconium while you are still in labor (a procedure called amnioinfusion), and will suction the baby's mouth and nose very thoroughly at the time of delivery. In this case, the obstetrician will ask you to stop pushing after the head of your baby is delivered so that she can suction the baby well. Once this is done, she will then ask you to push again to deliver the rest of the baby.

When the doctor sees signs of fetal distress, you and your baby will be assessed for the probable cause, and actions will be taken to correct it. The cause of fetal distress can't always be determined, however, even after the baby has been safely delivered. If at any point the baby is not responding, a C-section is performed, and the baby can be safely delivered incredibly quickly—within minutes.

LABOR INTERVENTIONS

Induction of Labor

Inducing labor means to use medical interventions to cause it to begin before Mother Nature does. This is an example of technology that's too often used just because we *can*, and not because we *should*. It's a growing trend: More than one in five births were induced in 2000, up from fewer than one in ten in 1989.

In my very strong opinion, inductions should be done *only* if medically indicated. Instead, they are often scheduled for the most inappropriate reasons: A patient is tired of being pregnant or wants her baby to have a certain birthday, or a doctor wants to clear his schedule before an upcoming vacation. Some doctors schedule inductions simply because a woman has reached her due date, even if she's still well within the window of expected full-term birth and both the woman and baby are doing fine.

There's a fundamental difference between these elective or "social" inductions, and a medically indicated one. I only do medically indicated inductions, with rare exceptions. (Once a woman's husband, a Marine, was due to be shipped overseas after her due date, so we induced her at 39 weeks so that he could be there for the delivery.) To have an induction is to override the whole process, body and soul, that leads up to labor. It's not known exactly what triggers labor to begin, but we do know that it's an intricate process, a complicated dance of hormones, physiology, and perhaps psychology between the baby and the mother that cannot be artificially duplicated. Especially if you've been working to have a conscious pregnancy, why voluntarily overrule your body's inner wisdom right at the brink of the main event?

An induction is typically beneficial to the mother and/or the fetus in the following situations:

- Your water breaks and labor does not start on its own. Ninety percent of women who experience premature rupture of membranes (before labor starts) once they are full term will go on to begin labor within 24 hours. If you don't go into labor, however, the ruptured amniotic sac opens the way for bacteria in the vagina to reach the sterile environment of the uterus. To avoid such infection, most doctors will induce labor within 24 to 48 hours (sometimes immediately after rupture) if it does not begin naturally. My own decision about when to induce in these circumstances hinges on my patient's desires and my intuition.
- You have preeclampsia and are full term.
- There is concern about the fetus's well-being (due to a nonreactive nonstress test or decreased fluid, for example).
- You have a medical problem, such as diabetes, that's not under control.

There's no one way of handling inductions. The main choices include the following:

1. Stripping the membranes. In this procedure, your doctor inserts a finger into your cervix and across the thin membranes that connect the amniotic sac to the uterus. This causes the release of prostaglandins, hormones that can help ripen the cervix. This is controversial and grounded more in folklore than in medical fact, though most obstetricians I know try it. It is typically done during an outpatient visit.

The next three options are done at the hospital once you have been admitted:

2. Ripening the cervix. This can be done by placing medicine (a tablet or gel) in or near the cervix to soften it and help it stretch for labor. It can also be done mechanically by placing a soft device known as a Foley bulb into the cervix.
3. Giving Pitocin. This is the synthetic form of oxytocin, the hormone that causes the uterus to contract. Given intravenously, Pitocin stimulates contractions (you may hear it referred to as "Pit" or a "Pit drip").

Your doctor must determine where your body is starting from in order to know the best way to induce your labor. Its readiness is usually assessed by calculating your Bishop score (a formula named after its creator). A Bishop score uses a point system of between zero and three points across five different criteria based on your cervical exam. The five criteria are:

1. How dilated you are
2. How effaced you are
3. How high or low the baby's station is in the pelvis
4. How soft or firm the consistency of the cervix is
5. How close to the front of the vagina the position of the cervix is

A woman with a high Bishop score (typically 8 or more out of 13), who is said to have a "ripe" cervix, for example, can go straight to Pitocin, or if the doctor is willing, she can have her water broken (an amniotomy or artificial rupture of membranes) and then wait for a period of time to see if labor begins on its own. If it does not, she can then be given Pitocin to stimulate contractions. A woman with a low Bishop score (typically 4 or less), on the other hand, will first have the cervix "ripened." Individuals respond to induction in very different ways. Some women need just a bit of Pitocin to get things going. (This is often the case with women who have given birth before and we refer to it as a "whiff of Pit.") Others' bodies seem more resistant. While it has never been studied, my belief is that working consciously with your body, soul, and baby—communicating, feeling prepared, doing all you can to understand and appreciate what's happening—can make a big difference in how readily you respond to induction.

FEAR: I've heard that an induced labor is more painful than a natural one.

FACT: No study has ever documented a difference between naturally occurring contractions and artificially stimulated ones.
Women commonly report such differences, however; they
very often describe the pain of contractions stimulated by
Pitocin as being more intense. Is it all imagined? Possibly.
But I also suspect that there may be a real difference of experience. It makes sense that there are subtle and complex
changes that occur when labor happens naturally that cannot be duplicated solely by Pitocin. It's also possible that
the actual mechanics of Pit-stimulated contractions are different than naturally occurring ones.

Whatever the possible physiological differences, there's
definitely a difference in the progression of labor. Rather
than the long, gradual roll-up of spontaneous labor, much of
which usually takes place at home, when you're induced it's
more of a forced march, which all takes place in a hospital
bed. And the contractions of induced labor can come more
quickly, with shorter recovery times between them, making
labor seem more intense and difficult.

Augmentation of Labor

If your labor stalls and the doctor determines that the reason is that
your contractions are not strong enough or frequent enough, Pitocin
is used to stimulate the contractions. This is called "augmenting" labor
and is different from inducing labor in that your labor started just
fine—it just didn't get where it needed to go. The strength of the contractions is closely monitored and the dosage is continuously adjusted
accordingly.

Forceps- or Vacuum-Assisted Delivery

These two mechanical aids help to pull out a baby who is low in the
birth canal and ready to be born. Neither should be used unless the
mother is too exhausted to push effectively, or the baby needs to be
delivered quickly. If the baby is not coming out easily because it is too
big, however, these are not good options. In these situations, there's a
very real risk of the shoulder getting stuck after the head is delivered.

Forceps are a curved metal instrument resembling two metal
spoons. The spoons cradle the sides of the baby's head as the doctor

> ✓ **REALITY CHECK:** Pitocin for "Speeding Things Up"
>
> Pitocin is one of the most unconsciously used tools in a doctor's bag of tricks. No one should be placed on Pitocin without a good assessment and clear rationale for its use, just the same as with any medicine, surgery, or device.
>
> Yet on labor and delivery wards around the country, Pitocin often seems to be administered like water—and with about as little forethought. Patients are routinely put on Pitocin if their labor is not fast enough for a care provider's liking, whether or not it falls within labor curve norms.
>
> If your doctor mentions starting a Pitocin drip, ask about the reasons behind this decision. "Just to speed things up" is not a good enough rationale. Ask to have the details explained. And keep asking until you feel comfortable with the explanation. One of the hardest scenarios, physically and mentally, is to have a long labor that stalls early in the active stage, to get started on Pitocin, and to eventually dilate completely, only to push for three hours and still wind up with a C-section because the baby won't come out (arrest of descent). If your care provider consulted with you about the decision to start the Pitocin and you felt comfortable with the decisions made and felt you were part of the process, you might still wind up disappointed—after all that, who wouldn't? But you'd be less likely to feel resentful, angry, and conflicted about the outcome. Women who wind up viewing labor as "horrible" tend to not be those who had long, hard deliveries, but those who ceded all control to the care team with little sense of involvement along the way.

pulls. A vacuum is a soft plastic cup that fits on the top of the crown of the baby's skull, and is held in place by suction. Both present some risk if not used exactly right. Forceps can bruise a baby's head, or if placed incorrectly can cause injury to the baby or tear the vagina or perineum. With vacuum-assisted deliveries, the risk of fetal injury is generally less, but the device can cause damage if positioned incorrectly, for example on the baby's face instead of the skull, or on part of the vagina. A vacuum also virtually always causes a temporary cone-head appearance. My colleagues who are craniosacral therapists feel this is *not* a good option. Because a vacuum provides a less secure grasp on the baby than forceps, the mother still needs to be able to push when the doctor pulls. And it may need to be tried more than once. If the vacuum hasn't extracted the baby in two to three tries, it's best to move on to a C-section. I have seen, however, my share of "cowboy" doctors who want to keep trying and trying, which rarely does mother or baby any good.

To use either forceps or vacuum, the doctor must be sure of two things: that the baby is low enough in the pelvis, and that the exact position of the baby is known (which way the baby is facing, for example) so the instrument can be placed safely. For a forceps delivery, anesthesia should be offered to the woman, because the forceps put additional pressure on the walls of the vagina. (If she has an epidural in place, more medication can be given if necessary.) Vacuum extraction requires less anesthesia because the vacuum is applied only to the top of the baby's head, not the sides. It doesn't stretch the vagina the same way forceps do, and it therefore causes less pain.

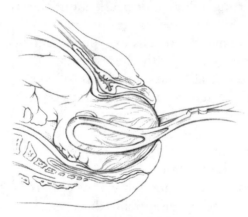

Forceps-assisted delivery

In the hands of someone experienced, both forceps and vacuum can be wonderful tools for a woman who is exhausted and wants to avoid a C-section. However, many physicians are increasingly reluctant to use either tool, particularly forceps, primarily because of fear of lawsuits and are moving right to C-section.

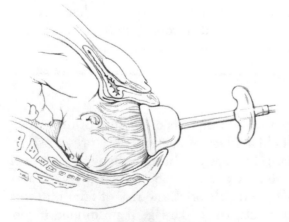

Vacuum-assisted delivery

Episiotomy

As the baby's head crowns, the doctor or midwife decides whether the vaginal opening is large and flexible enough to accommodate the baby. If not, an episiotomy is done. This is a cut made through the perineum (the area between the vagina and the rectum) to enlarge the opening of the vagina, usually because it looks like the tissue around the opening will otherwise tear. If you don't have an epidural, a local anesthesia is given so that you don't feel anything. The procedure is also used if the delivery must be hurried (such as in the event of fetal distress).

One in three American deliveries involve episiotomy, though the rate is dropping and there is a trend toward doing it only when clearly needed. I rarely perform the procedure myself. We've learned that the perineum is much more able to stretch than previously believed, and this natural process may also be facilitated by perineal massage before and during labor, and by doing Kegel exercises during pregnancy. (See "Third Trimester: Self-Care.")

To achieve optimal stretching of the perineum during labor, a slow and controlled delivery is best. When the baby's head begins to crown, it's important not to push or bear down too fast or too hard, so that the tissues can stretch naturally. Here's a great example of why you want to be able to give your attention to your doctor. As the baby's head begins to crown, the doctor will apply counterpressure on the perineum to help avoid a tear, and then instruct you to push slowly and gently (as opposed to making one massive, breath-holding push). Some midwives apply warm compresses to the area, though there is no evidence proving that this is effective.

Whether or not you are likely to have an episiotomy goes back to your choice of care provider and her or his philosophy about labor. Those who lean toward seeing birth as a natural process as I do will try to do everything possible to avoid an episiotomy. Other practitioners still do them routinely.

The argument for doing an episiotomy to avoid a possible tear is that some tears are so extensive and jagged that they are very difficult to repair (stitch back together) and can result in more blood loss and a longer recovery than an incision. Recent studies suggest that this reasoning is faulty, and that an incision increases the risk of additional tearing, including a tear all the way to the rectal area. This is rare, but possible. Postpartum recovery is slower and more painful when you have a lot of stitches, whether they are the result of episiotomy or a tear.

Cesarean-Section Delivery (C-Section)

Cesarean delivery is the surgical removal of the baby by making an incision through the abdomen and uterus and manually lifting it from the mother's body. C-sections save babies' and mothers' lives every hour of every day. If a surgical delivery is suggested to you, the most important question to consider is *why?* Understanding and accepting the answer can make all the difference in how you feel about the outcome. This is why every woman should bring consciousness to the possibility of having a C-section, even if there is nothing to indicate the need before you go into labor.

There are two categories of C-sections: those scheduled in advance (such as for a breech baby or because you've had two prior C-sections) and those that start as vaginal deliveries but wind up as C-sections because of developments during the course of labor (such as arrest of dilation, arrest of descent, or signs of fetal distress). Knowing in advance that you will have a C-section allows for a different mindset from having one unexpectedly. Ideally, you will have made this decision in careful consultation with your doctor and have had time to come to terms with and even embrace the decision. But even if you have an unplanned C-section, while you may be disappointed, you're less likely to be filled with remorse or to feel you have "failed" if you have brought consciousness to the possibility ahead of time. There are many reasons a last-minute C-section may be medically advisable, none of which have to do with any inadequacy or lack of preparation on your part.

If you are hoping for a normal, vaginal delivery—as in my experience most women are—you may not like to think about the possibility of C-section ahead of time. But it's hard to be fully conscious about birth if you ignore the realities of modern-day birthing practices. In the 1970s, C-section rates were around 5 percent. By 2004, a record 29.1 percent of births were by C-section—that's almost one in three! At some hospitals, including but not limited to those that provide care to high-risk patients, the overall rate approaches one-third. Several reasons are usually cited for the C-section boom:

First, rising medical lawsuits and soaring malpractice premiums make all kinds of physicians generally more inclined to err on the side of caution. On a related note, we have more monitoring in labor, which both saves lives and leads to more diagnoses of "nonreassuring fetal testing" (fetal distress), not all of which are warranted.

Second, the trend away from vaginal births after a previous Cesarean (VBAC) means that once a woman has had one Cesarean, her future children are more likely to be delivered the same way. And since first-time Cesarean rates are rising, a greater proportion of total births will be Cesareans.

Third, as with practices as diverse as hormone replacement therapy and removing tonsils, medical trends are influenced by new information as it comes out. As C-sections have been found to be less risky than vaginal delivery in certain circumstances such as breech deliveries, their use has risen.

I'm all for C-sections under the right circumstances. Thanks to the ability to whisk a baby out of the uterus through the abdomen, maternal deaths in childbirth have dropped a hundredfold over the 20th century. We are clearly saving babies that would have certainly died in childbirth as well. C-sections definitely save lives. I fear, however, that this good news has distorted our perceptions about just how benign this surgery is. Cesareans are major surgery, with all the attendant risks of any surgery. These risks include:

- infection in the uterus, pelvis, or incision
- significant blood loss and possible transfusion
- blood clots in the legs, pelvic organs, or lungs
- injury to the bowel, bladder, or ureters (this risk increases with each surgery)
- risks associated with anesthesia. These include: drop in blood pressure, which leads to drop in blood flow and oxygen to the baby (you are given extra fluids to try to prevent this); sore back from the epidural or spinal needle (this usually lasts only a few days); bad headache if the covering of the spinal cord is pierced (a spinal headache); and serious complications that are rare, including the drug entering your vein, making you dizzy or giving you seizures; the drug entering your spinal fluid, suppressing your ability to breathe; and death.

If the C-section is an emergency and general anesthesia is required (the fastest way to achieve anesthesia in someone who does not already have an epidural), then the biggest risk is aspiration (inhaling contents from the stomach into the lungs). If this does occur, it can be serious, and even deadly.

The recovery time from C-section is longer than from labor, because you have a series of incisions (from your abdomen to your uterus) that need to heal. Surgical deliveries are also more expensive than vaginal deliveries. Additionally, there are risks associated with future pregnancies after a C-section. A previous C-section increases the risk of placenta previa, placenta accreta, and uterine rupture, each of which also increases the risk of an emergency hysterectomy. Nearly 70 percent of women who require a hysterectomy at the time of their baby's birth have had previous C-sections.

As a surgeon, I want to stress that despite these risks, a C-section is by and large happy surgery. In what other situation does a doctor operate on someone who is fully conscious and aware of what is happening, with a family member in the room and an overall atmosphere of expectancy and excitement? I love it. These circumstances allow us to continue through this process together, and share in the birth of your child.

✓**REALITY CHECK:** Elective First-Time
                                    C-Sections

Here's one of those statistics that makes me shake my head: the rate of primary elective C-sections—that is, first-time moms choosing to have a C-section rather than a vaginal birth for no medical reason—rose by 36.6 percent from 2001 to 2003, (from 1.87 percent in 2001 to 2.55 percent in 2003) and it's getting higher. While this is still a small percentage of total births, the trend toward elective C-sections in first-time moms is alarming to me. The women are typically asking for these "patient choice" C-sections for the sake of convenience, out of fear of pain, or to be spared the risk of incontinence or pelvic floor problems associated with vaginal deliveries. (A colleague of mine jokingly calls this "vaginal bypass surgery.") As C-sections have grown safer and elective surgery in general has grown more commonplace, some women have the perception that the risks of vaginal deliveries and C-sections are comparable, and make their decision on the basis of this inaccurate understanding.

This, to me, is the ultimate in an unconscious pregnancy. Given the magnitude of the miracle of giving birth, the thought of actively avoiding this experience is difficult for me to comprehend. My guess is that women who are requesting C-sections have not brought much introspection to any aspect of the pregnancy journey, and are working with a doctor who is willing to go along.

What you should know about first-time (primary) elective C-sections:

1. They are medically controversial. The physician's credo is "First, do no harm." Doing invasive surgery where there is no medical indication to do so is difficult to justify.
2. They are not risk-free. You face all the risks of C-section described above.
3. You are much more likely to have a C-section with future pregnancies, and the risk of placenta complications increases with each subsequent surgical delivery (see discussion on risks of C-sections, above).
4. Perhaps most important, you deny yourself the entire experience of laboring and giving birth to your child, an experience that can be life-transforming. (It is interesting to note that there is even some research looking at the potential psychological benefit to the child of being delivered vaginally.)

Don't make such a choice lightly. Use your tools to figure out what motivates your interest in a C-section rather than labor: A fear of labor? Fear of pain? Fear of failure? Your partner's fear that your vagina may feel different sexually after giving birth? A desire to repress the whole idea of birth entirely? Explore it all. Use Dialoguing and Dreamagery. A strong interest in this choice could be a red flag for repressed or unexplored feelings or fears. Don't let such feelings cause you to make unconscious choices. Take the time and energy to understand your innermost feelings.

Note: A first-time (primary) elective C-section is not the same thing as a *repeat* elective C-section. A repeat means you have had a previous Cesarean and have been offered a medically based choice between a vaginal delivery (VBAC) and another Cesarean, both of which have risks that must be weighed. There is no medical indication for a primary elective C-section; it is purely a personal choice.

What Happens During a C-Section

Whenever possible, the anesthesia for a Cesarean is regional, either an epidural or a spinal. Under these circumstances, you will be aware of everything that is happening. Once you're in the operating room, if you do not already have an epidural catheter in place, this or the spinal will be done on the operating room table. You will then lie back and sheets will be draped across you to keep the surgical field sterile, and to create a visual barrier between you and the surgery.

After the anesthetic takes effect, the surgery can begin. This is the point at which I invite the woman's partner to come into the room where he or she can sit at her head and hold her hand (as well as stand up and see the baby being delivered). While the woman is fully conscious and can hear everything, she has no sensation below the waist except perhaps for some pressure at certain points in the procedure. For someone who has never had abdominal surgery before, the surgery is usually fairly simple and quick (30 to 45 minutes in total). If you have had abdominal surgeries, such as previous C-sections, scarring and adhesions can make the surgery more difficult and last longer.

As soon as the baby is delivered, it is handed to a pediatrician, who is always present in the OR for a C-section because the obstetrician is busy finishing the surgery and therefore unable to provide the usual newborn care. If the baby is healthy, it's usually shown briefly to the mother before being placed under a warmer to be cleaned and measured. Often once you have seen the baby, the anesthesiologist will give you some more medication to help you relax and even sleep. If you are comfortable and would prefer not to have this sedation, just let him know. Once the baby is dry and doing well, he or she will typically be given to your partner to hold.

C-Section Incisions

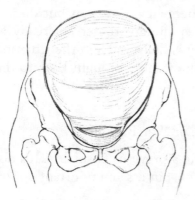

Low transverse incision

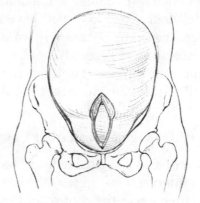

Lower midline incision

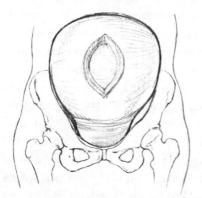

Upper midline or classical incision

With all the focus on maternal and fetal well-being and on finishing the surgery, operating room staff may neglect to allow time for the mother to hold the baby, make eye contact, and revel in the new life she has brought into being. If this is the case and you are eager to have your baby with you, your birth partner or spouse should feel free to follow the baby to the warming station and bring it to your side as soon as possible.

General anesthesia for a C-section is used only in emergencies, when there is no epidural catheter already in use and the baby has to be delivered immediately. That situation is always scary for the parents because everything happens so fast. The mood in the delivery room changes from mellow to urgent or even frantic (from the patient's perspective). The room crowds with people prepping the mother, administering medication, and then there's a dash to the operating room. In most hospitals, the patient's partner and other labor attendants are excluded from the OR when a C-section is done on an emergency basis. As unnerving as a sudden crisis may seem, it's reassuring to know how amazingly fast we can get a baby out—if necessary, in under two minutes. It can help for the mother in such a situation to focus on the fact that she is surrounded by people who are quickly and expertly doing what they are well-trained to do. If you have an emergency C-section but do not need general anesthesia (because an epidural catheter is already in place and can be used), once the baby is delivered and the situation quiets down, your family member will often be brought back to the OR to join you and meet the baby.

VBAC (Vaginal Birth After Cesarean, or "Vee-Back")

A VBAC is a vaginal delivery following a previous C-section. It's not an intervention—in fact it's the reverse—but it's an important option to mention in the context of Cesareans.

Not every woman is a candidate. Much depends upon the kind of incision that was made in your uterus for your Cesarean. Most C-sections done in full-term women are low transverse (side to side). This type of incision does not affect the part of the muscle that would contract during labor, which means these women are good candidates for future VBACs. (See illustration.) Women who have had classical (up and down) or "T" incisions, on the other hand, are not good candidates for VBACs because these incisions do go into the contracting part of the uterine muscle. Some low transverse incisions that had tears are also not recommended for a trial of labor. An important note: *The C-section scar that is visible on your belly does not necessarily indicate where the incision was made in your uterus.* You and your physician need to know your history (see diagrams) to be eligible for a VBAC, as there is no other way to be sure what kind of incision you had. This can be made clear by the operative notes from your first surgery.

The adage used to be "Once a C-section, always a C-section." It was thought that the risk of rupturing the incision in the uterus in a future pregnancy (because of the pressure of contractions and pushing) was too great to attempt a vaginal delivery. Then a body of data emerged in the 1980s indicating little added risk to subsequent vaginal delivery under certain conditions. From 1989 to 1996, VBACs steadily gained in popularity. The pendulum has since started to swing back because of a series of reports in medical journals about possible risks to mother and fetus. The primary concern, as before, is uterine rupture. Uncertainty about these risks, combined with the rise in malpractice suits (and spiking malpractice insurance rates), have made physicians wary of encouraging VBACs. In 2004, only 9.4 percent of women with a prior C-section delivered vaginally, down from a peak in 1996 of 28.3 percent.

Most physicians still offer a trial of labor or VBAC after one low transverse C-section. If you've already had two or more C-sections, however, VBAC is discouraged because the risk of uterine rupture rises with each subsequent C-section, as the repeated incisions weaken the uterine wall. My bias is to be very open to VBAC for a patient who qualifies and with whom I can explore the pros and cons in her specific case.

Keeping an open mind is key, because as with so many obstetrical questions, there's no clear thumbs-up or thumbs-down. But research results are encouraging. A recent large study reported that three-fourths of women who attempted VBAC were successful, with uterine tear happening in fewer than 1 percent of cases. Even in these situations both mother and baby did very well in almost every instance.

HOW TO MAKE A CONSCIOUS CHOICE ABOUT . . . TRYING A VBAC

If you've previously had a C-section, should you try for a vaginal delivery this time? Use the Feedback Loop to help you decide what's right for you:

First, reflection. What are your preconceptions about VBAC? What kinds of stories have you heard? What are your expectations?

How strongly do you feel about wanting a vaginal delivery? How would you feel if you did not have this baby vaginally? Explore the reasons you may want a vaginal delivery. Did you feel disappointed after your C-section? Was recovery difficult? Do you simply want to experience vaginal birth? How do you feel when considering a second C-section? Why did you have a C-section before? What were the circumstances surrounding that delivery? Was it a planned C-section? An emergency?

Do you plan to have more children after this one? Do you have strong feelings about how you would like to deliver them? (If you have another C-section now, it is nearly certain that all future children will also be born surgically; see section on C-sections and discussion of risks.) If this is your last child, what will you do for birth control afterward? Will you have your tubes tied at some point? (It is easier and less costly to do this while you are already in surgery for a C-section than to go back and have a separate surgical procedure.)

Second, information. Understand what a VBAC entails, and obtain more information if you still have questions. Make sure you are a candidate for a trial of labor; the obstetrician who handled your previous C-section can give you a copy of your operative report, which will document what kind of incision you had as well as other relevant information. What is her or his opinion based on your specific case? What are her or his biases? Different obs have different levels of comfort with risk. Someone who does not really want you to try VBAC can present the information in a skewed way.

What else do you need to know to better equip you to make this decision? Facts and figures? Testimonials? A refresher childbirth class? You should also review anything you feel you need to understand about vaginal delivery in general, as a first-time vaginal delivery and a VBAC are exactly the same processes.

Consider talking to someone who has given birth vaginally after a prior C-section. You can find many women's accounts on chat groups online.

Third, action. Consider living with the scenario for one option for a week (or a day if you are running out of time) and evaluating how that decision feels. Then switch and live with the other choice for a week. Notice how you feel when living with each choice. Then make your decision.

Then, re-reflection. Don't stop checking in about this choice even after you have made it. Continue re-reflecting.

Bringing Consciousness to Labor—No Matter What Happens

Louisa's Story: "We Did It!"

Louisa's pregnancy had been uneventful—a bit of morning sickness and a periodic backache were her only "issues." At 39 weeks, she noticed during her morning kick counts that her baby wasn't responding. She tried changing positions and moving around to wake the baby up. She even tried eating a cookie, as she noticed the baby always moved a lot more after she ate, especially sweets. She still felt nothing. Checking in with herself, she felt extremely anxious in a way she had not previously. I asked her to come in to be checked as a baby not moving is a serious sign.

Louisa did Dreamagery en route to the office. "I saw this big round head, which had been the same image of the baby that came to me all through my pregnancy, seeming cheerful and saying, 'It's okay, and I will see you soon,'" she reported. Although she felt slightly comforted, she was still worried. By the time she came in, Louisa still had not felt any movement and her nonstress test was nonreactive, a reason for concern. A biophysical profile seemed to indicate that the baby was all right, but as she was full term I discussed inducing labor with her. The nonreactive NST was worrisome, especially at term, and at that point in the pregnancy the risk-benefit analysis of leaving the baby in versus delivering led to a fairly easy choice. Louisa reflected on this, knowing it was not what she had wanted, but she understood the rationale and agreed with it.

Induction can be a long process when there are no other signs of labor, especially in a first-time mom who has never dilated before. It took 12 hours for her cervix to ripen, using first a Foley bulb, followed by Pitocin. Louisa spent this time in a hospital bed doing relaxation exercises and visiting with her husband, Lon, and her best friend, Kim. Since we were worried about the baby, it was monitored continuously.

Around 10 PM, we started the Pitocin. Louisa finally went into active labor around 4 AM. She decided she didn't find it helpful to have Kim present after all ("I felt kind of inhibited and Lon was being so great, I wanted just him"). Now tired and in pain from the rather intense contractions, she asked for an epidural. Although she had not made a firm decision about medical pain management before labor started, she decided after checking in with herself that she wanted that kind of help now. At 9 AM, her labor seemed to stall out at 8 cm. She really didn't want to have a C-section, and since the baby was tolerating labor very well, we gave her some more time. The nurses worked with her to try different positions to help get the baby aligned well with the birth canal, which we felt might be part of the problem. Louisa focused on relaxation techniques and imagery around letting go of her old preconceptions about labor and knowing that whatever needed to happen would.

At 1 PM, Louisa was ready to push. Three hours later, though, she had still not delivered the baby. "I think you're just exhausted and the baby is still slightly askew, which is making your pushing less effective," I told her. We discussed options. "If the baby were down lower, I would put forceps on him. They would allow me to correct the asynclitism [the technical name for the baby not being aligned properly]. But I don't feel comfortable doing that given how high the baby's head is. A vacuum will not allow me to correct the asynclitism. You've been amazing and I really think the best thing is to do a C-section. How does that sound to you both?" Despite her long, long ordeal, Louisa continued to ask questions and stay involved. We answered her questions and talked a bit more. She took some time to check in with her body, her soul, and her baby, and the feedback she got was unanimous. Wearily but with confidence, she said, "A C-section sounds good." Lon agreed.

Her son James was born at 5:22 PM, more than 31 hours after her induction began. "Physically, I felt pretty pummeled," she says. "Nothing went the way I had imagined. But I guess I feel really lucky that I noticed that the baby stopped moving and went in when I did. I still won the jackpot because James is here and perfect. Lon and I feel like we went through this tremendous journey to bring him here; he had the worst of it, I think, having to watch me struggling and keep mopping my forehead."

"We did it," Lon adds. "It was really hard but in a strange way the whole thing made us closer."

Labors like Louisa's are hard for me, too, because I'd like for every delivery to be a problem-free experience. When it doesn't go that way, I really feel for the woman and her family. Even then, however, the camaraderie, teamwork, and intensity of the ordeal becomes a bonding and transformative experience. You all—your body, your soul, your baby, your partner, your birth attendants—went through an incredible challenge together and met it. You came out the other side feeling even more connected, rather than less. And you never lost sight of that amazing soul who was entering the world. That's the real power of bringing consciousness to the experience.

Chapter 25

Labor and Delivery:
Self-Care

∞

Nurturing your Centers of Wellness during childbirth

Labor, to me, is largely about self-care. As a doctor, I certainly acknowledge that medical pain management can be very useful, and that medical interventions have made childbirth safer than ever in history. But paying attention to nurturing each of the five Centers of Wellness is the best way of helping your body to do what it was designed to do. Self-care is about supporting, rather than overriding, the natural process of childbirth.

The Mind, Movement, and Spirit centers play the dominant roles now in creating feelings of confidence and birth readiness as you approach labor. But as you will see, Nutrition and Sensation can greatly influence how you labor as well.

Remember to:

- consider each of these domains well before labor begins, and plan accordingly.
- discuss your plans and preferences with your birth partner so that you're on the same page.
- put yourself first. This is not easy for many women. But you're

the one giving birth. Your preferences—not your mother's, your sister's, your best friend's, or even your partner's—are primary.

- make sure your plans are in alignment with hospital policy. (It's rare that something isn't, but better to know ahead of time.)
- check in frequently with your body, your soul, and your baby—before, during, and after labor—to supply the information you'll need to make decisions about your care.
- be flexible. What feels good and provides support to you can be different from what you anticipated and can change throughout labor. You won't know in advance how you will feel when you're actually in the moment, regardless of whether this is your first labor or not. Frequent check-ins enable you to stay on top of these shifts and respond accordingly.

THE MIND CENTER

It's hard to imagine a more beautiful, satisfying, powerful, and effective illustration of the primal connection between mind and body than childbirth. The body is programmed to do it. The mind can help—or hinder—that process.

Mind Center goals for labor and delivery:

1. **To use the mind to actively support what the body is doing**
2. **To prevent the mind from interfering with the body**

These goals are slightly different from each other but the net result is the same: an easier, smoother, less painful delivery. Using your mental powers during labor doesn't mean that you can "think away" the pain. Nor does it mean that if you use mind-body techniques you will have a painless delivery. But you can set the overall tenor of the experience. You can make your mind your ally. You can relax and—yes—even enjoy labor more.

This is true whether or not you use pain medication and whether you deliver vaginally or surgically.

There are also medical benefits to feeling mentally ready. Your labor can progress more quickly when you are relaxed, in part because the relaxation response lowers the levels of stress hormones that work against the process of labor. Because energy is not being drained by anxiety and fear, you'll have more in reserve for when you really need it—pushing! And slow, controlled pushing is associated with a reduced risk of tearing. Feeling positive about your overall birth experience also reduces your risk of postpartum depression.

The Physiology of the Mind-Body Connection

First, let's look at the physiological pathways through which the mind can interfere with the body. When a woman is extremely anxious or fearful, those states trigger the stress response in her body: adrenaline surges, the heart rate increases, breathing becomes rapid and shallow. All of these actions are the reverse of a physical state that would ease labor—in other words, the relaxation response, which causes the heart rate to slow, breathing to become slower and deeper, and the pelvic and abdominal muscles to loosen and be able to work more effectively. A spike in anxiety may be one reason that labor often slows when a woman arrives at the hospital. There's usually a buzz of activity in this unfamiliar place full of new faces. Staff may be fussing over her, while she's struck anew with the reality that childbirth is imminent. Not surprisingly, a large study analyzing birth times found that most occurred in the wee hours of night and early morning, which is the time when things are much quieter on labor and delivery and visitors are usually absent. I would add to this the observation that night is also when people have a greater tendency to look inward.

Having some degree of anxiety about labor makes perfect sense—it's a rare woman who isn't revved up to a certain extent. After all, you're on the brink of a huge event that you have anticipated with some combination of excitement and anxiety for many months. The unknown can be frightening, even terrifying. Or it can be exhilarating, especially when one of life's most amazing mysteries is about to unfold both before you and within you. Which experience of the unknown will be yours? You get to choose.

Unfortunately, the only tools typically used to facilitate relaxation in the delivery suite are medical ones. Labor attendants make the correct assessment (this patient is stressed) and decide on the correct response (we need to help her relax). But then they tend to reach for the only kind of tool they are trained in using: drugs. (Physicians especially fall into this trap; often labor nurses will try other approaches.) In fact there are a number of proven mind-body tools that you can use to help yourself actively shift away from a stress response and toward a relaxation response:

• *The power of intention.* Believe in yourself. The power of intention in childbirth starts with your own sense that you can do this, that you are meant to do this, and that your body has been created to do this. Simply reminding yourself of this fact can alter your mind-set. Women have been giving birth since human life began—and you can, too! I have seen women write affirmations like this on cards that they look at during labor. Another option is for your labor partner to offer such prompts to you verbally.

• *Relaxation techniques.* Use your favorite relaxation technique every hour, whether you're feeling stressed or not. Being disciplined about this throughout labor is important because it helps keep you on an even keel. Throughout pregnancy, you probably discovered which relaxation methods worked well for you. Adapt them as needed. As your contractions grow closer together, you'll probably want to use a variation of one of the breathing or meditative techniques with each contraction. Ask your partner to prompt you from time to time to remember this.

• *Breathing patterns.* Breathing exercises are a wonderful, easy, and very effective way to relax and help your body work with the pain of contractions. By directing your full concentration to one sensation—breathe in, breathe out—you focus on something other than the pain and thus help to trigger the relaxation response, which allows your body to better work *with* the pain rather than fight it. There's no one magical technique that works best, but there are many different breathing patterns. Because being comfortable and familiar with a pattern tends to make it easiest to use, I recommend starting with patterns that helped you to relax during pregnancy (4/7/8 breathing works especially well for many women). Or practice those you learned in childbirth class. It's wise to learn and practice several different breathing patterns during late pregnancy, though you won't really know what works for you until your contractions begin. Take a cleansing or centering breath before and after each exercise (or each contraction).

- *Point of focus.* Find a place you can focus your eyes during contractions. Turn your full attention to this point as you breathe through the contraction. The target of attention can be your partner's face, an object you bring from home (such as a family photograph), something in the room, or even a randomly selected spot on the wallpaper pattern. Like breathing exercises, using a focal point enables you to mentally refocus. Here you are using vision to focus your senses. Most women have very powerful results when using breathing and point of focus at the same time.

- *Imagery.* Between contractions, take a mini mental vacation. Picture a favorite place (real or fictitious) and immerse yourself in its sights, sounds, smells, and general vibe. What matters most is that your mental picture of your chosen destination makes you feel at peace and rested. Throughout labor, revisit this place in your mind as a reward and resting spot between each contraction.

- *Mindfulness.* Stay present. If you find your consciousness shifting to the hypothetical future ("How painful is this going to be? How bad will it get?"), return to the present ("How are my body, soul, and baby doing with this right now? How can I respond to that?"). This is a form of practicing mindfulness. So when you hear your thoughts trending ahead toward the "what ifs," simply notice that your mind has wandered there and then come back to the present.

- *Flow.* Let the external world recede. Women deep in active labor often seem as if they are in a different reality—and they are. They're off on an inner journey that no one else in the room can share. During this journey they may lose their inhibitions, abandoning all sense of physical modesty, saying whatever comes to mind, not even noticing or caring who else is in the room. This altered state of consciousness can be a most beautiful and special experience, especially if you are working with it and not against it. Feeling supported and relaxed will help you to achieve this state.

- *Hypnosis.* If you have been working with a hypnotherapist during pregnancy to help you relax or prepare for labor, listen to the tapes during labor.

THE NUTRITION CENTER

Eating during labor is a controversial subject. Most conventional physicians prefer that once labor is under way, you take in no solid foods. Some doctors limit patients to ice chips; others allow Popsicles, too. If labor is long, electrolytes and sugar are supplied via IV. The reason behind the no-food philosophy is that in the event that you would need emergency anesthesia, aspiration (taking stomach contents into the lungs) is one of the biggest causes of surgical fatalities. (That's why you're ordinarily directed not to eat anything the night before a scheduled surgery.) What's more, the digestive system slows markedly during labor. Any food you eat even in early labor is liable to hang around a long time.

So from a purely medical perspective, it's simply a smart precaution to restrict food in a patient who might require surgery (by definition, any woman in labor). From a human perspective, though—and remember, labor is a natural human event, not (usually) a medical emergency waiting to happen—one questions the wisdom of withholding nutrition from a woman working so hard and who has no idea how long her labor might last. It could be a day or two!

This is why I tell patients to eat a light snack in early labor (once you are pretty sure you are in labor but before contractions become so intense that they require your complete concentration). Then once active labor begins, I, like most doctors, limit my patients to ice chips and Popsicles. Keep in mind that you're not liable to crave food once labor begins. You're likely to be too preoccupied by the work of labor to feel like noshing in between active contractions. That said, consult with your care professional. Some providers have a more lenient view about nutrition in labor.

Nutrition Center goal for labor and delivery:

To support your body nutritionally while minimizing risk
Here are some guidelines to help you achieve this goal.
Before labor:

- *Eat frequent small meals as your four-week window of delivery (the two weeks before and after your due date) approaches.* This will ensure that you feel continually well-fueled. Since it becomes uncomfortable to eat huge meals in late pregnancy, you're likely to eat this way naturally.

In early labor:

• *Start light.* When you think you are in early labor, eat a light, digestible snack such as yogurt or broth-based soup.

In active labor:

• *Once you're at the hospital, avoid eating.* It's better to err on the side of caution. Ice chips can keep you refreshed and slake thirst, which is why hospitals make these and sometimes ice pops readily available.

• *Even if you're not planning to eat, it's a good idea for your labor partner to have snacks available.* Labor may last awhile, and if your partner gets hungry and needs to run down to the cafeteria or find a vending machine, you may feel unhappy about being left for even 10 or 15 minutes. Store nonperishable snacks in your going-to-the-hospital bag. That way they won't get left behind. Include foods that you enjoy, too, in case you feel like eating after delivery but before the hospital offers a meal.

• *Avoid botanicals.* I do not endorse their use in stimulating labor, as there is no convincing evidence of either their safety or effectiveness.

After delivery:

• *Listen to your body.* You probably won't be hungry immediately after delivery.

• *Start small.* Assuming you had a vaginal delivery, there is no reason to restrict your choices, but take it gradually just to be sure you're feeling fine. If you had a C-section, you will be instructed on what and when you will be able to eat.

THE MOVEMENT CENTER

How you move your body in labor can influence your comfort and, in turn, your progress. In early labor you have the greatest ability to move about in ways that feel good to you. You can dance, rock in a favorite chair, take a stroll around your backyard, or lie down on the living room floor and stretch. In fact, being able to move around at will is another reason to stay home as long as feasible. By the time you reach active labor your options may be limited by fetal monitoring, by your own disinclination for movement due to feeling exhausted or in pain, or by an epidural. However, the days when every patient was given a dense epidural and positioned on her back for the duration are long gone. Today's epidurals, by and large, are light enough to allow for a fair amount of movement.

Throughout labor and delivery the way you position your body, and the movements you make can bring pleasure and nurturance to the process.

Movement Center goals for labor and delivery:

1. **To move your body in ways that support the natural process of contracting and pushing**
2. **To move your body in ways that release tension and provide comfort**

Here are my recommendations for achieving these goals:

• *Do as much as you can, but do it mindfully.* The first time you try to walk around your room or the delivery ward, you'll naturally want to take in all that you see around you. On subsequent laps, though, bring your attention to your body. How does it feel as it moves through space? Notice how it feels during a contraction and then afterward. How does walking or sitting or changing positions affect you mentally? Be mindful of the fact, too, that very likely these are some of the last steps you'll take while carrying this baby inside of you! Treasure that sensation as you move about.

• *Know that you can still move even when you are confined to bed.* It's even more important to be conscious of moving when you are attached to monitors. You can stretch, for example. Start at one end of your body and systematically stretch each muscle group that you can.

•   *Do progressive muscle relaxation every hour, or more often if needed.* Whether you are in bed being monitored or not, this technique will help you release unnecessary tension that you may not even be aware that your body is holding. See directions on pages 40–42.

•   *Choose the labor positions that are working for you.* I've sometimes seen zealous labor partners or even midwives urging women into particular positions that clearly are not working for them. Don't let yourself be guided by somebody else's idea of what your delivery should look like. Only you know how your body is feeling at any given time.

There's little good research on optimum labor positions. My best advice is simply to listen to what your body, your soul, and your baby are saying to you. Do contractions seem less intense? Do you prefer to assume one position during the contraction and then another during the rest afterward? What makes you feel more relaxed? Is the baby "happier" (as indicated by the monitoring) in one position compared with another? Labor nurses will often comment on the positions that "the baby likes."

Your preferences are likely to change quite a bit as your labor progresses. For example, you may find it comfortable to walk around for much of early labor, choose to spend active labor alternately rocking and lying down, and then squat or return to a position on your back for delivery.

•   *Vary your labor positions.* Even if one is working well for you, if your labor is long it's a good idea to change position every so often.

•   *Give a new position time.* Give yourself a few contractions to get used to a position before making a judgment. If you don't feel that a particular position works for you, don't discard it altogether; in a later stage of labor it may bring more relief.

•   *Use pillows and people to support you.*

Popular Labor Positions *Here are examples of common positions that seem to work especially well:*

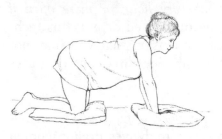

Kneeling

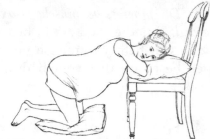

Kneeling, supported by a chair

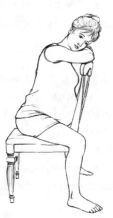

Sitting on a chair (rear-facing)

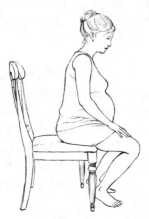

Sitting on a chair (forward-facing)

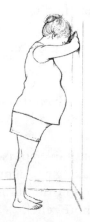

Standing, leaning on a wall
for support

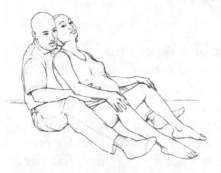

Sitting, supported by your partner

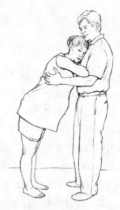

Standing, supported by your partner

Popular Delivering Positions

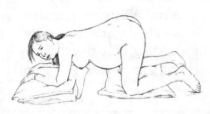

All fours

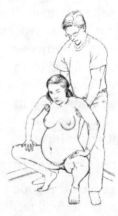

Squatting, supported by your partner

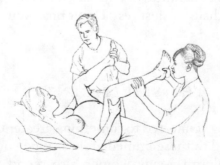

*Semi-reclining, supported by pillows
and others*

WATER BIRTHS

I have always loved the concept of a water birth—when the woman actually delivers while in a tub of water, often a whirlpool, a bath, or a special birthing tub. It is believed by some to ease the baby's transition to the outside world, since they are coming from a world of water. (Note: a water birth is different from occasional immersions in a bathtub or a whirlpool for purposes of relaxation during labor. See page 436.) While I find the concept interesting, not only have I never supervised a water birth, I haven't even witnessed one. This is simply because I have never practiced in a hospital where they were done. If you are interested in a water birth, find out if anyone does them in your area. Ask how many the doctor or midwife have attended; make sure that you are working with someone who has experience in these births. Someone willing to do it but with little or no experience would give me cause for concern. Whatever potential benefit there may be would be far outweighed by the risk of delivering your baby in a way and in a setting that the delivery team does not know well. Be aware that some facilities do not permit water births.

• In general it is good to begin to walk as soon after delivery as you feel up to it. This will facilitate your recovery. It's best to wait to do this in the presence of a nurse, who can both support you physically and observe you for signs of faintness or excessive bleeding. But listen to your body. If you are exhausted, just rest. Don't push yourself.

THE SPIRIT CENTER

Your sense of being connected to something greater than yourself, and of being connected to those immediately around you, are both intensified during childbirth. Many women also report feeling a sudden deeper connection not just to their own mothers, but to the generational parade of mothers who have come before them.

This sense of connection can bring surprising benefits. For example, studies show that laboring women whose partners are with them at delivery tend to have shorter, less painful deliveries. This is probably less because of anything they do than the effect of their reassuring presence, which is why it's so helpful to have your partner present in labor even if you are using a doula to handle the primary birth-support tasks. You can't underestimate the value of having your loved one holding your hand or looking into your eyes.

Bringing another life into the world also connects you to the miracle of creation. Whether your reference point is God, Mother Nature, or some other version of a higher power, and also or even if you have no belief in a higher power—if you are tuned in, you will feel awestruck by birth. There is now a new being in the room, and he or she didn't come in through the door.

Spirit Center goals for labor and delivery:
1. **To have a labor partner (or partners) to whom you feel deeply connected, and to be supported in whatever way works best for you**
2. **To remain mindful of the deeply spiritual dimension of giving birth**
3. **To have the experience of connecting with your newborn child, soul to soul**

To help you meet these goals:

Before labor:
• *Go over your labor preferences with your labor supporter.* Your labor partner plays many roles: making you feel more comfortable, confident, and relaxed; helping you through challenging contractions; speaking for you to hospital staff when you are unable; and supporting your preferences in every way possible. Prepare your labor partner for this role by sharing your birth philosophies long before labor actually begins. If you haven't yet thought about a birth vision statement, talk through one with your partner (even if you don't write one, this is a good guide to your discussion). If you have already written one give him or her a copy or be sure your partner is familiar with its contents.

• *Talk about specific things you would like your labor partner to be responsible for.* Do you want him or her to breathe through contractions with you? Be part of all discussions with medical staff? Ask guests to leave if their presence upsets you? Cut the umbilical cord? Also go over what you *don't* want your supporter to do: Watch TV? Use a cell phone? Leave the room?

• *Be sure that you feel good about who is present at your delivery.* Birth is perhaps the most sacred moment in the life cycle. There is no right or wrong answer about who should be in the delivery room with you, but it's incredibly important that you make this choice consciously. (See "How to Make a Conscious Choice About...Labor Witnesses," pages 316–319.)

After delivery:
• *Make a soul connection with your baby.* No matter how many thousands of deliveries I've witnessed, when I'm the delivering obstetrician I feel incredibly privileged and humbled to be the first person to touch and hold this brand-new life. At each delivery, I make sure to look into the eyes of the baby who has just emerged. I connect. There's only a few seconds to do this, because of course I want the baby to see his or her parents (and vice versa!), but a few seconds is all it takes. When I look into the baby's eyes, I get a real sense of the essence of this new human. It is an unbelievable gift.

Bring awareness to this opportunity. Let people know—in your birth vision statement and by means of reminders once you're in labor—that you want to see and hold your baby as soon as possible. If you've had an uncomplicated vaginal delivery, you'll probably be able to hold your baby immediately. If you've had a Cesarean and the baby is first handed to a pediatrician for assessment, ask your partner to inquire about your holding the baby as soon as he or she is stable and the pediatrician is finished. Typically everyone involved in your delivery will have this as a goal as well, but it never hurts to emphasize your desires. It can be particularly helpful during a C-section when the nurses have a lot more to focus on and the pediatricians are tending to the baby.

Don't just look at your baby; look *into* your baby. It doesn't take long to make a welcoming connection. While you will, of course, want to explore and touch every millimeter of your baby very soon, for now just look into the eyes of this new being. The eyes are indeed the window to the soul, and never will you feel the truth of this more keenly than during these first moments. This is a magical time.

- *Continue to foster this attachment in the hospital.* Among the ways you can build closeness:

  Bring your baby to your breast soon after birth. If your baby is awake and making mouthing movements, offering your breast can boost your confidence and help promote the let-down reflex for milk to eventually flow. A newborn is capable of suckling virtually immediately in a normal delivery, and can even creep up to the breast, an amazing instinct to witness. But be aware that many babies are drowsy or disinterested in nursing immediately. While suckling and rooting are inborn reflexes, successful breastfeeding is a learned art for mother and baby. Although your breasts don't yet have milk, they already contain a nutrient- and antibody-rich substance known as colostrum. Studies have found that breastfeeding is more successful when it is initiated within the first hour or two of life.

  Hold and talk to your baby. Your voice is already familiar and within days your newborn will be able to pick out your unique scent.

  Keep your baby in your room full-time if you feel up to it. "Rooming in" has become standard care in most hospitals (as opposed to putting all newborns in a general nursery). But if you're leveled by exhaustion, know that the nursery is there to help you, and your baby will be well looked after while you get some sleep. If you specify that you want to breastfeed, the baby will be brought to you for nursing.

  Revel in every aspect of your new baby. You can continue to nurture and deepen that soul connection that you established at delivery by doing what I call "soul gazing." In other words, look deep and long and often into the eyes of this child of yours. Encourage your partner to do the same.

Personally, I think the basis of bonding is attention. Love, at its essence, is attention. Focused, nonjudging, open-hearted unconditional attention. Whether or not you feel that open-hearted love toward your newborn from the very beginning, one of the best ways to cultivate it and further deepen it is simply by paying attention. The type of attention I'm talking about has no goal—it is not so you can take notes and learn the baby's patterns. It is not so the baby sees you paying attention. It is simply a time to be fully present, fully conscious, and fully aware of this living, breathing being.

Allow yourself to be amazed, to marvel at what you see. This little being truly is a miracle. Notice every detail of your baby. The way she looks, moves, smells, sounds, tastes. The way she interacts with the world. The way she holds her mouth when she sleeps. The way her ear curves. The shape of her head. The color of her eyes. What do you see when you look into those eyes? What sense do you get from her emotionally? Spiritually? Do this with a spirit of discovery, not with a feeling that you need to understand what you are observing. This being is brand-new. She is a link to worlds beyond this one. Gaze at your baby with your heart and mind open to the mystery and the wonder that is within her.

✔ **REALITY CHECK:** Bonding

Women often fear that if they do not get the opportunity to touch and hold their baby right after birth, they will somehow have "ruined" bonding. In reality, bonding—which is simply a term meaning parent–child attachment—is a process, not a moment. And that process began long before your baby was born. Remember, you have been in a relationship with this new life from the first time you began to think about it, whether this was before you conceived or as soon as you learned about the pregnancy. By being tuned in to that relationship throughout pregnancy and labor, guess what you've been doing? Bonding! If circumstances prevent your holding your baby in the first minutes or even hours after delivery, your future relationship is in no way jeopardized by the delay. If you have done the relationship-building work while your baby was still inside you, you have already built a strong foundation.

It's true there is a "sensitive period" in the first hour or so after birth during which the newborn is in a so-called quiet-alert state that makes for a wonderful opportunity to connect and say hello, face-to-face at last. Take advantage of this special time if you and your baby can. Keep the baby in the room; hold it skin-to-skin or in your arms.

On the other hand, the first hour is only an infinitesimal slice of what bonding is really about. If circumstances aren't ideal for this first leisurely hour together, don't worry that it will affect how much you love your baby, what kind of mother you will be, or whether you will have a strong parent–child attachment. According to bonding pioneer Marshall Klaus, 30 to 40 percent of new moms say they became attached to their babies in the first hour or two after giving birth. For another 40 percent, it takes a week to feel their baby is truly "theirs," and for the remainder it takes longer still. Many factors can color how the parent–child connection develops for you, including a difficult labor, sickness (yours or your baby's), colic, and sleep deprivation.

Give it time. If you have done the relationship-building work while your baby was still inside you, you are likely to feel connected and at peace, however your birth story unfolds. And you have plenty of opportunity ahead to continue connecting with your baby. Among the best ways:

- Breastfeeding
- Responding to your newborn quickly (such as picking him up when he cries; it's really true that you can't spoil a baby—at least not a newborn)
- Carrying your baby in a soft front-carrier
- Holding your baby
- Practicing "kangaroo care," an idea that originated as a therapy for preemies: holding your naked baby against your bare skin
- Loving your baby
- Reading about infant development, so that you know what is normal (which sets up realistic expectations) and you can feel more confident
- Having patience. Many moms for whom bonding is not immediate note that they feel it when their baby begins to respond—especially when the first "social smile" shows up at around four to six weeks.

THE SENSATION CENTER

Women labor more effectively when they feel safe and secure. What our senses pick up in the environment directly, unconsciously, and powerfully influence our perceptions of pain, and our overall ability to relax. This is part of the reason that today's birthing suites have been made more comfortable and homey than typical sterile clinics or standard hospital rooms. All the medical equipment a physician may need is there—but it's hidden away behind wood cabinets and concealed doors. The goal is to create an environment that soothes, one that speaks of health and life, not sickness or disease.

However, not even the plushest delivery room can meet every expectation of what constitutes "home" or "soothing" to you. Adding your own touches transforms the birthing space into a place that nourishes your personal sensation needs.

Sensation Center goals for labor and delivery:
1. **To create a birth environment that soothes, comforts, and relaxes you**
2. **To minimize distracting sensations**

To help you meet these goals:

Before and during labor:
*   *Bring things from home that make you feel at ease and safe.* Some women bring a special talisman (a small statue, a souvenir of a favorite place, or a picture) that they associate with feelings of inner strength. You may want to bring a photograph of someone you love who can't be with you that day or an object that symbolizes a loved one—your mother's shawl, your grandmother's rosary, slippers that your sister knit for you.

*   *Think about what fragrances appeal to you.* Hospital policy discourages lighting candles or incense, but there are other ways to introduce scent to your environment. Place sachets under your pillow. Bring a bowl of potpourri to set out in your room. Consider scented massage oil or scented beanbags such as are used in yoga classes or during massages to enhance relaxation. Calming scents to consider for

labor include lavender, geranium, vanilla, and eucalyptus. Choose what appeals most to you. Depending on where you are, simply opening the window can be refreshing.

• *Consider aromatherapy.* Essential oils derived from plant parts (flowers, resins, roots, seeds) release scents that create physical effects including relaxation. Aromatherapy is not well-studied, but many laboring women find it useful and there's no real risk to it. The idea is that these concentrated aromas move quickly from nose to brain, releasing helpful endorphins. The oils may be smelled from the bottle or applied to the skin. If this appeals to you, you might seek out a trained aromatherapist to work with you before labor to plan what to bring to the delivery room. Short of this, you can simply go to a store that carries essential oils (many health-food stores do) and smell them, buying those that appeal to you.

Before labor, get to know the scents more deeply. Spend a day with each one, smelling it and noticing how it makes you feel. By the end of the day, you will have a sense of whether this aroma is one that helps you feel relaxed or energized, positive or not. If you do this with several different essential oils, you will have a nice selection to use as you wish in the delivery room. You may choose to sniff one of the bottles every now and then, or leave a vial open for a while in your room—or you may never open a single one. Many women develop an aversion to certain scents in labor, so what was pleasing to you in pregnancy may not hold the same appeal later. As always, be conscious of what you want and need.

• *Avoid scents you find distracting.* Note that your sense of smell might be altered during labor, and strong odors may or may not appeal to you. If, for example, the odor of fast food distracts or upsets you, speak up if someone brings it into the room.

• *Bring sounds that comfort you.* Most birthing centers allow patients to play their own music, as long as it's not so loud that it disturbs patients in other rooms. Bring a portable CD or cassette player or your iPod to the hospital or birth center. Some women prefer to use a headset, especially if they are playing something that feels personal to them, such as a hypnosis tape. Up until the pushing stage when full connection with the birth attendant is important, this is great. Select your favorite music, burn a special disc, or make a playlist just for the occasion. Rock, jazz, country, chanting, New Age water-falls—how mellow or lively the sound depends only on what helps you feel at ease. It's wise to plan several different options as your mood will most likely change during labor.

• *Dim the lights.* Bright fluorescent lighting works against the im-pulse to create a safe cocoon for labor. Ask to have the lights dimmed or turned off, at least in the area of the room where you are. Dim lighting contributes to relaxation, and is also more welcoming for the baby.

• *Consciously surround yourself with stimuli that nurture you.* I of-ten see laboring women or their attendants turn on the TV or the ra-dio and just leave it on, even when they're not interested in what's playing. The sounds just become part of the background. Giving birth is not like any other day. Bring some consciousness to your decision about what to watch or listen to, if anything. Do you really want to listen to the news or watch a sitcom as your child is about to enter the world? You're not just biding time, after all. Whatever your prefer-ences, ask your partner and any birth witnesses to respect them, re-gardless of their own desires. This is a time when your wants come first.

• *Fill the spaces around you with tactile sensations that make you feel good.* You may want to wear a comfy old shirt rather than a hospi-tal gown during labor. If hospital policy requires standard-issue wear, consider bringing a pair of socks made of feather-soft cashmere or col-orful cotton. (Your feet are liable to get cold, and downy yarns that are attractive can warm as well as uplift you.) One woman brought a favorite throw blanket to touch during labor; after delivery, she tossed it over her shoulders like a shawl, and wrapped it around her and her baby. Another woman brought a favorite pillow. Be aware that deliv-ery is typically messy; save your best nightgowns for after delivery.

• *Let others move you.* Labor is a great time to allow your muscles and body parts to be massaged and stretched by those around you. I've even encouraged patients who have worked with a massage ther-apist throughout pregnancy and know they may have a long labor (for example, because they're induced or a first-time mom) to arrange to have a session while on L&D. Some women, however, find that they do not like to be touched while in labor. If this is the case for you, you might try:

- Foot massage; this may feel less objectionable and can make your entire body feel better.
- Therapeutic touch, a therapy derived from the ancient technique of laying-on-of-hands. It's based on the belief that the therapist can transmit a healing force, and many nurses are trained in this. The hands of the therapist can be placed lightly on the body or above the body, so it feels very noninvasive.
- Reflexology, a method of foot (and sometimes hand) pressure-point massage which some women find to be deeply relaxing in labor, and other women find to be uncomfortable.
- Reiki, an energy therapy that also involves very light touching or no touching. Many nurses are also trained in this.
- Remember perineal massage. Gently stretching the tissues of your perineum around your vagina, as recommended from the third trimester, can help reduce the possibility of an episiotomy. If you would like your nurse to do this in labor, just let her know.

After delivery:
- *Use all of your senses to get to know your baby.* Smell your baby, nuzzle and kiss your baby, touch your baby, listen to your baby, examine this incredible creature from every angle. Human beings have an instinctive need to be touched. Holding, stroking, and suckling your newborn is a way for you to get to know one another—a way to bond. It's also physically beneficial. Touch helps to regulate heart rate, lower blood pressure, and lower the level of stress hormones circulating throughout the body—important for your baby as he or she adjusts to life outside of you, and important for you as you begin your recovery.

WATER POWER

In the hospital where I deliver, we have whirlpool baths that many women like to use while they are laboring. There is something about water that is intrinsically relaxing to many of us, and you may enjoy the ability to regulate your body temperature in this way as well. It's best to wait until after a cervical exam to get in the bath, so you know where you are in your labor and so your obstetrician can decide if it is a good time for you to do this. You are also more likely to have a nice long window of time before you have to be examined again.

A warm bath (if you are still at home) or a shower can have a similar effect. Not all women like being in water during labor; some find it distracting rather than relaxing, so let your preferences be your guide.

Part Seven

Postpartum

---∽---

The Transition to Motherhood

Chapter 26

Postpartum:
Reflection and Observation

∞

Checking in with body, soul, and baby after giving birth

Medically and culturally, the first weeks after giving birth tend to be considered as pregnancy afterthoughts. We doctors typically send you home a day or two after your delivery—three or four after a C-section—and see you only once more, six weeks later, for about twenty minutes (and that's if you're lucky). Within the conventional medical framework, this short shrift is justified because the real medical and physical risks are behind you. There's little left for a disease-oriented doctor to do. Social convention takes a similarly brisk view of new motherhood. A new mom looks pretty "normal" compared to when she was visibly with child, certainly not in obvious need of assistance. Our society has few formal customs for acknowledging new motherhood. We simply don't pay much attention to the mother's well-being—especially not when there's a new baby on which to focus our collective energies.

But haven't you just had a huge, life-altering experience? To overlook this fact does a new mom a terrible disservice. Only by actively acknowledging the importance of this postpartum stage can she take the first step toward fully healing, body and soul, and achieve good health.

Between the demands of a newborn and a system that does not offer the new mother the time and space she needs to feel whole again, the road from mom-to-be to mom can be bumpy. "With each pregnancy and delivery I feel I've lost a bit more of my former self," a mother of three told me. If the birth is difficult, this transition can be even tougher. In fact, studies have found that 3 percent of women who had a "normal" birth and 33 percent of those who had a difficult or complicated birth met the clinical criteria for post-traumatic stress disorder. I believe that these women represent just the tip of the iceberg in terms of the total number of women who experience postpartum distress. Many, many others are not pathologically traumatized, but nevertheless are left feeling disappointed, confused, or "lost." Even when your birth experience was ideal, it takes time and attention to assimilate this big life event.

Interestingly, I've observed that cancer patients face a similar "reentry shock," even though you would not think that these two populations have much in common. Many of my nonobstetric patients are cancer patients who have sought out integrative medicine largely because they didn't know where to turn. At the end of their cancer treatment, the conventional medical system said, "Okay, we're done here. Go on your way, and come back for periodic checkups to make sure the cancer hasn't recurred." Stable health and remission are great news, yet alongside their relief these patients often feel alone, confused, bewildered, and afraid. They're unsure who they are now or how to live their lives. The only thing they do know is that they are not the same people they were before. Yet the system does not support them in this transition of integrating their recent experiences into the person they have become. Nor does the system offer any guidance to women who have undergone the experience of childbirth and are now fundamentally different as a result of having become mothers.

While this section of the book does not offer a lot of information about what is happening in your body right now, because physically not much *is* happening, an enormous change is taking place at the emotional level. I urge you not to skip over it. In the midst of competing priorities, minding our inner life is usually the first thing to fall from our to-do list. Being mindful of what your body and soul need during this time will revitalize you tremendously—which in turn makes you a happier, more effective mother to your new baby, and a whole and healthy woman.

HOW LONG IS "POSTPARTUM"?

Traditional Western medicine considers the postpartum period to last about six weeks—the length of time it takes for the uterus to revert back to a pre-pregnancy size. Sometimes postpartum is framed as a "fourth trimester," or roughly a three-month window to take time and adjust to your new life. Another adage advises that it takes nine months to make a baby and another nine months to get used to one (and to reclaim your body).

Though there is truth to all these views, I most like the model followed in some Asian cultures in which it is traditionally believed that the postpartum period is one full year long. Obviously a woman in this day and age in our culture can rarely take a full year to "recover" from childbirth, nor does she need to. But this perspective recognizes that while physical recovery from childbirth requires only a matter of weeks, the whole person requires a more generous span of time. Giving birth is a major transition to one's life—body *and* soul. It should be celebrated, not rushed.

OWNING YOUR BIRTH STORY

If you have been living consciously through your pregnancy, labor, and delivery, your payoff now should be a sense of peace. You might have had surprises or disappointments. But disappointment is a different emotion, and a healthier one than the bitterness or regret that often accompany a delivery that was framed by unconscious choices. Women who were fully engaged and present tend to feel happier about their delivery, whatever form it ended up taking.

I'm not saying that you'll find that new motherhood is a bed of roses simply by virtue of having approached childbirth consciously. Few moms who've had 24-hour labors followed by C-sections, for example, are going to be feeling perky, no matter how consciously they labored! Nor do I mean to imply that if you feel low, you've failed some kind of consciousness test. Every new mom feels low at times.

What bringing consciousness to pregnancy, labor, and delivery should have done, however, is help prevent feelings of devastation afterward.

I call it avoiding the "Oh-my-God-what-just-happened?!" syndrome. I've seen this again and again. It can occur regardless of whether the labor and delivery went exactly as planned, or was filled with unexpected interventions. The end result: a mom who's lying in bed (or back at home on her sofa) in a state of semi-shock and bewilderment. If it was a hard labor, these disoriented reactions can be even more profound. Typically, a woman in this situation tries to push the whole ordeal out of her head. She may feel that all of her worst fears about labor came true.

Processing your birth story, whatever it was, is key to integrating the experience into the fabric of who you are. Any really intense life experience, good or bad—a car accident, a rape, a wedding, a sudden promotion or move, the birth of a child—requires this effort. Talking, reflecting, and simply "sitting" with it allow you to "own" the event and weave it into the rest of your life story. Childbirth will continue to dramatically impact your life, whether you are aware of it or not. Now is your opportunity to embrace it and experience what it has to offer you.

Here's an example from my own life: My son, Ryan, is adopted. Before everything was finalized, when he was two months old, my husband, Rich, and I traveled to Haiti to spend time with him and see if we could help advance the endless paperwork. After a few days, Rich had to return to our home in the US while I was to stay a few extra days by myself. Instead, a political coup erupted and I got trapped there, at first unwilling to leave the country without Ryan and then unable to leave at all, even if I had been willing. In the end, I spent 12 weeks in Haiti after having planned to spend only one. The orphanage allowed Ryan to stay with me at a hotel. So there I was, with a new baby and few supplies or traditional forms of support (a partner, relatives, old friends) in the middle of a violent and unstable government overthrow in the poorest country in the Western Hemisphere. That experience was the most unique, stressful, challenging—and beautiful—of my life.

When I returned home, the life and job I had left behind were there, waiting for me to pick up where I had left off. But I'd just been through a hugely transforming life event. Not only had I become a mother, but I had lived in a very turbulent time in a very different culture, met amazing people, seen wonderful and scary things, and relied on inner strengths I didn't know I had. I could have just dropped back into my old life and cordoned off those Haitian months as a bizarre anomaly—but that would have meant minimizing a tremendous experience. Instead of compartmentalizing it, I worked to integrate that experience into my "old" life. Through Journaling and talking about my experience, through reflecting on it, I made it part of who I am. Having lived in a country where conditions are such that 30 percent of children die by age five, and yet the people have a depth and richness of spirit I have never encountered before, I see the world differently. I also see my place in it differently, and I am still in the process of discovering all that that means. How enriching, and what a blessing.

You have a similar opportunity now. What just happened to you in pregnancy and childbirth? And what does it mean for your life and who you are now?

AFTER DELIVERY: CHECK IN ABOUT YOUR CHILDBIRTH

Here are four steps that will help you capture the memory of your pregnancy and your childbirth—in a way that integrates the experience into the fabric of your being.

1. Imprint

Imprinting works the way a photograph does to capture a moment, but can be even more evocative because you use all of your senses to make a "snapshot" of the moment you don't want to forget. Do it as soon as you can after giving birth—it works best when you are right in the moment.

Stop and close your eyes. Recall the moment or moments about childbirth that you want to remember forever. It might be the instant your child was born, and/or other pivotal moments in your labor, such as arriving in labor and delivery, the room itself, the people attending you, feeling your baby inside you a last time before you pushed her or him out. Picture that moment in time, recalling as much as you can about it. Use all of your senses to bring it back to life. What did you see? What did the room smell like? Who was there and what were they saying? What else were you hearing? It's all there in your head, your heart, your body, and your soul. It's best if you can remember to do this while an experience is happening, and then do it again a while later to recall and preserve more of the memory. You can actually pull it into your consciousness in greater detail than you were aware of when you were living it. Take a still-life snapshot or "roll the camera" forward in time like a movie to imprint more of the experience.

By doing this, you will be better able to call up the memory whenever you want. You can keep it alive and come back to it again and again.

2. Document the "Outside Story"

As soon after delivery as you feel up to it, jot down key bits of the story of your labor. You don't have to use complete sentences. Simply capture any significant details of your experience that will help jog your memory later: key points, events, feelings, things said, and so on. That's the "outside story." It's another technique for preserving memories and will also help lay the groundwork for deeper processing of the event of birth.

Some women collect all this information in a baby book, along with photographs, a hospital ID bracelet, and other mementos of the birth. It's best to start by just jotting random notes on a piece of paper. The sooner this is done after delivery, the better you will be able to preserve the details. Don't censor this at all. If later you want to create a cleaned-up version for a baby book, that's fine, too. But first do it for your eyes only.

3. Journal the "Inside Story"

This related writing exercise involves deeper reflection on what transpired, and doesn't necessarily require the same immediacy as simply documenting the highlights. The "inside story" of your labor and delivery is akin to what was happening on the soul level. Birth is an amazing physical experience, but it also has a spiritual dimension. Capture as much of this dimension of your labor and delivery as you can.

Some suggestions: Reflect on your feelings about giving birth. How was childbirth for you? What did you love about it? What was the best thing about it? The worst? Was there a moment (or moments) that scared you? Was there anything that surprised you?

Remember to consider how both your body and your soul were affected. How do you feel about how your body was during labor? Are you amazed by it? Disappointed? Surprised?

An excerpt from Paula's journal
after delivery of her firstborn:

"Late labor was pretty grueling—but I was so afraid of drugs that I stuck it out. I completely depended on G for that time— squeezing his hand, following his breathing lead. When Susan [the labor nurse] said now I could push, I did think triumphantly way back in the recesses of my consciousness, that I had made it all drug-free, as I'd wished and hoped. It was a relief not to have to 'hee hee' anymore. Pushing was hard to get the hang of—they had a mirror set up but I couldn't really see anything. And it was no consolation to see a tiny glimpse of scalp, because that still made birth seem so far off. But then it happened so fast once he made it into position! I'll never forget the feeling of life shooting out from my body. I didn't believe them when they told me that in the next push or two the baby would be born. But they were right! Suddenly I felt this huge pressure (the head) and a long slither (the body and cord)! I clearly heard G say, "It's a boy!" as I saw a flash of pink and red and blue slide out from my legs. And when he was immediately placed on my chest it truly was a miracle—a moment of revelation that all the mystery and marvel of my changing body these past nine months truly *did* end in a baby. A human—a baby—my baby—our baby—from my body to my arms! I'd never felt anything like it in 32 years—that feeling of holding a baby—our baby—for the first time. I was too stunned to even cry, or smile."

4. Share

There's an old saying, "The world doesn't want to hear about the labor pains, it just wants to see the baby." Sometimes this feels all too true. In pregnancy, everybody focused on you. Now, they fuss and coo over your baby. Our culture doesn't have a tradition for sharing birth stories in a positive, mom-centered way. But the mom often needs for the world—or at least close friends or family members—to hear and share in the details of this experience.

Whether you were satisfied or disappointed by what happened during your labor, sharing your story is an important part of processing and integrating this into your life. I think part of the reason that pregnant women hear so many negative stories about birth (compared with relatively few blissful ones) is that some part of these horror-story-tellers have not fully processed their childbirth, and this is their "unfinished business," so to speak.

Share with people who understand the depth of you, those who will want to hear not just what happened, but how it changed you. You want listeners who can be nonjudgmental witnesses to your story. Let them know what you are doing and what you need from them—that is, simply to listen and be a witness to the story of this life event.

It's also a good idea to review at least the medical side of your childbirth story with your doctor or midwife. As a professional and participant in the delivery, that person can help clarify why things happened the way they did and answer outstanding questions you may have.

LABOR REFLECTIONS:
WHAT MIGHT COME UP FOR YOU

An Awesome Experience

Michelle had been apprehensive about labor and delivery throughout her pregnancy. She's nervous about medical procedures in general ("even getting my teeth cleaned at the dentist") and had little frame of reference for what giving birth would be like. During her pregnancy, she used many of the tools in this book, including Journaling and Dialoguing, to grow more comfortable with the prospect of labor. "I especially liked the check-ins," she reported. "More than anything else they were a reminder for me to slow down and really be aware of what was happening and what I needed. I think it's easy to submerge those needs when you're pregnant and just focus in an abstract way on the baby."

At 38 and a half weeks, Michelle began having regular contractions in the middle of the night. Although she was coursing with excitement, she tried to rest because she knew that since the contractions were still fairly far apart, it would probably be hours before it was time to go to the hospital and she would need all the rest she could get before labor. After falling back to sleep, she and her husband, Drew, awoke early, and she discovered that the contractions had slowed to every 15 minutes or so. She ate a light breakfast and tried to relax. Neither she nor Drew went to work, because Michelle felt the big moment was near.

Sure enough, by noon her contractions were every five minutes, and by 3 PM, they were coming every two or three minutes. When she called, I suggested she come to the hospital to be evaluated. Michelle was 5 cm dilated, and her contractions were beginning to require all her concentration. Drew held her hand and guided her through the breathing exercises they had practiced at home. Michelle wondered about pain medication and when to ask for it. She checked in with herself every hour, with Drew watching the clock and prompting her to do so since she quickly lost track of time.

"I felt really in sync with myself," Michelle says. "The contractions were really intense but nothing I couldn't handle. I guess I kept thinking it would get worse and I would wait to take drugs once that happened." At 4 PM, she was 8 cm dilated, progressing well. By late afternoon, Michelle was beginning to tire and relied heavily on Drew to breathe with her, massage her back, and feed her ice chips. Despite the intense activity, there was a sense of calm in the room. Soft jazz music played in the background, the lights were dim, and every nurse who entered the room couldn't help but smile at Michelle's bright pink wool socks with a kitten face and ears embroidered on them.

Eventually Michelle withdrew further and further into the work of labor. She stopped responding to conversation in the room as the duration of each contraction lengthened and the time between them shortened. At 6 PM she began to feel a lot of pressure and the urge to push, which surprised her because she had assumed she still had a long way to go. I checked and, sure enough, her cervix had dilated to almost 10 cm and the baby was very low, which was the reason she felt such intense pressure. "I can't make it!" she suddenly yelped after one really long contraction.

"You're almost to 10," Drew told her.

When Michelle realized that she had made it this far without an epidural or other pain relievers, she seemed to perk up. Later she said, "I kept thinking I would 'save' the epidural for when it was really awful—but by the time that point came, it was over and I was being told I could push! That was a surprise and kind of neat. When I checked in with my body—and by this point, it was like we were having a constant back-and-forth conversation—it was like the Little Engine That Could: 'I think I can, I think I can.' "

Although Michelle had practiced squatting positions and really wanted to deliver in this way, she found that when it was time to push, she was just too tired to sit up. Instead she pushed in a conventional supine position, and had a little difficulty. She required the support of Drew and a labor nurse on either side. She pushed for just over an hour, exhausted from having labored all day on a restless night's sleep. Then her daughter, Miranda, was born.

"After pushing so hard, she just seemed to slither out, and Drew shouted, 'It's a girl!' " Michelle says. "Tracy handed her to me the very minute she was born, and I guess at some point a nurse dried her off and bundled her in a blanket. I just kept looking at her, and at Drew, and she stared back at us with her big eyes, so calmly. I remembered to really focus on her, to look deep inside of her and welcome her to this big strange world. That's what I'll never forget, how all the pain was suddenly over and we were cuddled together staring at one another, a new family."

Michelle didn't even notice the quick stitching that was needed to repair a small tear. While the baby was being cleaned, weighed, and measured under Drew's watchful eyes, Michelle closed her eyes and tried to imprint the memory of her daughter gliding out of her, and then being placed in her arms, still coated with waxy vernix and blood, light as a feather and yet so warm and real.

Although it was midnight by the time they called their parents and then Drew went home to sleep, Michelle herself could not sleep. She reached for her journal and began writing down the day's events. Halfway through, exhaustion struck and she just jotted down the high points. But before she left the hospital, she filled in the rest. On the phone the next day she told all her girlfriends the details of her story. "It's as if I couldn't help myself," she reported. "What an incredible experience."

THE FIRST WEEKS AT HOME:
ONGOING CHECK-INS

Processing childbirth is one huge part of the postpartum experience. Adjusting to motherhood is the other. During pregnancy you reflected on how motherhood might be for you. Now it *is*. How does it feel? What do you love the most? Like the least? What is the greatest gift? The greatest burden? What do you need? Reflect on who you have become or are becoming in this new role as mother.

Ongoing check-ins with your body, your soul, and your baby continue to be important in the weeks and months ahead.

Some things to remember about checking in with yourself postpartum:

1. Commitment is key. You have to make a conscious commitment to continue this process. If you don't, it's too easy to let it fall by the wayside when your baby's crying, you're sleep-deprived, stress is high, and time is at a premium.

2. Give yourself a lot of time. Don't imagine that by your six-week medical checkup, all your feelings about childbirth and motherhood should be sorted out.

3. Expect the unexpected. Don't try to make your previous imaginings about motherhood fit what you're experiencing. This exercise is not about seeing whether you "got it right" in your earlier reflections. It's about what *is* right now, at this moment, in these circumstances. You may have planned on having your mother stay with you for the first six weeks, for example, only to discover that after two weeks you feel crowded by her presence and are ready for her to go home. That's perfectly legitimate, because you couldn't know ahead of time when you were making plans how you or your partner would feel once your baby was actually home with you. Or you may have waved off her offers to come and asked her to wait a couple of months, and then realized that you want her presence and her help much earlier.

4. Quiet the critical or analytical voice in your head. Accept what you're feeling without judgment. You might have expected that you

would bond instantly and joyfully with your baby, only to find that the baby's colic and your fatigue leave you feeling depleted and frustrated. Rather than blaming yourself ("I'm a terrible mother! What kind of mom would feel like giving her baby back because he won't stop screaming!"), acknowledge your feelings for what they are: frustration and exhaustion. And be compassionate with yourself.

5. Expect changes. How you feel at one week postpartum can be very different from how you feel at six weeks postpartum and at six months postpartum. For example, I've seen women who swore at their prenatal visits that they wouldn't be able to wait to get back to work, only to see them agonizing over this choice at their postpartum visit—and by the next annual exam having chosen to be at-home moms. And I've seen just as many women who planned all through pregnancy to stay at home, then decided that they'd really rather work part-time or full-time. Family and friends are often surprised by these shifts, sometimes because they seem "out of character." But that's all part of the mystery. Your character has shifted, and you can't know how until you're living it.

6. Acknowledge the disconnections and find ways to accommodate them. Sometimes there is a disconnect between what we want in our soul and what is possible. Work is a common example. If you are feeling inclined to stay home with your baby as your maternity leave ends, but for financial reasons this isn't possible, acknowledge that. If you're conscious about your true feelings, it doesn't change the reality but it does allow you to deal constructively with the disconnect between the ideal and the real. For example, you can take steps to protect the limited time you have at home with your baby and family by cutting back on other commitments. You can discuss your feelings with your partner and look for ways to make other adjustments to allow more time with your baby. It's useful to honor how you feel even when you can't "fix" it.

CHECKING IN WITH YOUR BODY

SUGGESTED TOOLS:

DAILY:

Body Scan (tool #2)

Continue to make this a start to your day. If you're too tired after a sleepless night of baby care, you might find it easier to shift Body Scan to the evening. Notice whether you hold tension in different places now. Pay particular attention to the parts of you that are in flux: your breasts, your abdomen, your uterus, your pelvis, and your perineum. How does each feel? What do you notice that is different?

Body Quick Pic (tool #1)

Your body has been through a tremendous enterprise in carrying and bearing a child. After delivery and while breastfeeding, it continues to go through rapid changes. Your body is really your underappreciated ally, healing while giving you the stamina and strength you need during the demanding phase of early motherhood. Show your thanks for all of its hard work by continuing to ask how it's doing and what it needs. Believe me, your body will appreciate the acknowledgment and attention.

WEEKLY:

Body Monitoring (tool #4)

The strange glamour of your giant belly has morphed into a dismayingly smushy midsection (*every* brand-new mom looks like this!), but don't let any surprise or disappointment over body image dissuade you from continuing this valuable tool. It's useful—and still a lot of fun—to really pay attention to what's happening with your body now. Give special notice to the fascinating changes taking place *each day* in the following:

- Your breasts. Also watch for signs of sore or cracked nipples, or signs of infection.
- Your abdomen.

- Your pelvis.
- Your perineum. If you had any tears or stitches in the area, look at them. Notice how rapidly these scars heal.
- Your discharge. (See page 460 in the next chapter for details on what to expect over time.)
- Your skin. Do you notice stretch marks or varicose veins? Are there any changes in the developments that might have appeared during pregnancy, such as spider veins or melasma?
- Your weight. This is a standard part of Body Monitoring in pregnancy that you should continue keeping track of now until you return to your baseline pre-pregnancy weight (or whatever you and your doctor agree is a healthy new baseline for you).

The following chapter will give you details about what to expect, and tips on dealing with problems.

AS NEEDED:

Dialoguing (with Your Physical Self) (tool #3)
Pick an aspect of your physical self that may be bothering you right now and have a conversation with it. It might be something very specific (your episiotomy) or more generalized (your overall postpartum appearance or your fatigue). Is there anything it needs from you? Is there anything you need from it?

BODY CHECKS:
WHAT MIGHT COME UP FOR YOU

- *Body pride.* Your body has just done a very awesome thing. Often women find that they think about their body in a new, more respectful way, like seeing a side of a friend that you hadn't realized existed before. I believe that women who have been connected to their bodies throughout pregnancy are less likely to experience the body-image dissatisfaction that troubles some new moms. Because a woman who has been consciously pregnant has a deep appreciation of how much her body has had to change and accommodate over nine months, she does not have the expectation that everything will immediately revert to baseline. She's able to call on greater compassion, patience, and support for a gradual return to her pre-pregnancy norms, a that which can take six to twelve months.

• *Fatigue like you've never known it*. Fatigue is your body's way of shouting at you to get your attention. It's depleted—and understandably so. On top of all it's just been through, the challenge of having to adjust to short, broken bursts of sleep is incredibly difficult. Listen to your body by sleeping when you can and work to replenish your depleted self across the Centers of Wellness. You'd be amazed how the small daily steps you take can help replenish you.

• *Weight worries.* Even when you have compassion for your body's remarkable achievements, it's not uncommon to have concerns about the sheer number of pounds you're still carrying. How long will it take to lose the extra weight? Will you be able to? When you're so tired and short of time that you don't always make the healthiest choices, this can add to the anxiety. Your best strategy is to simply stay aware of these concerns and to make a plan in your self-care that feels right to you.

• *Dislike of a particular pregnancy or postpartum development*. Stretch marks, varicose veins, a squishy midriff, or huge breasts may make you long for the body you used to have. Know that you are not alone in feeling frustrated about the changes pregnancy causes. Some of these changes will only be temporary; some you'll be able to alter with time and effort, while still others you can simply acknowledge. Talk to your doctor about your options and use the Feedback Loop to help you decide next steps, if any.

• *Diminished or absent sex drive*. Know that it is completely normal *and* understandable. Simply be aware of it and try not to judge it. Also be sure not to neglect the Sensation Center of Wellness just because you're feeling this way. It's actually all the more reason to pay attention to it and fuel it.

• *New feelings about your breasts*. Although women are prone to obsessing about many parts of their anatomies, breasts tend to get special attention. Some women love the voluptuous look they have while nursing, while others are dismayed by the added cup sizes. After weaning, some women will discover that their breasts have decreased in size, while others may never return to their former size. This could be a welcome change or an unwelcome one, depending on your perspective. Apart from size, some women feel great pride in their breasts because of the nourishment they provide to their baby, and may also feel pleased or surprised by how simple and enjoyable breastfeeding is. Other women may feel out-and-out fury at their breasts—fury for the pain they are "causing" during breastfeeding, or conversely, fury for their uselessness if for some reason breastfeeding is not possible. Hard as it may be to believe, this entire range of responses is completely normal. You don't hear much about the subject, however, which may leave you feeling embarrassed or conflicted. Don't be. Pay attention to what is true for you. And then try Dialoguing or Dreamagery to address these feelings.

CHECKING IN WITH YOUR SOUL

SUGGESTED TOOLS:

DAILY:

Soul Quick Pic (tool #5)
Be your own best ally by keeping tabs on how you're feeling now. Remember the Quick Pic doesn't need to take a lot of time. It's simply being aware enough to pause to ask: "How am I feeling? What do I need right now?" You can pair this with the Body Scan or Body Quick Pic at the start of your day.

WEEKLY (OR MORE OFTEN, AS DESIRED):

Journaling Your Journey (tool #6)
You may find it harder to use this tool now that the baby consumes so much of your day (and sleep whatever is left over!). After you've spent time processing your birth experience, it's useful to turn your attention to motherhood. A shortcut way to Journal is to simply jot notes, concepts, or even key words in your journal. It's amazing how

much just a few words can help you offload these emotions and even reconnect with them at a later time. If you can't get any reflections on paper, at least turn them over in your head. They can be great fodder for conversations with other women who have also given birth recently.

Some issues to explore:

• *Me as Mom:* Who are you now? Do you feel more aligned to motherhood or to the person you were before motherhood? Do you feel no different at all? There's no right/wrong, either/or answer. Your identity can fluctuate along a spectrum, and from moment to moment.

• *Me and My Work:* What's your soul drawn to now? Work? Home? Both? Neither? Is this the same or different from what you imagined in pregnancy?

• *Me as Wife/Partner:* How is your relationship with your partner since the baby's birth? How are your feelings toward your partner now? How is he adjusting to parenthood?

• *Me as Daughter and Mother:* Has your relationship with your mother changed since your baby's arrival (whether or not she is living)? Has your perception of her shifted at all? In what ways?

AS NEEDED:

Dreamagery (tool #9)
Use this tool to further explore issues where you feel especially conflicted or ambivalent now. Work, or your feelings toward your body, for example, are common issues. Or try doing Dreamagery with an image that represents your feelings toward your partner. What does your partner need from you? What do you need from him? How can he help you, and how can you help him? This can be a fun and illuminating way to get at the heart of what you're feeling and explore your options.

SOUL CHECKS:
WHAT MIGHT COME UP FOR YOU

Know that all of the following emotional responses are normal during this time, even if you feel you "shouldn't" have them.

• *Anxiety.* Your baby can seem so fragile and small, and your own experience caring for newborns so minimal, that you may be afraid you'll do the wrong thing and hurt your baby. Knowing how to mother is not an inborn skill or one that develops the instant you give birth. But you'll be amazed at how quickly the comfort with this kicks in!

• *Uncertainty.* You might feel self-conscious about your mothering skills or simply not yet comfortable in the role of parent. A baby who is fussy or sick can further undermine confidence. The fact that opinions abound about how you should dress, feed, and carry your baby can be particularly demoralizing to a new mom. Try not to take such comments personally. If you can breathe and distance yourself a bit, you can listen to what's being said to see if there's anything you would find useful, and discard the rest. Jettison the idea that you will be a "perfect mother," since there is no such thing. When you stop aspiring to perfection, you're freer to take each day as it comes. Your competence will grow along with your baby.

• *Sensitivity.* It may seem as if your emotions are more on the surface, and more erratic, than ever before in your life. Sometimes I liken the postpartum phase to a super-duper case of PMS. This is completely normal. Every aspect of your life is undergoing transformation. Give yourself space for the full range and intensity of these feelings, and that includes the special level of sensitivity you now have.

• *Bliss.* A feeling of contentment and happiness may permeate your day and make the sleepless nights more bearable.

• *Mood swings.* You may feel happy one minute and depressed the next. Try to go with it.

• *Irrational fear.* It's normal to be a little obsessive about your baby's well-being at first. Many a new mom has stooped over the crib to check breathing every time her baby sleeps. Or you might be afraid to let others hold the baby, lest they drop her or make her sick. These fears are quite primal, a reflection of how deeply you care about your baby and your responsibility for her.

• *Loneliness.* Being home with a new baby can be isolating in our culture. New parents often live far from family members and may have little firsthand experience with babies. If you have a lot of companionship in the immediate postpartum phase (such as a partner on family leave or your mother visiting), you may be vulnerable to feelings of isolation after they return to their everyday lives and leave you alone. Other factors that can contribute to this feeling include inevitable changes in your relationships with childless friends.

• *Second thoughts.* Now that you've gone through pregnancy and labor and are finally home with this baby you have been waiting for all these months, it's not uncommon to be questioning why you wanted a baby in the first place, or whether this was really the right choice for you at this time. Again, don't turn away from these feelings, turn into them.

• *Detachment.* If there are parts of the birth that you still haven't fully processed, it can take a while to get to know and love your baby. Maybe the baby is a boy and you were sure you were going to have a girl, or the baby has a birth defect you were not aware of during pregnancy. Maybe you have unresolved issues about the delivery itself, or motherhood isn't as fun as you'd imagined. All of these are complicated, highly emotional issues. You can even feel disconnected if everything seems terrific. How easily one steps into motherhood is colored by many factors—fatigue, changing hormones, colic, the presence or lack of practical as well as emotional support, outside stresses, confidence, and expectations, just to name a few.

• *Pervasive sadness.* Many new moms feel unbelievably sad, and don't know why. It is very important to pay attention to these feelings and not dismiss them, because while your current mood could be just a transient and harmless phase, it could also be a sign that you need help. Postpartum blues and depression are very real and common phenomena. (See next chapter.)

CHECKING IN WITH YOUR BABY

SUGGESTED TOOLS:

∞

DAILY:

Baby Quick Pic (tool #8)

Before conception, in pregnancy, and during labor, you did this exercise with an abstract vision of your baby. Now you can do it with the real thing. Take a few minutes every day, apart from baby-care duties, to look into your baby's eyes and simply be with him or her. What is the essence of this brand-new being? How is he or she changing each day? I believe that when babies first come into this world, they have a very unique receptivity and openness of the soul. Be sure to take advantage of this magical interlude by devoting as much focused attention as you can on getting to know your newborn.

∞

BABY CHECK-INS:
WHAT MIGHT COME UP FOR YOU

For many moms, the whole day is one big baby check-in. You can't stop holding your baby, touching her, smelling her, loving her. Protect and treasure this time as much as you can. In fact, checking in with your baby can actually raise your confidence about your mothering. No matter how inept or inexperienced you may feel, your newborn isn't judging your skills or criticizing you. She is just happy to be here, content to be cared for, held, fed, and loved.

Chapter 27

Postpartum:
The Inside Scoop and Medical Care

∞

An integrative medicine perspective on postpartum

WHAT'S HAPPENING WITH YOUR BODY

Your baby's out—but inside your body a cascade of changes continues, beginning within seconds of delivery.

Your uterus begins to shrink (involute) immediately after the baby and placenta are delivered. During pregnancy, it grew to 10 times or more of its starting size. In pregnancy the weight of the uterus itself—not counting the baby, placenta, membranes, or amniotic fluid—is approximately 1,000 grams, or 22 pounds, compared with just 50 to 100 grams when not pregnant. Rapid involution stops excessive bleeding by closing the blood vessels where the placenta separated from the uterus.

What you may notice: Contractions known as *afterpains* cause involution. They tend to be strongest right after birth in the delivery room, and then diminish in intensity in the hours and days after delivery. Afterpains feel most intense during breastfeeding because oxytocin, the hormone responsible for causing milk to flow, also causes the uterus to contract.

While involution happens amazingly fast at first, it doesn't happen overnight. Right after delivery, the uterus is still large enough to fill your lower abdomen and can be felt right at or below your belly button. By two weeks, it is contained within the pelvis, but it's not back to normal size until six weeks postpartum. Afterpains usually subside within the first few weeks.

What to do: Breathing exercises during an afterpain help make the discomfort more manageable. If pain is severe, try over-the-counter acetaminophen, which is fine if you are breastfeeding.

The lining of the uterus is shed. The bleeding that results from the shedding lining is called *lochia*.

What you may notice: Its appearance follows a distinct pattern. For the first several hours after delivery, lochia is a steady blood flow. It then quickly decreases to a reddish-brown discharge through day three or four postpartum (this can be even heavier than a menstrual period). After that it's a more watery and blood-colored discharge that still requires several pad changes a day and may smell like menstrual flow. Lochia continues for an average of 22 days after delivery, although some women still have discharge at the six-week checkup. In most women, the flow gradually becomes a thin, yellow-white discharge before disappearing completely within about two months of delivery. The lining of the endometrium is fully restored by the 16th day postpartum.

What to do: For the first week, absorb lochia with pads, not tampons. After that you can use tampons if you are comfortable doing so. Use them only during the day, however, and change them frequently. They should never be in place for longer than a few hours at a time, in order to avoid the possibility of infection or toxic shock syndrome. If you need to change pads more than once or twice an hour for several hours, call your doctor. Don't worry if you see clots in this discharge; this is perfectly normal.

Your abdominal wall readjusts. Because the tissue has been stretched significantly, the way it looks in the weeks (and months and years) following childbirth is largely an issue of genetics and tone. In some women the abdominal muscles that run from the chest to the symphysis pubis separate, a condition known as *diastasis recti*. Abdominal exercises such as pelvic tilts can help remedy this.

What you may notice: Immediately after giving birth, every woman sees a loss of abdominal tone—the infamous "jelly belly" of new motherhood. Indeed, most brand-new moms leave the hospital looking as if they are about six months pregnant, a point of great surprise to many. As involution continues, the poochy look tends to disappear, and women who were fit before pregnancy generally return to near their former profile by the six-week checkup.

Stretch marks that developed during your pregnancy will change in appearance, becoming more silvery and faded. This is normal. While most stretch marks do not go away completely, they will continue to become less noticeable as time passes.

What to do: As far as stretch marks, I am sorry to report that no creams, vitamins, or lotions in the world have been proven effective in making them disappear completely. There's better news as to your slack midriff. Working out, particularly with routines that do core strengthening such as Pilates or weightlifting, can make a big difference. Do remember, however, that your belly was very extended for a long period of time. Depending on your age, your genetics, and your commitment to working those muscles, you may never quite return to your pre-pregnancy abdomen. Remember why that is, and have compassion for your body that serves you so well.

The vagina begins to heal. Your birth canal had a major role during delivery, expanding enough to allow a baby to travel through it. After delivery the vagina essentially returns to its pre-pregnant shape and form, and does so remarkably quickly.

What you may notice: Some women report feeling "stretched out" and sore after giving birth; others do not notice any changes. The accordion-like walls of the vagina are seldom permanently altered by childbirth.

What to do: Kegel exercises can help improve overall pelvic muscle tone. You can begin them a day after giving birth.

Many women who breastfeed experience vaginal dryness. That's because of the associated hormonal changes. This effect can last as long as you continue to nurse, but is easily remedied by the use of a water-soluble lubricant (such as K-Y Jelly) or, in more severe cases, a prescription estrogen cream.

The perineum begins to heal. There's a small risk of infection at the site of an episiotomy or vaginal-tear repair. Although there are many bacteria present, this area has an excellent blood supply and heals remarkably quickly.

What you may notice: If there was no trauma from delivery requiring stitches, you may experience only mild swelling and tenderness in the first days after delivery. But soreness even to the point of being afraid to urinate or have a bowel movement is very common. If pain is severe, though, tell your doctor. Occasionally pain and swelling make urination difficult; if this is the case a catheter can be inserted. Your doctor will also want to rule out infection and other potential causes.

What to do:

• *Keep the area as clean as possible.* Since the usual wiping can hurt, instead use a plastic spray bottle filled with room-temperature tap water to rinse the area.

• *Try a sitz bath.* This is a small, shallow tub that fits over the toilet bowl so you can sit down and soak your perineum in warm water. (You can also use it in any chair; it's just more convenient and comfortable to do it in the bathroom in case of spills.) There are two schools of thought on sitz bath temperature. Some like it hot, while recent research finds that cold provides immediate pain relief and reduces swelling and spasms. For a cold sitz bath, start in a tub of room-temperature water, then add ice cubes, so the cold is less sudden and unpleasant. Try both and see which one your body responds to better. Sit for 20 to 30 minutes.

• *After a sitz bath or rinsing, try applying witch hazel.* This is a liquid plant extract available over the counter that reportedly relieves swelling. Soak a clean cloth in witch hazel and gently pat the area. Then blot dry with the softest toilet paper you can find, and then use a clean menstrual pad to protect the area. For a lot of pain, try freezing small gauze pads soaked in witch hazel to place next to your menstrual pad.

• *Take an over-the-counter pain reliever.* Ibuprofen (Motrin, for example) is more effective than acetaminophen (Tylenol) or aspirin and is safe for nursing moms.

• *Resume Kegel exercises to tone muscles.* If these increase your discomfort or pain, though, wait until they are comfortable to do.

Your breasts prepare for breastfeeding. By the time you give birth, your breasts are filled with a substance called colostrum, a high-protein, antibody-rich pre-milk. Within two to four days, the actual breast milk, which is higher in fat and calories, comes in. This happens whether or not you plan to nurse.

What you may notice: When milk first arrives, breasts can feel overfull: hot, hard, and painful. This engorgement is a temporary condition—not what you have to look forward to once a normal breastfeeding routine has been established. Engorgement usually subsides within 48 hours.

What to do: The best way to manage engorgement is by feeding your baby on demand, around the clock; once your milk supply is established and regulated, your breasts will look and feel more like pillowy balloons than hot rocks. A warm compress between feedings (such as a washcloth dampened with hot water) can also encourage milk letdown and ease pain. You can also take acetaminophen or ibuprofen.

Hormone levels change dramatically. As soon as the placenta is delivered, estrogen and progesterone levels, which were 10 times higher than usual during pregnancy, begin to drop back to their pre-pregnancy baseline. By the third day postpartum they are back to normal.

What you may notice: Mood swings are the most apparent effect, with many moms experiencing short-lived feelings of sadness called "baby blues" around the time of hospital discharge or within a day or so of going home.

What to do: See "Baby Blues" on page 478.

FEAR: Having a bowel movement will hurt!
FACT: If you have stitches close to the anus, general soreness, and/or constipation, the prospect can be a little unnerving. Moms used to remain hospitalized until they'd had their first bowel movement, but this isn't always the case now. Sometimes a laxative is prescribed after birth. If you've had a tear that has gone into or through the anal sphincter, you will most definitely be sent home with stool softeners. Always let your doctor know if you haven't had a bowel movement by your fifth day postpartum.

To help avoid hemorrhoids, wipe the area gently after each bowel movement or use a soft medicated pad (Tucks). If you had a lot of trauma to the area, your doctor may recommend stool softeners, an over-the-counter rectal suppository (such as Preparation H), as well as supplementary fiber (such as Metamucil or ground flaxseeds) to help stool pass easily. Drink plenty of liquids and avoid straining.

HEADING HOME

Vaginal Delivery Recovery

Your doctor or midwife will provide detailed care guidelines when you leave the hospital. Here are some of the whys behind commonly given advice (along with my own reality checks):

- *Don't use tampons for the first few weeks.*

  WHY: To allow any lacerations to heal and the cervix to close completely. Until the cervix closes, bacteria can pass easily from the vagina to the uterus. A tampon absorbing the vaginal secretions and blood—a haven for growing bacteria—increases the risk of infection.

- *Abstain from sex.*

  WHY: Caution and common sense are behind this guideline. Usually the arbitrary length of four weeks is given. This is long enough for any tears or an episiotomy to heal, and for the cervix to close completely. Check in with your body and listen to what it tells you; you might feel ready for sex sooner—or much later. In one study of women three months after delivery, 20 percent of new moms had little desire for sexual activity and another 21 percent had a complete loss of desire for or aversion to sex. Don't feel you have to hurry up or slow down; your body and your soul will tell you what is right for you.

- *Don't drive.*

  WHY: New moms are often told not to drive for a few weeks after delivery for reasons of safety. The fear is that a woman who's had a C-section or episiotomy may have slowed reaction times because of pain—or the anticipation of pain. Some women are temporarily anemic after giving birth, which can make them very fatigued. And nobody is sleeping very well. *However,* if you had an uncomplicated delivery, it's okay to drive when you are feeling up to it. Again, follow your body's cues.

- *Don't climb stairs or overdo activity.*

WHY: To prevent strain on stitches. Again, if you had an uncomplicated vaginal delivery with no episiotomy, you probably feel great and this advice does not apply to you, but it's still smart to limit your efforts to short periods of activity for the first few days. On the other hand, if you had complications, your body may require extra TLC. Listen to your body. If you've had an abdominal incision, lift nothing heavier than the baby until your postpartum checkup. Another commonsense rule of thumb for any new mom: if something causes discomfort or pain, don't do it.

- *Don't worry about swelling of the legs, hands, and feet.*

WHY: It's a normal occurrence during the first few days after delivering and is caused by fluid shifts. After being on the alert for swelling for so long, you may find it difficult to let go of this vigilance. Most of the postpartum swelling in the extremities will disappear within the first week.

C-Section Recovery

Since a C-section is major surgery, recovery takes longer than for a vaginal delivery. Your body goes through the same steps in reverting to a pre-pregnancy state (except there is no healing necessary in the perineum or vagina), and the same general care advice applies. On top of all that, however, your body must also cope with healing multiple incisions (even though you only see one) from the skin down through the uterus. Therefore you may experience more pain postpartum.

In the immediate postop period, as with any surgery, you will be observed very closely. Your vital signs will be taken regularly, and your incision dressing, catheters, and uterine tone will all be checked. Most likely, you will sleep through most or all of this. Once you're alert, you can still spend time with your baby, even though you're unlikely to be able to lift him or her just yet. As you gain strength and mobility, your time and actions around the baby can increase.

In the next several days, you will be encouraged to begin to move around and walk as much as you can.

What you may feel:

• *Disorientation, headache, or nausea from anesthesia.* Though most women do not have lingering aftereffects, if you do, let your postpartum nurse know. Acupressure bands or electroacupressure bands worn continuously can ease postop nausea. Wear them for as long as you have any nausea. This usually resolves by the first day after your surgery.

• *Fatigue.* No matter how elated you are about having your baby at last, you may feel too wiped out to receive visitors or to interact a lot with your baby. Sleep as much as possible in these early days, especially while you're still in the hospital. Getting plenty of rest is a crucial part of your healing process.

• *Constipation.* Sluggish bowels are a common aftereffect of surgery, which is why you may be prescribed a stool softener. It's also a good idea to slowly begin to introduce fiber into your diet. Don't expect to have a bowel movement within the first few days postpartum.

Remember that stress slows healing, and activating the relaxation response speeds it. Being a brand-new mom and simultaneously recovering from surgery is a double-dose of stress. The great news is that you can counterbalance this by using relaxation and mind-body approaches daily. These include breathing exercises, visualization, Journaling, and hypnosis. All can help significantly with recovery from surgery, particularly with pain management, nausea, vomiting, return of bowel function, and general healing. Do at least one, and preferably two, techniques every day. Once you are in a relaxed state, simply envision your body continuing to heal. Do some Dialoguing and ask your body if there is anything it needs or that would help in its healing. Give positive suggestions such as "I will continue to heal well. My body will gradually and easily return to its optimal healthy state. My incision will heal thoroughly. My energy will grow stronger each day. My sleep will be deep and replenishing." (Individualize these affirmations according to what you most need.) If you are having any particular challenges, do Dreamagery with these issues.

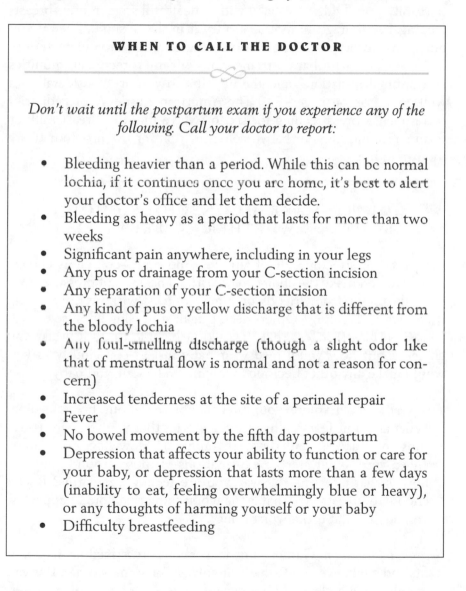

WHEN TO CALL THE DOCTOR

Don't wait until the postpartum exam if you experience any of the following. Call your doctor to report:

- Bleeding heavier than a period. While this can be normal lochia, if it continues once you are home, it's best to alert your doctor's office and let them decide.
- Bleeding as heavy as a period that lasts for more than two weeks
- Significant pain anywhere, including in your legs
- Any pus or drainage from your C-section incision
- Any separation of your C-section incision
- Any kind of pus or yellow discharge that is different from the bloody lochia
- Any foul-smelling discharge (though a slight odor like that of menstrual flow is normal and not a reason for concern)
- Increased tenderness at the site of a perineal repair
- Fever
- No bowel movement by the fifth day postpartum
- Depression that affects your ability to function or care for your baby, or depression that lasts more than a few days (inability to eat, feeling overwhelmingly blue or heavy), or any thoughts of harming yourself or your baby
- Difficulty breastfeeding

BREASTFEEDING

After working so hard in pregnancy, your body now has one more opportunity to provide your baby with a healthful start in life—breastfeeding. I encourage all mothers to try it in the hospital. Even if you
nurse only for a few days, or for only the duration of your maternity
leave, you give your baby a tremendous gift in protective immunities
and optimal nutrition—and the benefits to you are considerable as
well. (See box on page 473.) The American Academy of Pediatrics
recommends breastfeeding for six to twelve months. Breast milk or
formula should be your baby's sole nutrition for the first four to six
months of life.

HOW TO MAKE A CONSCIOUS CHOICE ABOUT . . . WHETHER TO BREASTFEED

I am pro-breastfeeding. But I am even more pro–conscious choice.
Some women make the choice to breastfeed because of pressure from
their doctor or from friends or other sources, without considering
their own real feelings. Others decide against nursing because of preconceived biases or fear that they won't be able to do it. Make the
choice about how you'll feed your baby just as consciously as you
would make any other decision involving body, soul, and baby.

First, reflection. Explore your preconceptions about breastfeeding.
What are your fears? What are the stories that you've heard (both
those of "success" and those of "failure")? How have they influenced you? What are the expectations of those around you, and
how is that affecting the way you are feeling about this? If you
choose to breastfeed, what is the worst thing that could happen? If
you don't, what is the worst thing?

Second, information. Gather some facts about breastfeeding, its benefits and challenges, and what it involves. For some women this can
entail taking a class while pregnant or reading books or websites,
while others may feel they get enough information from talking to
their care provider, a lactation consultant (professional breastfeed-

ing adviser), or experienced friends. Try not to limit your information to just one perspective.

Third, action. Make a choice. Realize that it is much easier to start breastfeeding when nature intended it—from birth—than to decide you won't nurse and then try to restart your milk supply after it has begun to dry up. Because of this fact, if there is any part of you that is considering it, even if you are unsure, start by breast-feeding.

Then, re-reflection. It is perfectly fine to start down one path and then, listening to your body, soul, and baby, take a different path. If you have fears or concerns that you want to explore more deeply, consider doing Dreamagery.

Here are some guidelines for breastfeeding success in the first weeks of motherhood:

Feed Early

Ideally your baby will be put to your breast within an hour or so of delivery when he begins to make mouthing movements and to root for the breast—another reflex a baby is born with. Some newborns are drowsy at first and merely seem to lick at the nipple and fall asleep. If this happens to you in the delivery room, don't panic; wait 15 minutes or so and try again. Nothing bad will happen to your baby if he does not suckle in the first hour. Ask a nurse to help you get started.

A baby who needs special care and can't nurse right away can still be breastfed. Ask for a pump so that you can provide milk that can be fed through a tube or bottle until he is able to nurse on his own. Hospitals have electric pumps on hand for this purpose. At home you can use a manual or electric pump, which can be purchased or rented from hospital supply stores and other sources.

Feed Often

The first feedings are not actually breast milk but a substance called colostrum, a pre-milk rich with the protective substances that bolster the newborn's immune system. Offer your baby the breast every two to three hours, or 8 to 12 times per day. Frequent feedings are necessary because breast milk is quickly digested. Breastfeeding advocate, pediatrician, and mother of five Marianne Neifert recommends that you try to get your baby to suckle 5 minutes per breast per feeding in the first day, 10 minutes the second day, and 15 minutes or more per breast per feeding thereafter. Feedings may last longer on the second breast, but offering both is important in order to stimulate milk production on both sides and also to avoid discomfort by distributing the pressure points affected.

Bottle-fed babies also need to be fed every two to three hours at first. Over time, however, they require fewer feedings per day because formula is less quickly digested.

Your baby won't feed by the clock, however. Sometimes she'll be hungry sooner than you expect and sometimes she'll sleep right through the planned feeding interval. The AAP advises waking your baby for feedings after three to four hours until your milk supply is well established, generally for the first two to three weeks. The more often you nurse, the more milk your body will produce. Demand feeding is best in the early weeks—that is, feed your baby anytime she shows the signs of being ready: moving her mouth or smacking her lips, nuzzling your breast, sucking fingers or blankets, rooting (turning her head as if looking for your nipple). Don't wait until she's crying—that's actually the last hunger signal in a baby's repertoire. A crying baby is also harder to settle down to the nipple; she may become so frantic that she's unable to take it in her mouth properly. If this happens, try to squeeze a little breast milk onto your clean finger and offer it first. As your baby begins to suck it, she usually calms slightly, enough to then be placed at the breast and latch on to it properly.

How do you know if your baby is getting enough to eat? Once you're home, look for at least five to six wet diapers a day and one stool a day. If you still think she's not getting enough, let your pediatrician know. It's normal for a baby's weight to slip below birth weight by a few ounces after delivery.

Expect a Learning Curve

You'd think it would be so easy. After all, women's breasts are designed to manufacture milk, nature's perfect baby food, and newborns are born with the reflex to suck. Alas, this natural act doesn't come naturally to all mothers—or all babies. In fact, there's a learning curve involved for both parties. Women who go into the experience expecting this, and who approach breastfeeding with equal measures of patience and good humor, tend to be the most successful over the long haul. Many moms and babies experience few problems. But if you encounter great difficulties, try not to get discouraged. It takes at least three weeks for your milk supply to become established and to develop a mutually smooth feeding routine.

Attach with Care

The number one cause of pain in breastfeeding is a baby who doesn't attach properly to the breast. Master this step and you're on your way to breastfeeding success. When you bring your baby to your breast, line up his nose with your nipple. The more of your lower areola (the pigmented skin around the nipple) that's in his mouth the better; he's less likely to clamp his mouth on the nipple itself. Get your baby to take in as much of the nipple and areola as possible by tickling his chin or upper lip, which encourages him to open his mouth widely. When he does, bring him to the breast. Avoid the opposite move—bringing your breast to the baby—as this causes you to hunch forward, a position that's uncomfortable and bad for your shoulders and back.

If your baby doesn't seem to latch on exactly right (for example, you can feel your breast tissue pulling or he doesn't have enough areola in his mouth), don't let the feeding continue. Stop and try again. Never pull your baby off your breast. First break the suction by gently inserting your (clean) pinky into the corner of his mouth.

Don't Be Shy About Getting Help

Belief that she ought to just know how to breastfeed—and embarrassment if she's having trouble—often prevents a woman from getting the very simple thing she needs: advice. Whether you have a quick question or need a hands-on tutorial, don't hesitate to consult a nurse (if you're still in the hospital), your pediatrician, an experienced friend, or a lactation counselor (a woman who is trained in providing breastfeeding support). Not only will solving your problem ease your stress and anxiety, you'll boost your overall level of parenting confidence and feelings of connectedness to your baby. That in turn may enable you to continue breastfeeding longer.

If you can find one, a structured class in breastfeeding is the most effective way to learn, according to the US Preventive Services Task Force. Its review of 22 studies on breastfeeding education found that it didn't matter what size the classes were or whether you took the class prenatally or after the baby was born. Many hospitals and local La Leche League groups offer classes; they're a terrific way to connect with other new moms near you as well. One-on-one instruction from a lactation consultant can be most convenient for new moms as these experts make house calls; ask your childbirth educator, doctor, or hospital.

Create a Nursing Space

Since each feeding session lasts a minimum of half an hour, make the experience a relaxing one by setting up a comfortable, pleasant spot in which to do it. This is especially useful when you're first getting the hang of breastfeeding and being calm and undistracted is so helpful. A rocker or other comfortable chair is ideal, with a footstool so that you can slightly elevate your feet. This makes it easier for you to hold your baby close to your breast without straining. A pillow in your lap and under your arm also help; look for a special nursing pillow (Boppy, for example) shaped to do the trick.

Every morning, fill a large sport bottle with water and keep it in your nursing space. Breastfeeding makes you thirsty and you'll want to replenish liquids after every session. Consider your other Sensation needs, too: Do you want to have music or the TV available? A phone? A nice view out a window? Some potpourri or an essential oil in a scent you found relaxing during labor? Keep a favorite shawl draped over the back of the chair to wrap around you and your baby.

Here are some common breastfeeding challenges:

Nipple Soreness

During the first days of nursing, it's not uncommon for the nipples to be painful to the touch or even to crack. Fortunately this is a short-lived problem caused by skin irritation, and will disappear as your nipples "toughen up" and grow accustomed to their new use. Rotate which breast you offer first at each feeding (when suckling is

REASONS TO TRY BREASTFEEDING

Benefits to your baby:

- Transfers protective antibodies to fight infection while his own immune system continues to develop
- Reduces the incidence of diarrhea, ear infections, respiratory infections and pneumonia, urinary tract infections, and meningitis
- Associated with reduced chance of sudden infant death syndrome
- Helps protect against diabetes, many types of allergies, some chronic digestive diseases
- Provides skin-to-skin closeness; touching is associated with better weight gain and, in some studies, higher IQ

Benefits to you:

- Helps the uterus return to normal size more quickly and decreases vaginal bleeding by releasing the hormone oxytocin
- Reduces risk of osteoporosis and some forms of breast and ovarian cancer
- Convenient (no bottles to tote or clean)
- Enables you to feed your baby faster (nothing to mix or heat)
- Free
- Provides an extra skin-to-skin closeness
- Can speed weight loss as nursing burns calories

strongest); as a reminder, some moms pin a safety pin on their bra on the side they plan to start the next feeding with, or shift a rubberband or bracelet from wrist to wrist. Also shift the way you hold your baby so that the same part of your breast is not compressed in the same way at each feeding. For example, you might lie down side by side for the day's first feeding and for the next feeding use a football hold (holding the baby like a football, with your hand supporting his head and his feet tucked into the crook of the same arm, pointing behind you).

Let your breasts air dry after feedings and apply lanolin (available in drugstores or ask your doctor) afterward. Use breast pads to absorb leakage between feedings; always change these as soon as they are wet, since prolonged moisture will further irritate the nipple. You can buy disposable breast pads or washable cotton ones; some women fashion their own out of fabric. While some women leak constantly between feedings, others experience very little leakage.

Nipple Confusion

Suckling a human nipple requires a different positioning of the lips and tongue than sucking an artificial nipple for a bottle. Some babies get "confused"; they will accept the artificial nipple, which requires less effort, and reject their mother's. For this reason, it's best to avoid offering your baby a bottle (whether pumped breast milk or supplementary formula) until your milk supply is well established, which is usually within two weeks. If your nipples are inverted or seem to be hard for the baby to latch on to, talk to your doctor or a lactation consultant about ways to help protract the nipple to make it more accessible.

Mastitis (Breast Infection)

Signs of a breast infection include fever accompanied by areas of pain or redness on either breast. It's most common before the end of the second week after delivery, but can occur at any time. The interesting thing is that not only do you not have to give up breastfeeding, it's better if you don't. Your doctor will give you a course of antibiotics that are safe for your baby and the infection will almost always be quickly and easily cleared. The baby cannot become infected through nursing. A new mom most vulnerable to mastitis is one who is generally run-down, a good reason not to neglect self-care now.

If You Don't Breastfeed . . .

Very few women are physically unable to breastfeed. But there are many women for whom it is problematic. These include, for example, women who have had reductive surgery on their breasts and may have impairments to their nipples or milk ducts, women with hepatitis, or those taking certain medications. Check with your doctor if you have any concerns or preexisting medical conditions, or are taking any medications.

If you cannot or choose not to breastfeed, what you need to do is avoid suckling your baby or releasing milk manually. The hormone prolactin, which keeps the breasts producing milk, is naturally inhibited when there is no breast stimulation, and the production of milk stops. Any kind of stimulation can interfere with this process, though, including sexual foreplay or even water from the shower. You may experience breast engorgement (hot, heavy, painful breasts as the milk comes in) for 24 to 48 hours; this should then disappear. To alleviate discomfort, wear a supportive and tight bra (some women prefer to wrap a towel tightly around them to bind their breasts, which prevents straps from digging in), apply ice packs, and take a pain reliever such as Tylenol. If this method does not resolve your symptoms, medication may be given (typically a two-week course) to dry up your milk supply.

THE POSTPARTUM CHECKUP

Typically you will not see your doctor again until six weeks after delivery, which can be a shock to you after the frequent checkups of late pregnancy and the continuous care throughout delivery. It can seem especially long if the doctor who attended your birth wasn't your regular ob-gyn, for example, in the event of a rotating practice or an emergency.

I think the lag in medical care between birth and the six-week follow-up tells you two very interesting things:

On the bright side, it's further confirmation of how well-designed a woman's body is for childbirth. On its own, it makes the transition from a pregnant state to a nonpregnant one quite efficiently and effectively. It does this no matter how many invasive procedures (such as induction, epidural, episiotomy, or C-section) you may have had. It does this even when the pregnancy had been threatened by a dangerous condition such as preeclampsia, gestational diabetes, or preterm labor. Very few women have medical problems postpartum.

On the other hand, the long lag from hospital discharge to postpartum visit is another reminder of where the medical system's focus lies: on the body, and only the body. Although it's true on a physical level that you tend to heal rapidly after childbirth, on a psychological and soul level, the adjustment is a much longer process. Sleep deprivation, anxiety over baby care, breastfeeding, and the new stressors that come from living in a heightened state of change (in your day-to-day life, in your identity and self-image, your relationships, your work, etc.) can all affect your body. Caring for your whole self is critical and can impact everything from the rate at which your wounds heal to how well you weather stress. Don't hesitate to ask your doctor about any question or challenge you face in the postpartum period. There are many resources available for virtually any issue you may encounter. And, remember, there is no reason you can't make an appointment to see your obstetrician anytime you feel the need. See also the Centers of Wellness modifications for postpartum in the following chapter.

Why is six weeks after giving birth the arbitrary date usually set for the follow-up exam? That's the point at which we expect the body to be back to its baseline. Bleeding has pretty much stopped, the uterus has returned to its pre-pregnancy size, hormonal levels have returned to pre-pregnancy levels, and any incisions or repairs should be healed.

The exam is much like an annual gynecological exam to assure that everything is on course in the recovery. Remember that most doctors are trained to focus on the body. They may not address the rest of your life or ask about it in any depth. Do take the initiative to bring up what's on your mind, particularly if you have any concerns or problems. Resist giving the automatic "Fine" in response to being asked how it's going. Even if your doctor does not practice integrative medicine, she is still connected with counselors and other professionals to whom you can be referred for more support.

Postpartum Contraception

Ideally you will have made a decision about this during your pregnancy. Be sure to re-reflect after giving birth to make sure your feelings about this haven't changed. Whatever your choice, you will need to use some form of contraception, virtually from the start of motherhood as ovulation can resume function as early as 27 days after delivery in nonlactating women. Technically, you could ovulate and conceive even before you have your first postpartum period. So unless you want *very* closely spaced children or you opt for complete abstinence, you need to have a contraception plan in place. Even if you do want another child very soon, it's ideal to wait a cycle or two in order to give your body time to fully recover, and to enable you to establish baseline LMP and due dates. Also, be very mindful of what your soul needs or desires. To become pregnant soon after delivering can be incredibly stressful, and rob you of a very precious time in your life.

The average time for ovulation to resume after delivery is between 70 and 75 days (and menstruation would begin two weeks later). In breastfeeding women, the average is 190 days. But don't count on breastfeeding alone to protect you against unintended pregnancy. How long you stay anovulatory (not ovulating) depends on how often you breastfeed, the duration of each feeding, the proportion of supplementary feedings, and your unique makeup. In women who are exclusively breastfeeding, the risk of ovulating within the first six weeks is 1 to 6 percent, probably due to the hormone prolactin, which remains at high levels in lactating women until the sixth week postpartum. (If you're not breastfeeding, prolactin falls back to the normal range by the third week postpartum.) Some breastfeeding women do not menstruate until their babies are weaned, but others resume periods within the first couple of months postpartum even if they are exclusively nursing.

If you chose tubal ligation: If you had a C-section, this procedure was done during the surgery, after the delivery of your baby. If you had a vaginal delivery with an epidural, typically the catheter will remain in place and you will have the ligation done under epidural anesthesia the day after delivering your baby. (They will simply redose the epidural.) If you didn't have an epidural, the procedure is typically done the day after delivery under spinal block. The reason for doing it so close to delivery is because the uterus is still so large that it is easy to reach the tubes through an incision around the belly button.

If you chose the Pill or other hormonal method: If you are not breastfeeding, you can start oral contraceptives or the Patch about the fourteenth day after giving birth. The reason for the delay is that during the first two weeks postpartum there is an increased risk of blood clots for every woman; starting the Pill or Patch increases this risk significantly. Often doctors wait until the postpartum checkup to begin a prescription, on the assumption that most women do not feel ready for intercourse until then.

Nursing moms can take an estrogen-progestin pill, but this can slightly decrease milk production. Alternately, a progestin-only pill (such as Micronor) can be used. It does not affect milk production but can result in breakthrough bleeding. If you don't want to use a pill while breastfeeding, condoms, a diaphragm, or an IUD are good choices.

If you chose the diaphragm: Your diaphragm should be fitted (or refitted if you used one previously) at the six-week checkup.

If you chose an IUD: IUD insertion should not take place until as many as eight or more weeks after delivery. At your six-week checkup, your doctor will evaluate the size of the uterus and determine whether you're ready to have the IUD inserted or need to wait a few more weeks. Though IUDs are perfectly safe and a good choice for women who have given birth before, there is an increased risk of uterine perforation if the device is inserted before eight weeks after delivery.

If you haven't chosen anything yet: Use these immediate postpartum weeks to review your choices, and use the Feedback Loop to help you decide. (See "How to Make a Conscious Choice About . . . Postpartum Contraception" on page 286.) Remember that this decision isn't yours alone. Contraception affects both partners, and ideally you should come to a consensus. If you are sure this was your last child, don't forget to include vasectomy in your considerations.

"Baby Blues"

As many as 80 percent of new moms experience a roller-coaster of highs and lows or a marked dip in mood in the days immediately following birth. Moms often wonder: *What's wrong with me? What kind of mom cries or feels sad when she has a beautiful new baby?* These feelings can be troublesome if you don't know to expect them, since most new mothers want to be deliriously happy now that their baby has arrived. The result can be guilt, feelings of inadequacy as a mom, or worries that there is something seriously wrong.

In fact, these "baby blues" or "maternity blues" are normal and common. Unlike postpartum depression (see below), the condition is short-lived and thought to be due to the abrupt declines in progesterone and estrogen after delivery. Baby blues are not necessarily related to stress in your life or to a lack of support, although sleep deprivation and stress can exacerbate them. Crying is the classic symptom, although in addition to weepiness you may experience mood swings, headache, confusion, forgetfulness, irritability, insomnia, anger or other negative feelings toward your baby, and increased sensitivity to criticism and advice. (Most women experience some combination of these, not all of them.)

Baby blues require no medical treatment. The best thing you can do is nurture your Centers of Wellness (talk, do stress reductions, exercise as you can, rest when your body is tired, and get support and proper nutrition). These strategies can help you weather the condition better. Symptoms typically peak about three to five days after giving birth and often last only a day or two, usually resolving completely on their own by the tenth day after delivery. If your moodiness and irritability persist for more than two weeks, those can be signs that you could use more help with the baby or an indication that you are experiencing depression. (See below.) Tell your doctor and ask for a checkup before the six-week mark.

Postpartum Depression (PPD)

One in ten new mothers experience postpartum depression. Some estimates are as high as two in ten, or 20 percent. PPD is not simply a "bad case of baby blues"; it's a different mood disorder and one beyond your ability to manage by yourself. Don't sit back and wait to "snap out of it." Postpartum depression can be doubly challenging for a woman to get help with because she must set aside feelings of secrecy, shame, or denial, all of which are very common. Though all women with PPD can be helped, fewer than one in five receive treatment. Fortunately, some of the confusion about PPD is lifting as more research is done about depression and as those who have struggled with it, such as the actress Brooke Shields, come forward to share their experiences.

Like many doctors, I explore the possibility of PPD at the postpartum exam, even though this is far later than it should be. The conversation often goes something like this:

Me: *How are you doing?*

New Mom: *Fine.*

Me: *How are you adjusting to motherhood?*

New Mom: *Okay.*

Me: *Tell me, what has been the hardest part for you?*

At this point, her lower lip begins to quiver and a tear spills down her cheek, followed by a shower of them. With encouragement, she shares a picture of many challenges, including overwhelming sadness and insecurity, crying jags, loss of energy, an inability to sleep whether or not the baby is sleeping, and irrational fears that the baby might fall or she might drop her. Sometimes she has corresponding physical symptoms, such as rapid weight loss, palpitations, or headaches. Some mothers feel detached from their babies as well and question what bonding really means and whether they have experienced it. The details of postpartum depression vary (see box), but the essence of the story is the same. I see a new mother struggling to present a competent and happy face to the world, a face that most of the world expects, while a frightening cauldron is simmering right below the surface. Those who struggled with infertility confront a triple-whammy: the PPD itself, a reluctance to admit it, and tremendous guilt over feeling so ambivalent or unhappy now that they have their long-desired child in their arms.

Symptoms of PPD usually appear within the first four weeks, though they can occur anytime during the first year. (See box.) Many doctors don't routinely probe about possible symptoms at your six-week checkup as I do. If you feel something is not right, or someone else has suggested this possibility to you, don't feel embarrassed about bringing it up with your doctor or midwife first. This is another critical place where being conscious of the state of your body and soul can result in very effective care and treatment. The condition is no reflection on what kind of mother you are. In fact, talking about it means that you are doing the right thing to take the best care of yourself and your baby. By sharing your observations and concerns early, rather than repressing or denying them, you ensure that you will get the support you need to heal, for you and your baby.

Though a great deal of research has been done to try to understand the cause of PPD, it's still not well understood. Estrogen, progesterone, prolactin, and cortisol levels all shift after delivery, but do not seem to be any different in women with PPD compared with women without. It may be that women who develop depression are particularly sensitive to the hormonal fluctuations, or they may have other hormonal differences.

A history of depressive illness puts you at particular risk. Almost 24 percent of women with a history of depression develop postpartum depression, compared with 2.6 percent of women with no history of depression. Other risk factors include prenatal depression in this pregnancy, postpartum blues in a previous pregnancy, a history of alcoholism or substance abuse, a difficult pregnancy, being young or single, having marital or financial problems, and having a seriously ill baby.

IS IT POSTPARTUM DEPRESSION?

The signs of PPD are the same as in major depression. If you experience five or more of the following symptoms in a week, tell your doctor or midwife:

- Internally disturbed sleep. This refers not to disruptions by an external factor (such as a hungry newborn who can't tell day from night) but to being unable to sleep even when you have the opportunity, sleeping restlessly, or awakening frequently and not being able to get back to sleep.
- Fatigue. Of course all new moms are bushed. But if you are tuned in, one good clue is that the "normal" fatigue of the postpartum state will be significantly relieved after a great night's sleep, a decent nap, or a break from the baby, whereas the fatigue of depression often doesn't seem to respond to any external measures.
- Irritability or anxiety for no apparent reason
- Feeling despondent and hopeless; loss of enjoyment in activities that previously gave you pleasure
- Feeling inadequate about your ability to care for your child
- Feeling worthless
- Sluggishness or restlessness
- Inability to make decisions
- Obsessive concern about baby care and safety; blaming yourself when any little thing goes wrong
- Excessive weight gain or loss
- Persistent feelings of ambivalence about your baby
- Suicidal thoughts and/or thoughts of hurting or killing your child

If you are in a risk group, it's a good idea to be seen and evaluated for PPD one to two weeks after delivery rather than waiting until your six-week postpartum visit. In addition to the immediate risks of depression, elevated levels of cortisol (a stress hormone) are found in both depressed mothers and their babies, setting both up for chronic health problems. There's even evidence that children whose mothers had PPD may experience behavior problems, have lower IQs, and develop depression later in their life. PPD also strains marriages. You can see how an unfortunate cycle can be easily created, especially if the problem is not diagnosed or treated.

Whenever PPD is suspected, the mom needs a full evaluation and a treatment plan that addresses her whole person. Options for treatment include:

1. *Antidepressant medication.* SSRI (selective serotonin reuptake inhibitor) antidepressants are typically prescribed. This is an active area of research, and I would recommend that you be evaluated and treated by a psychiatrist who deals with PPD and will be up-to-date on the latest research.

2. *Talk therapy.* Psychotherapy provides an important adjunct to medical treatment. I encourage my patients with PPD to continue in counseling long after they are feeling better, as this is such a stressful period. Having a committed time during which you can explore all of your feelings and thoughts is invaluable for any new mom. Together with your therapist, you can decide when it is right to discontinue your sessions.

3. *Hormonal medication.* Estrogen therapy is currently being researched, with one study showing success with an estrogen patch. Estrogen can interfere with breastfeeding, however, and raise a woman's risk of blood clots. This approach will be considered by your psychiatrist, and often in conjunction with your ob-gyn.

4. *Adequate time to adjust to this major life transition.* One study of nearly 2,000 working mothers found that those who take at least three months off after childbirth show 15 percent fewer symptoms of depression after they return to work than those who take six weeks or less. Also pay attention to getting adequate help during this time. Look into using volunteers or paid help to assist with your baby and your household (such as preparing meals, cleaning house, running errands, and caring for older children).

5. *Ongoing consciousness.* Although it's unlikely that you can avoid depression simply by being conscious of your health, I do believe that mindfulness can make a huge difference in how soon you become aware of the problem and seek treatment. One of the scariest and most dangerous aspects of PPD can be the isolation and denial that anything serious is happening.

6. *Self-care across your Centers of Wellness.* Any treatment should include a multidimensional plan for care that involves all Centers of Wellness. Paying attention to these aspects of your health can shorten the course of the depression, minimize its severity, and help you to cope with the symptoms. Reflect on your own life in each of these areas and focus on the ones that you feel are most out of balance. The more dimensions you can fuel, the more resilient you become.

CENTERS OF WELLNESS SELF-CARE PLAN FOR PPD

Movement: Prioritize an exercise routine with emphasis on an aerobic activity that you love. Aerobic exercise has the greatest effect on depression, and in nonpregnancy-related depression it has been shown to be as effective as antidepressants. Often the hardest aspect of this is motivating yourself to go— especially when you have a newborn at home and are feeling depressed. One of the best approaches here is to ask someone to be your workout buddy and commit to working out with you. Also ideal is a gym with baby care; alternatively ask your partner or another friend to watch the baby while you work out. This is advisable for any new mother but especially if you are combating PPD. It's central to recovery.

Nutrition: Because caffeine, sugar, and alcohol can cause mood swings and affect sleep, avoid them completely. Also be sure to get plenty of omega-3 fatty acids. Preliminary findings suggest that decreased omega-3s may be related to postpartum depression. More research needs to be done on this, but in the meantime, I recommend increasing omega-3s in your diet and supplementing with fish oil capsules.

Mind: Do one stress-reduction technique religiously at least twice a day. In addition, take one mini mental vacation daily. Journal about your darkest thoughts and feelings in a confidential and safe place.

Sensation: When well-wishers ask how they can help, request such sensory aids as fresh flowers (have them around your home all the time), favorite foods, or regular massages. Ask your partner to support vigilance about this underemphasized domain.

Spirit: Reach out to those who love you; lean on them and let them help you. This assistance can be practical (child care or household errands) or tactical (listening to you when you need to unburden yourself). Be candid about your struggle. Simply sharing this information aloud demystifies it for everyone, making you feel freer to ask for help and making friends and family all the more eager to lend it. Draw on the strength you derive from your spiritual practice as well; you may wish to seek out your minister or other spiritual leader, and share your situation with them. Ask friends to support you by watching the baby so you can attend services or a meditation group.

Postpartum Psychosis

A more extreme and rare situation is postpartum psychosis (postpartum mania), which affects only 1 in 1,000 women. As with the other psychological reactions postpartum, the role that hormones or biochemicals play is not well understood. Women at the highest risk are those who have a known bipolar disorder (25 to 35 percent of these women will develop postpartum psychosis), as well as those who have postpartum thyroiditis (a thyroid condition that can occur postpartum), and vitamin B_{12} deficiency.

Postpartum psychosis appears within the first six weeks of delivery.

Symptoms are dramatic, including delusions, hallucinations, sleep disturbances, and obsessive behavior toward the baby. Because of this, family members are typically much more aware that something is not right with PPD. The mother often appears extremely disoriented, agitated, and emotionally unstable.

This is a serious psychiatric disorder that warrants getting help quickly. Risks include harm to one's self or one's baby, including suicide and murder. If you or anyone in your family is noticing these kinds of changes, you need to be evaluated immediately. This condition requires initial hospitalization and medication.

Note, though, that postpartum psychosis is not a severe form of postpartum depression. Mood disorders in postpartum don't develop along a spectrum, beginning with baby blues and then progressing to psychosis. Each of the conditions I've discussed is a separate concern. Thankfully, postpartum psychosis is very rare, and can be treated when it is recognized.

Chapter 28

Postpartum: Self-Care

⸂⸃

Nurturing your Centers of Wellness during recovery

Balance is the key to self-care, but I wager most moms feel more *un-balanced* after giving birth than at any other time in their lives. Make time to keep your Centers of Wellness a priority in your life even when days and nights are upside down and your newborn consumes so much of your energy. You will feel better physically, and you will feel better mentally. You'll be more likely to have a speedy recovery and have more to give this time in your life. A bonus to continuing your good pregnancy health habits now: You'll be much more likely to maintain them in the years to come. Of all the things we teach our children, how to love yourself, find balance in your life, and optimize your health are certainly among the worthiest goals!

That's not to say it's easy. It is very, very challenging to do self-care on top of baby care. So remember this:

1. *Be conscious of that challenge.* Awareness is always the starting point and makes you less likely to let healthy habits slip away.
2. *Don't put off getting started "until things are calmer."* They may never be. It's easy to follow the path of least resistance when you're stressed. A new mom who is operating on little sleep and feeling demoralized about the way her body looks may be tempted to say, "Forget it!" and concentrate only on her baby.

Trouble is, then it becomes much harder to ever get started and find your way back to great health. Don't throw the calming bathwater out because of the baby.

3. *Look for shorter, faster ways to nurture each center.* Maybe you can't do the whole ritualistic, bubbles-and-candles bath you loved when you were pregnant. You can still turn a quick shower into a sensual, nurturing experience. Suggestions follow in "The Sensation Center," below.

4. *Keep the momentum.* When you can't work out for an hour, try to stretch for five minutes. That's something. Big steps are hard. But small steps are much easier and are the key to long-term success. Taking even one small step works better than taking no step at all, because it gives you immediate success. Small successes keep the momentum for change going. Each small effort becomes a mental placeholder for a time in the future when you are capable of taking a larger step.

THE MIND CENTER

Postpartum is one of the most mentally vulnerable times in a woman's life. The stressors, which may include shifting hormones, disrupted sleep, the unfamiliarity of caring for your baby, and a strained relationship, can be tremendous. Fueling your Mind Center will enhance everything else.

- *Be aware of what your stressors are now.* Chances are, they are very different. What is hardest for you? When the baby cries? Lack of sleep? Having your parenting skills criticized? A lack of help with the baby when your partner is at work? Just notice what is difficult. Even aspects of life that have always been there can be stressful now in a way they weren't before. Whatever your stressors are, just notice them, without judgment.

- *Find ways to unplug when your baby sleeps.* If you can tie your relaxation strategies to your baby's routines, you'll be more likely to do them. When my son was an infant, I figured that every time he napped, I could either take a shower or meditate. I chose to meditate because that was something I could not do while he was awake, while I could put him in his infant seat in the bathroom with me while I jumped in the shower. Showers, of course, are a form of self-care, too—an important one—but meditation is something for the mind. Think about what kind of mind strategies work for you now. Maybe spend five minutes doing a breathing exercise or a visualization before you take your own nap. Mental vacations are great for new moms.

• *Keep your expectations realistic.* Among the mind-sets that trip up new moms: A strong sense of what new motherhood is "supposed to" be like, how your baby is "supposed to" act, how you're "supposed to" feel, or what you or your partner is "supposed to" know or do. Remember there are many ways to be a great mom. You and your child can learn from each other.

• *Give yourself lots of space for the entire spectrum of feelings.* If you feel like crying, go ahead. Don't repress it. It's not unusual for all emotions to flow more freely now—don't be surprised if you start laughing uncontrollably at a sitcom and end up bawling at the sappy commercial break. That, in turn, might get you laughing again!

• *Discover your baby's rhythms and work within them.* Rather than imposing a schedule onto your baby's life, learn to read her cues and patterns and respond to them. Use the same skills of observation and awareness that you have been learning over the last nine months. You'll find that frustration lessens when you try to work with these natural rhythms for sleep, feeding, and alert times. Having a general structure to your day and a routine is useful; just don't be a slave to it.

• *If you are interested in pursuing more mind-body techniques, consider seeing a hypnotherapist or an expressive arts therapist.* These approaches can help you not only offload stress, but can help you make the transition to this next phase of your life with greater ease and awareness.

THE NUTRITION CENTER

You don't need to follow a special postpartum diet. Better to simply continue the general principles of nutritious eating that you followed throughout pregnancy. Eating well gives you the energy that you'll need to recover and to care for your baby, and fuels breastfeeding.

Two extremes of behavior are common postpartum, neither of them particularly healthy. Some women are preoccupied with, even fixated on, losing weight immediately. Others rationalize that extra pounds don't matter at all now, using frustration over pregnancy weight gain and fatigue as excuses to ignore nutrition entirely. Women in the former category often wind up denying themselves optimal nutrition during this physically demanding time, putting them at risk for problems ranging from inadequate milk production to osteoporosis later in life. Those in the latter category risk overeating and gaining still more weight postpartum on top of the pregnancy gain, feeding a cycle of depression, fatigue, and poor self-image.

• *Continue reflecting on your relationship with food now.* Has it changed since giving birth? Are there foods that you find yourself craving, such as coffee, sodas, or other things that you stopped consuming in pregnancy? In times of stress, we're apt to revert to old patterns (snacking, skipping meals, overeating, etc.). Know that now that you no longer have the motivation of "eating right for my baby," you may be especially vulnerable to falling back on old habits that are less than optimal.

• *Eat mindfully, even on the run.* Because you may have less time to cook, making nutritious choices can be challenging. Unconscious eating tends to be unhealthful eating, however. Notice what your body wants before you grab something. Check in briefly: Something salty? Sweet? Protein? Grain?

• *Give weight loss time.* Returning to your pre-pregnancy weight is a worthy target—and it doesn't all have to happen within the first two to six weeks. Indeed, for many women, it shouldn't. Remember that much of the weight gained in pregnancy is lost immediately due to the combination of the baby's weight, amniotic fluid, and so on, so the total you have to lose postpartum is not as daunting a figure as the number of pounds you gained in pregnancy.

• *Don't skip meals.* If you're too tired to make a full meal yourself, rely on healthy snacks or even a healthy frozen meal rather than skipping it altogether. If people offer to bring you food when you're first home from the hospital, don't dissuade them. If you don't need it right then, you can always freeze it.

- *Keep up consumption of omega-3 fatty acids.* In the last trimester of pregnancy, development of the fetal nervous system uses these nutrients in increasing amounts from the mother's system. It is possible that these essential fatty acids can be depleted by the time you head into postpartum. Omega-3s are thought to possibly have a protective effect against postpartum depression. I believe that women today are at added risk because many shun all fish during pregnancy out of fear over mercury contamination; in fact, as I point out in the Centers of Wellness dietary guidelines, it's safe to eat many kinds of fish, which are an excellent source of omega-3s. Other good sources include flaxseed and omega-3 eggs (special eggs from chickens who have been fed flaxseed). (See Omega-3 chart on pages 51–52.)

- *Keep nutritious snacks on hand.* You probably won't have as much time to shop daily, wash and cook fresh produce, and plan elaborate meals. But if you always have access to nutritious choices and foods that you like, eating right becomes less of a chore, and you're less likely to grab heavily processed, quick foods. Examples of healthy choices include string cheese, peanut butter and carrots, pre-mixed salads, hummus, fresh fruits, pre-cut crudités (raw carrots, celery, pepper strips), canned fruits in natural juices in individual-sized servings, almonds and sunflower seeds, hard-boiled eggs (especially omega-3 eggs), lowfat or non-fat yogurt.

- *Limit your alcohol and caffeine consumption.* You don't need to eliminate either beverage, just don't overdo them. Be sure you're not using them to self-medicate. For example, I often see women who have a glass of red wine to help them relax from the stress of a crying baby, or sip Starbucks all day to keep going. Not only are alcohol and caffeine mere Band-Aids to the real problems (stress and fatigue, for examples), they can actually make things worse. Alcohol can contribute to insomnia, for example. And if you're breastfeeding, these substances can pass through your breast milk to your baby. It takes about three hours for a glass of wine or a beer to pass through your system, so the best time to have a drink is immediately after a feeding. That way, the alcohol will be metabolized before the next feeding.

- *Be aware that in order to lose weight you need to eat less than you did during pregnancy (unless you're breastfeeding—see below).*

Additionally, if you're breastfeeding:

• *Don't diet.* You need an additional 600 calories per day over pre-pregnancy norms, or about the same as you needed in the third trimester to meet your added energy needs. Women who breastfeed partially need only an extra 400 calories per day. Many women can lose weight while breastfeeding, but don't count on it; you have to do the math and make your nutritional choices consciously.

• *Continue taking your prenatal vitamin.* The extra iron is beneficial. In fact, iron and calcium are about the only nutrients you really need to supplement now; almost everything else you need is provided in a well-balanced diet. Your doctor may prescribe supplemental iron if you lost a lot of blood in childbirth. If you are a vegetarian, you also want to be sure to get enough vitamin B_{12}.

• *Be sure you consume adequate calcium.* Your stores are taxed by breastfeeding. You should consume approximately 1,000 mg a day total. That's more than in a typical prenatal vitamin, so you may need a supplement if your diet doesn't contain enough. If constipation is a problem, take 200 to 400 mg of magnesium a day along with the calcium.

• *Go outside!* Vitamin D is absorbed through the skin. Sometimes infants of dark-skinned mothers are vitamin D–deficient. Brief daily strolls outside replenish your supply.

• *Drink water.* To stay well-hydrated, have a glass of water every time you nurse your baby. Keep a water bottle handy next to the chair where you usually nurse, and at your bedside table. Some moms like to carry a sports bottle with them at all times during the day. Pay attention to your thirst level when you do check-ins. Thirst is your body saying, "I need water."

• *Don't eliminate any foods arbitrarily.* While it's true that newborns can be allergic to certain foods or be sensitive to foods through their mother's milk, most have no trouble. If you suspect an allergy, always consult a nutritionist and work with your baby's doctor before removing important sources of nutrients from your diet.

THE MOVEMENT CENTER

Most women think of postpartum exercise in terms of weight loss. In that regard, make like a tortoise, not a hare: slow and steady wins the race. Your body is still recovering from childbirth. While this recovery process is more or less invisible to you (except for the lochia), your body still needs TLC, especially right away. Do remember, though, that movement isn't just about burning calories. It also lifts spirits and restores energy and can be a very effective antidepressant.

• *Check in before and during exercise.* Really listen to what your body has to say about what it's ready for and what it needs. Loose joints and altered balance can continue for a few months after delivery. Fatigue is a very real signal that your body needs sleep; don't push it and power through a workout. Also pay attention to how your body feels when it moves. What has changed from when you were pregnant? What is different from before you were pregnant?

• *Begin early.* You may hear admonishments not to exercise until the second, fourth, or sixth week postpartum. But remember, Movement means any kind of movement. And you should begin this as early as the first day postpartum. Get out of bed and shuffle to the bathroom if you can. If you can't, stretch in bed and practice a few Kegels.

• *Move a little every day.* Once you are home, take a short walk with your baby—even if it's only to the end of the driveway because your healing episiotomy is still sore. Some days you may feel only like stretching. That's fine. Just do something.

• *Use exercise to combat fatigue.* It seems counterintuitive, but movement actually results in more energy overall. Walk, dance around the house (with or without the baby), do some stretching, practice yoga or Tai Chi. Your body is freer to move than it has been in many months—bring your attention to this new reality and have fun with it!

• *Walk consciously.* Walking is a great activity postpartum because it's gentle yet beneficial, aerobic as well as strength-bearing, requires little preparation, and can be done with your baby, either in a stroller or a soft front-carrier. Pay attention to each step, to your surroundings, to the weather. Leave your stressors behind. If you've worked all your adult life, these mid-day walks with your baby during maternity leave can be a revelation and a great mental refresher.

• *Look into exercise classes for new mothers.* If you're feeling self-conscious about your post-baby body, you'll find kindred shapes—and spirits—here. Ask at local gyms, health clubs, and YMCA/YWCA programs. Some programs (such as Strollercise) incorporate babies into the routines. Many such classes offer child care.

• *Convert an out-of-home exercise program to an at-home plan.* If you find it difficult to get to the gym, consider ways to adapt. Instead of working out on weight machines, buy simple hand weights. Try an exercise videotape if you can't make it to a step or spinning class. Look into jogging strollers if you're a runner, but be sure to get one that's safe for newborns—some models are only designed for babies six months and older.

THE SPIRIT CENTER

While I consider all five centers necessary for balance, the Spirit Center takes on particular resonance postpartum. One example of the advantages of connectedness is that it has been shown to reduce depression. When I was in Haiti all alone with my two-month-old son, a wonderful woman I had never met before (a Canadian reporter covering the coup that had me trapped in the country) came to my rescue at the hotel where we were both staying. It was 5 PM, the time Ryan always seemed to get fussy, and I was exhausted and feeling frustrated with him. She spotted us walking around the lobby. "May I hold him?" she asked. She mentioned that she was missing her own children. When she took him, I realized with surprise and relief that it was the first time he had been in someone else's arms in the many weeks since I'd been there. She went on to tell me that all babies get fussy at this hour. I hadn't heard of "the witching hour," as this veteran mom called it, and was hugely relieved to understand that his fretfulness was normal. "That's why they invented the cocktail hour!" she said, and she sat me down and ordered me a drink! (Needless to say, we've been great friends ever since.)

• *Make conscious choices about the kind of support you need and want.* That means seeking out and accepting the kind of support that you want and declining "support" that isn't truly supportive. Asking for help or accepting it when offered can be hard for some women. "What's the big deal about having a baby?" you might wonder. But all the little assists that are offered—meals, errand running, someone to check in on you or babysit while you nap—add up. Keep revisiting your needs as time goes on. What's working? What isn't? What do you need now?

• *Arrange for support after the first week.* There comes a point where the calls and cards start to peter out, your partner goes back to work, maybe your mom who came for the homecoming has gone back to her life—and there you are, all alone with seven or eight pounds of uncommunicative, peeing, pooping, sleeping, squalling baby. Don't be left alone with your baby day after day. Get out into the world. Arrange for phone buddies to check in on you every day. Have meals delivered, if that makes your day simpler.

• *Expect a time of adjustment as you move from partners to parents.* The birth of a baby is considered by family therapists and researchers to be the biggest challenge of marriage. Increased irritability, conflict over finances or child care, postpartum depression, and a lack of intimacy, all of which are common postpartum events, can lead to disconnection and even infidelity. In one study by University of Washington psychologist John Gottman, two-thirds of 82 newlywed couples who were tracked for four to six years (before and after the birth of their first baby) reported marital dissatisfaction within three years of the child's arrival.

Among the preventive strategies: protect "couple time" even though you are in a very child-centered life phase; keep up communication to resolve conflicts and negotiate new responsibilities; and respect your differences. Each of you brings different things to parenting that deserve to be honored and respected. And above all, share your feelings with each other.

• *Connect with other new moms.* If you don't know any in your immediate circle, consider looking up women you met at prenatal classes or finding a local mothers group. Look online for chat groups at the many parenting sites. The goal is not necessarily to become friends for life; you might not even have a lot in common other than your babies. But this space of time is such a unique one in life and you'll have that experience in common. Comparing notes can be of terrific help practically as well as psychologically.

• *Spend social time in those relationships that fuel you.* Now is not the time for the coworker you can't stand to come visit the baby. Politely and firmly say "Not now" to people with whom you have less-than-supportive relationships. Protect time each week with someone to whom you really feel connected, time when you can really be yourself (with or without the baby in tow).

• *Get out of the house.* Newborns sleep so much in the very early weeks, and they weigh so little even in their car seat, that they're more portable than they will be in a few months. You can go out to eat or watch a movie along with your baby. It's also not too early to start hiring babysitters. If you time short outings between feedings while the baby naps, he or she won't even know you're gone.

• *Consider how you might want to explore your spiritual side now that you're a mother.* This often becomes highlighted as new parents begin to think about how they will raise their child with regard to religious or spiritual beliefs. Going through childbirth is also a profoundly spiritual experience for many women. Spend some time reflecting on your beliefs about things larger than yourself, whether your mode for this is prayer, meditation, reading spiritual writings, attending services, or something else. If you don't have such a framework for spiritual reflection, consider whether this is important to you now or not.

THE SENSATION CENTER

Both dimensions of this center—sexuality and sensuality—deserve focus postpartum, even if having sex is the farthest thing from your mind right now!

Sexuality

Sex—or the lack thereof—is a huge opportunity for consciousness. Most couples don't resume intercourse until about six to eight weeks postpartum. But because most people weren't having frequent sex in the last trimester, there can be pent-up desire (usually coming more from the male partner than the one who has just delivered a baby).

For many women, libido can remain low to nonexistent for months. Hormones and exhaustion can create this feeling. If you're breastfeeding, the vagina can feel dry and thin, because the hormone prolactin, which stimulates milk production, inhibits estrogen, which in turn decreases lubrication. And while stitches in the perineum will heal in three to four weeks, generalized soreness or sensitivity in the area can persist much longer. Sleep deprivation and stress don't feel very sexy, either.

Some strategies for postpartum:

• *Recognize and honor how you're really feeling regarding resuming intercourse.* Resist jumping back into old routines just because you feel sorry for your partner or you feel you "ought" to. The first time, especially, can be fraught with nervousness. Check in with yourself.

• *Accept that your body has changed—and that you may have changed feelings about your body.* One reason sex may feel different now is that your image of your body as a sexual being has been altered. Your breasts are not just breasts—they're milk machines. Your midriff may feel mushy and unsexy. Your vagina has just had a different kind of traffic in it—a baby. It can be hard to wave these images out of your head during sex. And your perineum may be sore. Some women feel "touched out" from holding and suckling their babies all day. Honor your feelings and share them with your partner.

• *Then, reflect on what you DO want in this domain.* For many women now, the answer is "just cuddling." Are there parts of your body, that if you knew it wouldn't lead to sex, you actually might like to have touched sensually and sexually? I usually recommend for the first several weeks, once you are ready to explore your sexual relationship again, that you and your partner agree that you will *not* have intercourse. (I tell my patients to feel free to blame it on me.) Knowing this up front can relieve a lot of the anxiety that can come from the above physical considerations, and thus allow you to relax so that you can actually *enjoy* the interaction! That then begins to build a great foundation. While this may seem like cruel and unusual punishment for your partner, there's certainly no reason he can't have a fulfilling sexual experience. It's far better to approach it this way than having a situation that is uncomfortable or painful for you, resulting in fear and anxiety about the next time. It is also better than avoiding "the whole sex thing" altogether, which can really damage your intimacy. This can create the beginning of a negative cycle that then becomes self-fulfilling.

• *Carve out intimate time. (It's not the same as "time for sex.")* Realize that many, many women complain of low libido for years after they deliver. Here's the good news: this doesn't have to be you. For many such women, low libido is rooted in exhaustion and lack of intimacy with their partner. Sexually, women are typically wired differently from men. A man uses sex to feel close to his partner, while a woman wants sex *when* she feels close. It's easy to see how a common postpartum scenario unfolds: New Mom is exhausted, harried, and can't remember the last time she spent uninterrupted romantic time with her mate, a time when she spoke from the heart and felt heard and embraced. She's not even thinking about that as she crawls into bed after a feeding; she's calculating the precious number of hours she hopes to sleep—and then New Dad rolls over and hugs her, his erection unmistakable. The prescription here is to create a real connection with your partner. Commit to scheduled time together where all focus is on *emotional* intimacy. This has been a huge life transition for you both. You can each process that individually and in parallel, or you can share it with each other and deepen your emotional connection.

• *When you do resume intercourse, go gently.* Give yourself help in the form of lots of foreplay and lubrication (such as K-Y Jelly or Astroglide). Especially if you're nursing, the vagina can be drier than usual. If these creams aren't working, you might want to consult your physician, who may suggest a prescription cream.

FEAR: I'm all "stretched out" since having my baby.
FACT: The vagina is an elastic organ and shrinks remarkably after

delivery. But the best way to rebuild pelvic muscle tone is to work at it. Remember your pregnancy Kegels? (Firmly tense your vaginal and anal muscles, hold for a count of five, then relax.) Do up to 50 reps at a time, as often as you can.

Sensuality

Late in the third trimester you probably discovered how rewarding it can be to turn inward and cosset yourself a little. Respecting your sensuality is even more important in new motherhood, when the impulse is to focus on your baby and put your own needs second. You may feel that you barely can manage sleeping, let alone taking the time to pamper your sensual side. Here are some strategies for postpartum.

• *Check in to discover what really nourishes you now.* The heightened sensitivity to smells that some women experience in pregnancy has disappeared. Different, stronger odors may appeal to you now, everything from the smell of your tea to the flowers in your home. Go through each of your senses and get an idea of what, if anything, has changed for you since giving birth.

• *Do something each and every day to be kind to yourself.* No matter how rough a night you've had, do something that pleases you. While walking your baby, stop at a neighborhood café for a smoothie. My favorite new mom indulgence: Ask someone who wants to come and see the baby if he or she is willing to watch your child while you have a massage therapist come to the house and give you a massage. You can offer for them to get one next (preferably while the baby is napping!).

• *Don't wait until you fit back into your old clothes to dress with care.* The no-mom's-land between maternity clothes and your pre-pregnancy wardrobe is an awkward place. Most moms make do with some combination of maternity stretch bottoms and loose tops. Look for little ways to lift and personalize your look now—your favorite earrings, a new pair of shoes, a shawl in your favorite colors or textures, your signature scent. Nursing mothers have a huge array of attractive and convenient nursing clothes to choose from. Buying a few shirts or nightgowns with hidden flaps or openings is not only convenient, it's a pick-me-up that celebrates this special time.

• *Turn routine self-care into tender-loving care.* If you don't have time for a long bath, you'll probably take a shower. But be fully present for it. Notice how great it feels—the hot water running over your shoulders, an invigorating loofah scrub on your arms and legs, the clean smell of soap. Things you're going to do anyway can become ways to meet your Sensation Center needs simply by really tuning in to them with all your awareness rather than considering them another rushed thing to check off your to-do list.

• *Make sleep pleasurable.* Keep a soft, cheerful throw and small pillow on the sofa for when you catnap there. In your bedroom, simply changing the sheets and opening a window can make rest more refreshing.

• *Enjoy your baby.* Your newborn learns through his senses. You can't touch or hold him enough, especially in the newborn period. Get to know him (or her) with each of your senses, and allow him to do the same with you. To be sure, there's a lot of drudgery involved in caring for your baby. Make time, within that, to be really aware of the miracle before you. Sniff her clean, fresh hair and skin. Massage his roly-poly limbs. Sing and talk to her. Enjoy the sensation of his skin against yours during feedings. All of these activities reinforce the connections between mother and baby, promoting bonding and teaching your child trust and love. And notice that they are all sensual acts for you.

If you're really aware and in the moment, you can make even ordinary interactions with your child into special events that stoke your own body and soul. Whether you felt madly intoxicated by this beautiful new life the minute you saw him or her, or need more time to adjust to this incredible change in your life, simply enjoying your baby is healthy for both of you.

Internet Resources

Acupuncture

    American Association of   www.aaom.org
    Oriental Medicine

    North Carolina Association   www.ncaaom.com
    of Acupuncture and Oriental
    Medicine

    Tai Sophia   www.tai.edu

    American Academy of Medical   www.acupuncture.com
    Acupuncture   www.medicalacupuncture.org

American Holistic Medical   www.holisticmedicine.org
Association

Botanicals

    American Botanical Council   www.herbalgram.org

    Consumer Lab   www.consumerlab.com

Cochrane Collaboration   www.cochrane.org

Counseling and Communication

International Family Therapy   www.ifta-familytherapy.org
Association

Gottman Institute   www.gottman.com

American Association for   www.aamft.org
Marriage and Family Therapy

eMedicine.com Consumer Health   www.emedicinehealth.com

Guided Imagery

Academy for Guided Imagery   www.academyforguided
imagery.com

Health and Wellness   www.instincttoheal.org

Hypnosis

The American Society of   www.asch.net
Clinical Hypnosis

Integrative Medicine

Duke Integrative Medicine   www.dcim.org

Duke Health System   www.dukehealth.org

MD Anderson Cancer Center   www.mdanderson.org/
departments/CIMER

National Center for   www.nccam.nih.gov
Complementary and Alternative
Medicine

Lactation Consultant

International Lactation   www.ilca.org
Consultant Association

Massage

American Massage Therapy   www.amtamassage.org
Association

National Certification Board for   www.ncbtmb.com
Therapeutic Massage and
Bodywork

Mind-Body
    American Society of Clinical   www.asch.net
    Hypnosis

Natural Standard Collaboration   www.naturalstandard.com

Nutrition
    Consumer Lab   www.consumerlab.com
    Isodisnatura   www.isodisnatura.net
    NIH Office of Dietary   www.dietary-supplements.
    Supplements   info.nih.gov

U.S. Food and Drug   www.fda.gov/opacom/
Administration News   hpnews.html

Yoga   www.himalayaninstitute.org
    www.kripalu.org
    www.yogadirectory.com

Index

TRACY W. GAUDET, M.D., is the executive director of Duke Integrative Medicine at Duke University Medical School and a practicing, board-certified Ob-Gyn who is a fellow in the American College of Obstetrics and Gynecology. She was the founding executive director of Dr. Andrew Weil's Program in Integrative Medicine at the University of Arizona in Tucson.

Her first book was *Consciously Female: How to Listen to Your Body and Your Soul for a Lifetime of Healthier Living.* A noted expert on women's health issues, she's appeared on *Oprah, The CBS Early Show,* and the PBS series *New Medicine,* and she writes a column in *Body & Soul Magazine.* She has a son, Ryan, and lives in Durham, North Carolina.

PAULA SPENCER is a writer and mother of four in Chapel Hill, North Carolina. She's the "Momfidence!" columnist in *Woman's Day* magazine and a contributing editor to *Parenting* and *Babytalk.* She's also the author of *Momfidence! An Oreo Never Killed Anybody and Other Secrets of Happier Parenting* (www.momfidence.com) and *Pregnancy Journal: A Week-by-Week Guide to a Happy, Healthy Pregnancy.*